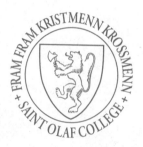

THE HEALTH
OF NATIONS

THE HEALTH OF NATIONS

Public Opinion and the Making of
American and British Health Policy

LAWRENCE R. JACOBS

Cornell University Press | *Ithaca and London*

To Julie Schumacher

Contents

Part IV *Bold Innovation in Ongoing Policy Discussions*

Preface

The first of two purposes in this book is to use extensive primary research on the formulation of the American Medicare Act of 1965 and the British National Health Service Act of 1946 to explain the sources of contemporary health policy in each country. The Medicare and the National Health Service (NHS) acts were critical legislative landmarks: in important respects, they established today's access to and reimbursement of doctors and hospitals. A history of these acts also accounts for policymakers' seemingly inexplicable failure, especially in the United States, to ensure cost control over the new health programs.

I could have compared different countries. The United States is often compared with Canada because the two countries share a federal government structure as well as a history of introducing government insurance by selectively focusing on a population group (e.g., the aged) or a service (e.g., hospital care). Instead, I chose to emphasize variation. Not only does Britain have a unitary government structure, but its NHS Act was formulated (during a war) two decades earlier than the American legislation and was characterized by quite different administrative arrangements. These differences are analytically useful: they raise critical but often neglected research questions by identifying the "silences" in each country's development—why, for example, policies evolved in significantly different ways or altogether failed to materialize.

An American-British comparison is especially attractive because the differences in the NHS and Medicare acts developed in countries with broad similarities. The United States and Britain share legal customs and liberal commitments to individual freedom and minimum government. Moreover, this health care legislation emerged from similar political times. The making of each act was characterized by parallel developments in both the political process (analogous periods of deadlock broken by electoral landslides) and the policy process: each country discovered the health problem as an agenda issue, pursued consensus, and enacted bold solutions. These similar progressions produced landmark legislation that expanded access. My specific intention, then, is to use a comparison of the origins of Medicare and the NHS to better understand contemporary health policy issues related to access, provider reimbursement, and cost escalation.

My second purpose is to present an alternative way of understanding policy making in liberal democracy. I use the investigation of why two broadly similar countries produced different legislation to rethink prevailing approaches to policy making.

In weighing liberal democracy's dual commitment to individual liberty and popular consent, theoretical inquiry has traditionally feared excessive public involvement in decision making. A persistent theme in liberal democratic theory is that the citizen's role should be limited to selecting the elites who will do the deciding. Empirical research within diverse traditions—such as those associated with the pluralists, rational choice practitioners, Max Weber, and V. O. Key—suggests that the mass public's influence is in fact limited to the broad boundaries of government decisions; elites are given free rein to determine the details of policy making. The study of comparative public policy has also tended to focus on elites, the leadership of organizations such as trade unions and political parties who are assumed to express or reflect the objective interests of workers and other classes. Similarly, health care research has portrayed the NHS and Medicare acts as the almost exclusive work of a small circle of elites: these legislative programs are believed to illustrate the comparative irrelevance of public opinion and the significance of medical professionals, labor and business groups, and other influentials.

The empirical research on American and British health policy presented here suggests, in contrast, that public preferences and understandings have extensive influence on detailed policy making. My central analytic concerns are to explain policymakers' relationship to major relevant interest groups and to examine two stages of the policy-making process—the placement of health care on policy-making agendas and the formulation of detailed policies. Existing research, especially by Weberians, anticipates that policymakers become locked into an insulated and highly cooperative relationship with interest groups, and that elite judgment of organizational capacity determines the setting of agendas and the formulation of detailed administrative changes. I find, however, that strong public sentiment produced both weak influence on the part of interest groups (despite their fierce opposition) and administrative arrangements that ignored or defied the technical assessments of elites. In short, government decision making is coupled to public preferences and understandings.

I challenge two central assumptions of the prevailing approaches to policy making in liberal democracy. First, policymakers and scholars have assumed that the moral and instrumental knowledge of elites is far superior to that of the mass public, the so-called ordinary people. It has seemed reasonable to equate detailed policy making with elites because they alone appear to possess objective, scientifically ascertainable knowledge of the most efficient means to achieve universally recognized policy ends (human happiness and well-being). This assumption of elites' superior competence is, however, one-sided. Not only is the competence of elites exaggerated, but ordinary people—not unlike legislators and chief executives—have sufficient knowledge, if not to master all policy details, then to offer general principles that can guide policy making.

Second, observers have assumed that the mass public's involvement in policy making has been limited to staking out broad and permissive parameters within which a small minority have been free to make detailed decisions. In contrast, I demonstrate that, despite sheer population size and institutional arrangements that limit democratic involvement, the mass public has a significant impact on broad policy goals and administrative details. In part, political competition and electoral contests motivate bureaucrats and officeholders to anticipate voter reactions. The public's impact also stems from the all-encompassing nature of culture, which ensures that socially constructed values and assumptions seep into even insulated policy deliberations.

I do not claim that the type or degree of American and British democratic influence is either optimum or desirable. Certain social groups are disproportionately favored by the limited scope of politics and public participation as well as by inequalities in financial and organizational resources. Indeed, the general tendency of government policy to reproduce the power of dominant social groups was evident in the medical profession's privileged position in American and British policy discussions: while other important organized groups were deliberately excluded and still other interests remained unorganized, the medical groups enjoyed multiple points of access and disproportionate attention.

Nonetheless, the relations between dominant and subordinate groups, and between policymakers and the mass public, do not typically involve the unilateral exercise of power. New government policy is not simply something that happens to people but something that the mass public, within real constraints, helps to make. Whereas previous conceptions of policy making overemphasize the insularity and capacity of elites, I emphasize the degree to which agenda setting and policy formulation are penetrated by the preferences and understandings of the mass public. My objective, though, is to assign analytic importance to the mass public without over-emphasizing it. In particular, I argue that ordinary people have conditional relevance to detailed policy making; this claim provides a basis for reversing the process of experts displacing the public.

This book has four parts. The first introduces the analytic framework and national settings. In Chapter 1, I synthesize existing interpretations of institutions and culture in order to develop an analytic framework for ex-plaining interest group influence and the policy-making process. In partic-ular, I draw on recent studies of culture to conceptualize public preferences and understandings; I integrate this culturalist analysis with Weberian inter-pretations of institutional change, which assume that policymakers' deci-sions are largely a function of objective administrative capacity. My aim is to build on, but push forward, these two previously separate areas of re-search. The result is an approach that incorporates public opinion into an analysis of institutional and political processes and provides a framework for investigating whether and how culture influences government decisions.

The second and third chapters outline the American and British national contexts for the formulation of the Medicare and NHS acts. In Chapter 2 I examine the disposition of government elites toward the mass public and provide a historic account of policymakers' growing preoccupation with public opinion. In Chapter 3 I discuss the evolution of enduring public understandings of health care and the state's involvement in its provision; I examine culture by using social historical evidence to identify enduring public understandings and public opinion polls to capture more temporary preferences.

Subsequent chapters, based on interviews with major policymakers as well as each government's published and archival records, explore the im-pact of public sentiment on health policy discussions. In Part II I examine the agenda-setting process and the public's impact on moving the health care issue from the margins to the mainstream of national debate. Part III is a study of the ways public influence was refracted through political and policy processes—namely, the pursuit of consensus by Britain's wartime government and by the Kennedy administration. Part IV is an analysis of the aftermath of historic electoral landslides. American and British policy-makers' perception of a transformation of public opinion led to bold in-novations in Britain's postwar Labour government and in Johnson's administration. Although the differences between the Medicare and NHS acts have often been stressed, in these chapters I emphasize the similar process by which these two pieces of legislation were formulated.

In the concluding chapter I marshal evidence from the NHS and Medicare acts to address critical theoretical issues. These two cases supply a starting point for a more general argument concerning the conditional relevance of public opinion to policy making in areas outside health care. In particular, I suggest that whether and how public opinion influences policy making are affected by critical political and policy processes. In short, I offer an empirical and theoretical critique of the existing analyses of policy making in liberal democracy.

In conceiving, researching, and writing this book, I have accumulated many debts. As my work on this project has drawn to a close, I am struck not only by the sheer number of contributors but by the range of contributions, professional, intellectual, and personal.

The argument developed in this book is the product of many conversations and letters. Paul Addison, Lawrence Brown, Frank Dobbin, Daniel Fox, John Freeman, Virginia Gray, Fred Greenstein, Charles Hamilton, Jennifer Hochschild, Ira Katznelson, W. Phillips Shively, Rosemary Stevens, and Charles Webster read the entire book or sections of it. Raymond Duvall, Joel Krieger, Richard Pious, and Robert Shapiro read and reread the book as it worked its way into final form. My research on health policy has benefited enormously from the contributions of a group of exceptional and broad-thinking scholars. I am grateful, in particular, for the contributions of Theodore Marmor, who generously drew on his encyclopedic knowledge of Medicare and comparative health policy, and James Morone, who pushed me to address the broad implications of my case studies. I owe a special debt to Robert Shapiro, who encouraged this project at the beginning and supported it unfailingly at every point along the way; his generosity, given at all times and in many different forms, has been unsurpassed.

I have relied on the following organizations for assistance in conducting archival research: the John F. Kennedy Presidential Library in Boston, the Lyndon B. Johnson Presidential Library in Austin, the Public Record Office in London, and the Mass Observation Archive in Sussex, England (especially Dorothy Sheridan and her friendly staff). Moreover, financial support from Oberlin College, the John F. Kennedy Foundation, the Lyndon B. Johnson Foundation, and the University of Minnesota Graduate School and Department of Political Science helped to keep this project afloat. I would also like to thank my editors at Cornell University Press. Roger Haydon was a steadfast supporter and proposed the book's title. Elizabeth Holmes was gentle but firm in preparing the book for publication. Finally, with permission of the publishers, I have used material that appeared previously in my articles in *World Politics* (January 1992) and *Comparative Politics* (January 1992).

I also acknowledge a more general intellectual debt—for the four years

I spent at Oberlin College. More than a decade after graduation, I still feel an enormous respect for the community at Oberlin; it instilled in me a deep respect for the importance of original and critical thought.

Finally, this book would not have been possible without important personal contributions. My parents, Henry and Judy Jacobs, have always been in my corner. More than their unfailing support, it is their political and intellectual integrity that has shaped me to the core. No contribution can be more profound. I also thank my sister and brother, Mai and Paul Jacobs, and my young daughters, Emma and Isabella, for being patient when I needed patience most.

This project is dedicated to Julie Schumacher. It is a testament to Julie's own analytic powers and perseverance that she made significant contributions on all levels—professional, intellectual, and personal. All aspects of our lives have been thoroughly and joyously intertwined. Dedicating this book to Julie is both the least and the most that I can do to express my thanks.

LAWRENCE R. JACOBS

Croton, New York

Abbreviations

ACT	Government's Actuary, Public Record Office, London
AHA	American Hospital Association
AMA	American Medical Association
BHA	British Hospital Association
BIPO	British Institute of Public Opinion
BMA	British Medical Association
BOB	Bureau of the Budget
CAB	Cabinet file, Public Record Office, London
CF	Confidential File, Lyndon B. Johnson Presidential Library, Austin
CP	Cabinet Paper, Public Record Office, London
EHS	Emergency Hospital Scheme
GP	General practitioner
HEW (DHEW)	Department of Health, Education, and Welfare
HPC	Home Policy Committee, Public Record Office, London
INF	Ministry of Information file, Public Record Office, London
JFK Library	John F. Kennedy Presidential Library, Boston
LBJ Library	Lyndon B. Johnson Presidential Library, Austin
MH	Ministry of Health file, Public Record Office, London
MO	Mass Observation Archive, Sussex
NHI	National Health Insurance
NHS	National Health Service
OASI	Old Age and Social Insurance Program
PIN	Official Committee on the Beveridge Report file, Public Record Office, London

POF   Presidential Office Files, John F. Kennedy Presidential Library, Boston

PREM   Prime Minister's Office file, Public Record Office, London

RG   Ministry of Information file, Social Survey: Reports and Papers, Public Record Office, London

RP   Committee on Reconstruction Problems file, Public Record Office, London

SIC   Interdepartmental Committee on Social Insurance and Allied Services file, Public Record Office, London

TC   Topic Collection file, Mass Observation Archive, Sussex

Cohen Interview Interview with Wilbur Cohen, Austin, Texas, 4/1/87, by L. R. Jacobs

Godber Interview Interview with Sir George Godber, Cambridge, England, 12/13/86, by L. R. Jacobs

Mills Interview   Interview with Wilbur Mills, Washington, D.C., 6/18/87, by L. R. Jacobs

Nestingen Interview Interview with Ivan Nestingen, 1966, Social Historical Research Office, Columbia University

Pater Interview   Interview with John Pater, South Croydon, England, 12/15/86, by L. R. Jacobs

Note on Documentation. All file dates are given in the American style: month/day/year.

PART I

*Theoretical and
Empirical Contexts*

1 | Institutions and Culture

Comparative analysis of political and policy development across Western countries has tended to concentrate on general structural characteristics and broad generalizations. Thus, the processes of industrialization and class relations in capitalist societies have been used to analyze comparative public policy (Wilensky 1975; Esping-Andersen 1985; Korpi 1983) and specifically health policy (Hollingsworth 1986; Doyal 1983). The comparative study of political development has similarly pursued a broad-gauged approach to researching and generalizing about administrative capacity: the "strong" and intrusive states of the European continent are typically contrasted with their polar opposite—the "weak" or antistate legacy in the United States and Britain (Almond and Powell 1966). Neglected, though, in broad-gauged political and policy analysis has been the variation in the content of government decisions.

An alternative tradition of analysis uses detailed empirical research on policy content to develop theoretical generalizations (Allison 1971; Heclo 1974; Marmor 1973). I draw on this tradition of intensive analysis to develop an explanation for institutional differentiation—the differences between, and the specific features of, the NHS and Medicare acts.[1] My central research question is, why did two broadly similar countries produce health legislation that differed significantly in terms of administrative arrangements

1. Fox (1986) pursues an alternative approach to comparing the development of American and British health policy—he organizes his comparaison in chronological terms. For instance, Britain's formulation of the NHS could have been compared with America's rejection of national health insurance (NHI) during the 1940s. While I do discuss the defeat of NHI in chapters 3 and 5, my central focus is on the differences between and specific features of the institutions that are established.

and basic principles (e.g., universal vs. more selective coverage)? The British NHS Act established government provision of a comprehensive range of medical services to the entire population free of charge at the point of delivery.[2] The American Medicare Act, in contrast, funneled government money into a privately run health system for selected groups; it established a means-tested program for the indigent as well as two related insurance programs for social security recipients.[3] These American programs provided money to a limited segment of the population—the aged and the means-tested indigent—to purchase a limited range of services from nongovernmental providers.

My argument is that these two acts were produced by a common process in which public preferences and understandings took precedence over interest group demands and state actors' concerns with administrative capacity. Despite this similarity, and despite shared legal and cultural customs, the distinct nature of the American and British relations between public opinion and policy making produced the dramatic differences in each country's health policy.

This chapter offers an analytic framework for explaining two central issues: the specific direction of administrative changes and the variation in interest group influence. To develop analytic frameworks that are relevant to other policy areas, I do not explicitly concentrate on existing theoretical debates about the history of the NHS and Medicare acts.[4]

THE NATURE OF POLITICS

Institutions without Subjects

Although several research traditions have relegated the mass public to a limited role in detailed policy making, I focus on a single currently influential mode of institutional analysis, one motivated by Max Weber's theoretical insights. Because general reference to the "Weberian" approach exaggerates the degree of consensus among a diverse group of scholars, I concentrate on one especially prominent variant that is closely associated with the work

2. Although I refer to the British NHS Act of 1946, this act formally applied to England and Wales; Scotland was not incorporated in the health service until the passage of the 1947 NHS Act.

3. In formal terms, the American legislation enacted two amendments to the Social Security Act, which were subsequently referred to as the Medicare insurance program and Medicaid program for the indigent. In this book I use the term "Medicare" as it was understood by Americans at the time, to refer to one major reform package that encompassed both an insurance and a public assistance program.

4. For an important tradition of health policy research that does build theoretical frameworks relevant to different policy areas and broader political developments see Marmor 1973; Eckstein 1958 and 1960; Hollingsworth 1986; and Hollingsworth et al. 1990.

of Theda Skocpol.[5] This variant has particular theoretical relevance here, because it explicitly analyzes both the variations in the relationship of government elites with interest groups and the making of detailed policy decisions. It asks, how much free rein do elites have and why do they choose one specific policy direction when altering administrative arrangements?

This variant of institutional research has tended to draw on one dimension of Weber's writings, which stresses that "the advance of bureaucratic organization" is due to its "purely *technical* superiority over any other form of organization." Weber emphasized the "objective" nature of this advance in modern organizational forms by drawing direct parallels to the advent of mechanical modes of production: the introduction of machines to the process of production and the bureaucratic mechanism to modes of organization both ushered in impersonal routines that were cheaper, faster, and more predictable. Modern bureaucratic organization enhanced our physical capacity to achieve our ends by structuring state activity to conform to "purely objective considerations," which were guided by "*calculable rules* and [were] 'without regard for persons' " (Weber 1978, 214–16).

Contemporary Weberians have analyzed the state's "technical" organizational attributes by examining the two related concepts of "capacity" and "autonomy." This technical interpretation of institutional change has developed the concept of capacity from Weber's analysis of two organizational attributes, specialization and hierarchy. An important part of bureaucratic development involves the definition of specialized tasks performed by full-time, salaried experts.

Contemporary institutional research especially concentrates on the emergence of differing degrees of hierarchy. American and British institutions have been interpreted as failing to develop fully along bureaucratic lines because of the dispersal of authority; no one group of officials is able to take the lead in formulating policy. Neither state, then, has established a firmly ordered system of authority in which a relatively small number of higher officials can dominate policy formulation by supervising their subordinates. Weberians, though, emphasize the exceptional degree to which the American state has historically defied authoritative control and direction because of its federal structure and its fragmentation of authority within the national government. Using organizational attributes to assess objective capacity, this techno-Weberian interpretation concludes that the American state is characterized by structural weakness (Skowronek 1982; Orloff and Skocpol, 1984).

5. Weberian research has developed in multiple and diverse directions; I am concerned with one variant, which emphasizes the technical organizational attributes of states. Other Weberian accounts emphasize the role of nontechnical factors such as mass public attitudes. For examples, see Katzenstein 1986 and 1985 and Stepan 1978.

Weberians expect an institution's existing administrative capacity to be a primary factor in determining the direction of change. In general terms, several studies on the United States conclude that the nineteenth century's "statelessness" and reliance on political parties for distributing patronage distorted subsequent institutional changes, causing incoherence and an incomplete development of impersonal and rule-governed routines (Skowronek 1982; Orloff and Skocpol 1984; Orloff 1988). In a more detailed analysis of the significance of existing state capacity for institutional change, Skocpol and Finegold examined the New Deal's establishment of two new executive branch offices—the National Recovery Administration and the Agricultural Adjustment Administration. Emphasizing its high degree of specialization and hierarchical control, they argued that the Agricultural Adjustment Administration was an "island of state strength in an ocean of weakness" (1982, 271). Its administrators' specialized skills and hierarchical control over policy formulation equipped a small group of officials to design and implement agricultural policies characterized by clear priorities and minimal internal contradictions. In contrast, National Recovery Administration efforts to regulate industry suffered from the weak capacity more typical of the American state; its policies for industrial coordination were characterized by fragmentation and uncertainty about basic goals. Weberians hypothesize, then, that an institution's existing organizational attributes prefigure the direction of policy departures.

A second critical concept of Weberian analysis is that of autonomy, the potential of state actors to define and pursue distinctive goals that are independent of, and often in opposition to, the interests of leading societal groups and individuals. In particular, Weberians claim that the autonomy of state actors, who are defined to include bureaucratic officials and elected politicians, is a function of administrative capacity. Drawing on research into "policy networks" (Katzenstein 1978), Weberians suggest that certain groups are granted the privilege of multiple points of access and disproportionate attention. Thus, in the context of private control of economic activity, state actors incorporate interest groups, which represent producers of critical goods and services (e.g., business and labor associations), into "patterned interrelationships" of bargaining (Atkinson and Coleman 1989). New policies emerge from state actors' continuous bargaining with representatives of relevant producers.

Weberians expect state actors to exercise autonomy from relevant interest groups when the execution of new policy by existing institutions is perceived to be administratively feasible; but the pursuit of distinctive policies that would require the costly and uncertain development of new state capacity is unlikely, and state actors are expected to be especially responsive to interest group claims (Orloff and Skocpol 1984). Thus, Skocpol and Finegold (1982) argue that the Agricultural Adjustment Administration's institutional capacity equipped it to exercise an administrative will independent of the claims of farm groups. The National Recovery Administration's comparatively weak capacity for either hierarchical control or specialized knowledge, however, made its officials unwilling and unable to intervene autonomously in industry; to have expected otherwise "asked too much of the government machinery of the time" (1982, 268). Similarly, Orloff and Skocpol (1984) claim that British policymakers' confidence in the government's capacity to implement social policies led them to take the initiative in formulating pathbreaking social insurance legislation, Whereas the American state's weak capacity made comparable policies seem neither feasible nor desirable. In short, Weberians claim that policymakers' decisions to alter institutional arrangements and to respond to interest group demands are largely a function of objective administrative capacity.

Culture without Institutions

Cultural explanations of politics challenge the Weberians' central assumption, that it is possible to ascertain the objective status of administrative capacity. All members of a society are *enveloped* in culture, ensuring that elites' "technical" assessments are socially constructed and imbued with socially shared values.

Research on culture is extensive and has developed in many directions; I pursue one of these approaches, which treats culture as a representation of socially shared meanings produced from the interaction of ordinary people. Traditionally, historic approaches to culture have traced the development of ideas among politicians, policy experts, and scholars. Louis Hartz (1955) traced Lockean values of individualism in order to study Americans' liberal tradition; in health care, Daniel Fox (1986) largely concentrated on doctors, hospital managers, public officials, and social scientists to study the emergence of new ideas about the organization of health care. I depart from the traditional approach to culture by shifting the focus from the ideas of elites to the understandings and preferences of the mass public.

To analyze the ways ordinary people think and behave, anthropologists, social historians, and social scientists have come to argue that culture is grounded in social relations: in the actions and interactions among members of a society as they attempt to make sense of their contexts (Geertz 1973; Giddens 1979; Thompson 1978a, 1978b, and 1966; Berger and Luckman 1967; Douglas 1982 and 1970; Wildavsky 1987). It is through social interactions that the core of culture—meanings and understandings—comes to be shared and reproduced. Equating culture with social relations and shared meanings has encouraged a growing emphasis on the competence and extensive (explicit and tacit) knowledge of ordinary people about the society of which they are members.[6]

According to this view, institutions embody or represent culture's organized existence. Institutional arrangements organize social relations and social interaction among society's members. Shared meanings and understandings come from, and are formed through, institutions. Culture, then, is not an attribute of a lone individual: it is not locked inside his or her head as part of an isolated consciousness. Rather, it appears at the individual level largely as a reflection of institutions (Wildavsky 1987).

A broad consensus has emerged among both Marxists and non-Marxists that culture is a mediating factor or "middle term" between environmental conditions (such as administrative capacity and economic or class forces) and human behavior; it represents the subjective orientations by which members of a society can understand and respond to their environment.[7] Culturalists directly challenge Weberians' theoretical expectations that state actors can and do measure the state's objective administrative capacity.

Two aspects of culturalist analysis are particularly relevant here: its empirical investigation of culture and its implications for analyzing policy making. Culturalist investigation of the mass public is at odds with most American social scientific research. The typical empirical analysis of culture is exemplified by the "political culture" tradition, which uses polling data to measure "things that exist within individuals" (Inglehart 1977, 4, and 1990; Almond and Verba 1963). According to this approach, culture is equated with an individual's immediate preferences, and a country's culture is equated with the pattern produced by aggregating individual responses to polling questions. But, by narrowly using polls to track individual preferences, this analysis disembodies culture into isolated and temporary parts; meaning-centered approaches insist that culture is an attribute not of individuals but of organized social interactions. It is not sufficient, then, to simply paste into institutional analysis the conventional approach of treating culture as synonymous with polling results.

To avoid operationalizing culture at the individual level, I tap both the

6. Social actors' knowledge is based on their explicit monitoring of their environment as well as their tacit understanding of their society. With explicit monitoring, individuals can give reasons and rationalize their conduct; tacit understanding includes one's stock of unarticulated knowledge, which one uses implicitly to orient oneself and to interpret the acts of others (Giddens 1979; Brown 1980; Hochschild 1981; Page and Shapiro 1992; Ortner 1984).

7. Both neo-Marxists and non-Marxists agree that it is not possible to decode and trace human behavior back to its real material essence (e.g., Thompson 1978a, 1978b, and 1966; Katznelson 1986; Hunt 1984; Eckstein 1988). The neo-Marxist argument that human behavior is not simply the product of material forces has been roundly criticized, alternately for abandoning the orthodox Marxist concern with economics and for continuing to overemphasize material conditions: for an example of the former, see Johnson 1978; for examples of the latter, see Hunt 1989 and Jones 1983.

enduring aspects of culture and the more explicit (often transitory) preferences of the public. To capture public preferences, I examine published as well as previously unpublished (government) polling data. These polls provide evidence of both interest in major reform (such as the extraordinary salience of Britain's social planning document, the Beveridge Report) and support for specific policy directions (like American respondents' support for attaching Medicare onto Social Security's financing mechanism). To explore culture's enduring and more general aspects, I use social historical evidence. The arrival of social history over the past three decades has shifted the analysis of the past from the activities and intellectual concerns of elites toward the perceptions of ordinary people; the result is a vast literature on ordinary people's enduring knowledge or understanding about themselves and their institutional contexts (see Chapter 3; Jacobs and Shapiro 1989).

I use such evidence to supplement survey data on the assumption that general aspects of culture, which are widely shared and transmitted down generations, pattern or underwrite the public's more specific preferences. Individuals draw on or reference already formed and socially shared understandings to reach and articulate judgments about particular policies; in this way, an individual's perceptions are organized by and embedded in trans-individual values. Thus, in both the United States and Britain, enduring understandings offer individuals a slim but important cue in organizing their immediate preferences.[8]

Social historians modify conventional generalizations about national character by investigating the content of, and change in, the public's understanding of the state and different types of health care. Of particular importance is the dynamic process by which the public's understanding of the state intermingles with its perceptions of hospital and general community-based care in such facilities as infirmaries. I trace the emergence in Britain of a widespread expectation of both hospital treatment by specialists and community care by general practitioners; Americans, in contrast, came to associate health care largely with hospitals. Because a tradition of general medical care never emerged in the United States, community-based care never gained the foothold it found in Britain. Moreover, partly as an emanation of different experiences with poor-law institutions, public understanding of the state's role diverged in the two countries. Whereas in Britain centuries of experience accustomed the public to state provisions and made direct state involvement in hospital and general health care seem

---

8. Various research traditions have—from different analytic perspectives—addressed the issue of general public understandings orienting an individual's specific preferences: Conover and Feldman 1984, Feldman 1988, Feldman and Zaller 1992; Wildavsky 1987; Hall 1988. For a recent debate about some of these issues see *American Political Science Review* 85 (1991): 1341–80.

conceivable and necessary, in the United States the public was comparatively unfamiliar with this type of direct and extensive state role. Nevertheless, Americans' understanding of the state was not as monolithic and unchanging as suggested by conventional portrayals of American national character; the public's understanding of the state combined a long-standing uneasiness with a gradual recognition and acceptance, which was spurred on by Social Security's development after 1935.

The enduring meanings associated with health care and the state pattern the formation of specific public preferences. The danger of divorcing the interpretation of specific individual preferences from that of culture's enduring, more general patterns is illustrated by political observers' use of polling data as evidence of unambiguous American support since the 1940s for a comprehensive national health insurance program. The focus is on individual preferences for the objective of national insurance; this attention, however, ignores the long-standing (even if changing) meaning that Americans have conferred on health care and political institutions—namely, an uneasiness about governmental provision of social welfare (Payne 1946; Schiltz 1970; Hirshfield 1970; Marmor et al. 1990).

A second aspect of meaning-centered analysis that is particularly relevant in this book is culture's impact on state capacity and elite negotiating patterns. The first theoretical expectation is that policy discussions on altering state capacity are enveloped within culture. Weberians assume that political development is detached from the broader societal culture. Culturalists claim that meaning is conferred on institutions and that the knowledge of society's members is necessarily involved in, and directly relevant to, institutional change. Because culture is all-encompassing, controlling the conceptual tools and emotional repertoires of all members of a society, socially constructed values and assumptions seep into even insulated policy deliberations. It is not possible, then, for institutions to operate and change behind the backs of social actors: even if state actors attempt to concentrate on considerations that seem detached from culture, institutional change cannot be separate from, or external to, what all members of society know about such institutions.

Culture's impact on specific institutional changes is confirmed by recent quantitative research on the covariation between opinion poll results and policy decisions. Several studies report that public preferences have substantial effects on American policy making when they are sustained, substantial, and directed at a salient issue (Page and Shapiro 1983; Shapiro 1982; Erikson 1976; Monroe 1979; Weissberg 1976). In perhaps the most comprehensive study, Page and Shapiro demonstrate that policy tends to move in the same direction as opinion changes as much as 90 percent of the time; additional evidence suggests that changes in public preferences *cause* changes in policy.

Nonetheless, previous analysis of the mass public's relevance to policy making has persistently failed to focus on (let alone explain) specific changes in state capacity. The quantitative analysis of poll results and final policy decisions does represent an important corrective to the tendency among culturalists to exaggerate culture's causal significance. Thus, culturalists expect that socially shared meanings and public preferences affect political and institutional outcomes; this expectation assumes, though, precisely what must be empirically investigated—culture's specific impact on politics and institutions. For instance, during the formulation of the NHS and Medicare acts, electoral competition and political divisions obstructed government responsiveness, creating a four-year lag between the formation of strong public preferences for health reform and actual policy change; these acts were not inevitable in the absence of major political developments. As Marmor convincingly argues in his analysis of Medicare's origins, legislative activity is never just a matter of ratifying public opinion polls (1973, 3).

But even quantitative research obscures the policy formulation process and the influences on it; the problem lies in its level of aggregation (see especially Monroe 1979; Page and Shapiro 1983). As a result, this quantitative analysis does not examine culture's actual impact on the multitude of issues that are addressed *before* any final policy decision.[9] In short, culturalists pose the important (but untested) theoretical expectation that public understandings and preferences toward existing institutions are a primary determinant of specific changes in administrative capacity.

Moreover, culturalists imply that state actors' negotiations with powerful interest groups cannot simply be expressive of self-evident administrative capacity. Because of state actors' reliance on culture to render their environment intelligible, it is not possible for state actors to construct objective accounts of institutions. This means that state actors' relations with interest groups cannot merely reflect the technical capacity of institutions. Rather, the decisions of politicians and bureaucrats during their bargaining with interest groups are conditioned by prevailing understandings and preferences. Culture is the medium for, and therefore an influence on, state actors' assessment of interest group demands.

Culturalists, though, neglect policy networks and state actors' strategic

9. To quantify governmental policy decisions, investigators of the relationship between public preferences and policy making have counted the votes of legislators or the overall vote or decision of a collective political institution (e.g., congressional passage of a bill). The problem is that, by aggregating multiple policy decisions, this research has ignored policymakers' decisions during the *prevote* stage.

calculations in weighing interest group pressure. As the Weberians empha-size, state actors have the potential to autonomously define and pursue distinctive policies. Thus, culturalists again posit an important (but largely untested) theoretical expectation: the development of strong public pref-erences and enduring cultural patterns affects the state's autonomy from interest group pressures. Interest group claims are unlikely to be influential when they confront strong public preferences and understandings; but claims are more likely to win government concessions when such preferences and understandings are relatively unformed or potentially supportive of pressure group appeals.[10] Culturalists, then, expect the mass public to be a primary influence on policy making and elite negotiations with powerful interest groups.

FORMULATION OF THE NHS AND MEDICARE ACTS

The NHS and Medicare acts were formulated in central states whose administrative capacities are often portrayed as weak in comparison to those of continental European countries; the American and British states are not expected to be up to the task of coherent, detailed intervention in domestic affairs (Almond and Powell 1966; Heclo 1974; Skowronek 1982; Orloff and Skocpol 1984). Although the United States and Britain are clustered together as administratively weak, the two countries do differ, with the British state enjoying more extensive institutional capacity.

Consistent with the general pattern of comparatively weak American and British states, both the NHS and Medicare acts were designed in policy-making sites that lacked (to differing degrees) the strong hierarchical or-ganization of European institutions. Authority over Medicare's formulation was dispersed among the lawmaking branches. Instead of dictating policy, the president and the Department of Health, Education, and Welfare (HEW) were generally left to provide encouragement and technical assistance to a decentralized legislative branch and, in particular, to finance committees in the Senate and, especially, the House. In formal terms, the British state's hierarchical structure had no parallels in the United States: the prime min-ister's office was at the apex of a unitary government structure, which centralized the country's health policy in a single agency—the Ministry of Health. During the NHS's formulation, though, the British state's formal

10. Although they emerge from different theoretical traditions, culturalist expectations are consistent with Schattschneider's (1960) thesis regarding the socialization and privatization of conflict.

lines of control were partially compromised by the dispersion of authority within the executive branch. Major decisions were made before legislative consideration, but the prime minister could not dominate the deliberations of the Ministry of Health, the cabinet, or the cabinet's unusually active committees.

The development of specialization, though, enhanced (to differing degrees) each state's capacity in the area of health policy; it equipped American and British civil servants with the expertise and experience to design policy options aimed at harmonizing competing claims. In the United States, policy discussions drew from an isolated area of strength—the Social Security Administration and its expert, experienced, and committed staff of civil servants (Derthick 1979). British capacity was enhanced by the contribution of national health insurance's development to the Ministry of Health's "policy learning" and by the input of the department's medical officers. Generally, given its longer experience with health policy and stronger position in cabinet-centered government, the British state had a more extensive institutional capacity than the American state.

During health policy formulation in each country, politicians and bureaucrats in authoritative positions assessed their prevailing institutional and political environments. The relevant state actors in Medicare's formulation were the president, critical members of Congress, and officials in HEW. In Britain, the important state actors were officials in the Ministry of Health as well as elected politicians who were active as cabinet members and department heads. The active intervention of politicians provided the critical thrust for pursuing major new policy objectives; policy experts generated the alternatives from which authoritative choices could be made. Under Britain's wartime coalition government of Labour and Conservative parties (Spring 1940–May 1945) and the Democratically controlled White House (November 1960–November 1964), politicians attempted to pursue health care reform but were constrained by political deadlock. After the landslide electoral victories of the Labour party in July 1945 and Lyndon Johnson in November 1964, politicians pushed for bold innovations and quickly enacted new legislation: NHS became law in November 1946 and Medicare in July 1965.

In later chapters, I use American and British innovations in health policy to explore contending theoretical expectations. The cluster of decisions that are packaged in final legislation are dissected in order to identify the primary focus of and influence on policymakers. In particular, I analyze culture's impact on two aspects of decision making: variation in state actors' autonomy as they formulated basic principles and state actors' decisions to make specific changes in administrative capacity.

State Autonomy and Basic Principles

During serious government discussions of the NHS and Medicare acts, policymakers not only framed new arrangements but also debated whether to adopt previously designed arrangements.[11] Each government's decisions emerged from policy networks that organized continuous bargaining between relevant state actors and interest groups representing powerful health care producers—the American Medical Association (AMA), the American Hospital Association (AHA), and their British counterparts.[12] In particular, the NHS was the subject of nearly four years of organized discussions between leading interest groups and the Ministry of Health, and Medicare was formulated within a network that incorporated health care producers into congressional deliberations.

What is analytically significant is the variation in interest group influence on policymakers' formulation and acceptance of basic principles, such as the degree to which services and the population would be covered. Although the organized incorporation of health care providers did enable them to exercise significant influence on some issues, state actors nonetheless protected and used their jurisdictional position to reject interest group claims on other issues. Thus, neither the Medicare nor the NHS acts were simply the by-products of interest group competition: on important policy issues, politicians and bureaucrats defied even fierce opposition to pursue their own distinct calculations concerning their careers and the interests of their departments and nation.

To what extent, and under what conditions, did state actors exert independence from medical interest groups? For Weberians, the state's autonomy is a function of its administrative capacity: they expect the moderately weak American state to generally exercise minimal independence, establishing a relationship with producer groups that is dominated by cooperation and concessions to private interests. Research on the NHS and Medicare acts confirms Weberian expectation: the preferences of interest groups are identified as the single best predictor of policy (Marmor 1983, chap. 6, and 1973; Hollingsworth 1986; Eckstein 1958 and 1960).

Culturalists, though, attempt to explain the variation of interest group influence within a single policy area:[13] they expect state autonomy to vary

11. An illustration of a policy designed before serious government discussions is Medicare's use of Social Security's financing mechanism: though it was initially formulated by a small group of governmental and nongovernmental officials, authoritative policymakers still vigorously debated whether to address it when serious discussions began.

12. See Hollingsworth 1986 for a systematic discussion of American and British representatives of health care providers.

13. Marmor's classic study (1973) of Medicare illustrates the tendency to neglect the variation in interest group influence: it does not systematically explain the swings between interest

according to policymakers' perceptions of public preferences and understanding. In particular, policymakers' sensitivity to strong and weak public sentiment is expected to be inversely related to interest group influence. Accordingly, policymakers should readily dismiss even fierce interest group pressure when they perceive strong public support for such basic principles as Medicare's Social Security financing and the NHS's universal coverage.[14] Conversely, medical producer groups should exert significant influence when the public is seen as apathetic or as potentially supportive of their claims.

In this book, I present evidence that confirms the culturalists' conceptions of state autonomy and modifies Weberian expectations. The Medicare and NHS cases pose a difficult analytic puzzle for Weberians: under stable administrative conditions in one policy area, interest group pressure produced concessions on some issues but proved ineffective on others. Some Weberians recognize that state autonomy from interest group pressure may vary within one national state (e.g., Skocpol and Finegold 1982), but these cases suggest that variation can occur within a single policy area. Thus, evidence of medical producers simultaneously exerting both strong and weak influence challenges attempts to monolithically categorize state autonomy in terms of either an entire state or a single policy area. Moreover, the degree of state autonomy is not simply a function of its administrative capacity; state actors' balancing of public sentiment and interest group claims produced complex negotiating patterns, which were not directly tied to the state's organizational attributes. The extent to which the state's continuous interaction with health care producers translated into actual influence varied according to policymakers' perception of public preferences and understandings. Contrary to Weberian expectations, moderately weak administrative capacity was associated with high state autonomy on specific policy issues.

State Capacity and Administrative Arrangements

Policy discussions regarding the design of administrative arrangements for the Medicare and NHS acts concentrated on altering the state's capacity—its specialization in, and hierarchical control over, health care. According to Weberians, technical administrative attributes are the focus and primary determinant of elites' decisions to change existing state institutions: existing capacity is expected to prefigure the specific direction of institutional

---

groups winning permissive remuneration arrangements and the exclusion of hospital specialists, and their ineffectiveness in preventing the use of Social Security's financing arrangements.

14. The weakness of major interest groups in the face of popularly embraced principles seems consistent with findings that interest group positions on salient issues, as transmitted through television news, can push public opinion in the opposite direction. Faced with this negative response to interest groups, policymakers can be expected not to accord much weight to interest group views in cases of salient issues (Page et al. 1987).

change. The Weberians should anticipate that the American state's moderately weak administrative resources in the area of health policy would produce new administrative arrangements characterized by weak hierarchical control and low specialization; the British state's relatively greater capacity would be reflected in stronger administrative arrangements. Existing research on the NHS and Medicare acts similarly connects institutional change to elites—the expertise and rational actions of civil servants and influential politicians as they assess the capacity of existing institutions (Hollingsworth 1986; Klein 1983; Eckstein 1958). Culturalists, however, lead us to expect that public perceptions and understandings should dominate policy discussions and account for policy decisions.

I explore these contending theoretical expectation by analyzing American and British discussion concerning the state's administrative structure. Thus, this book closely examines the decisive influences on debates over whether and to what degree the Medicare and the NHS ought to establish direct central authority over new programs. In later chapters, I argue that these detailed discussions are largely consistent with culturalists' expectations: politicians and specialists focused on and were primarily influenced by their perceptions of public sentiment.

LINKAGE MECHANISMS

An important reason for synthesizing culturalist analysis with institutionalist accounts is to avoid the tendency of treating policy making as an epiphenomenon of public opinion. A critical research question involves explaining how policymakers come to perceive and incorporate public understandings and preferences. After all, congruence between the values and preferences of elites and those of the mass public is neither natural nor inevitable in liberal democracies; a disjuncture can develop because state actors misperceive, fail to recognize, or outright defy public understandings and preferences. I argue that the mass public had extensive influence on the NHS and Medicare acts not simply because its concerns naturally (and unintentionally) seeped into discussions among elites but also because policymakers had come to feel politically pressured to take an explicit interest in tracking and incorporating public preferences. Examination of culture's relevance to policy making must incorporate, then, analysis of politics and institutions.

Here I concentrate on two especially critical mechanisms that link public sentiment to the policy-making process, institutional developments and political dynamics.[15] In both the United States and Britain, a public opinion apparatus developed during the twentieth century to perform two functions: to conduct public relations in order to manage public perceptions, and to track public sentiment, largely through the use of polls.

The institutional development of a public opinion apparatus created both direct and indirect links between the public and policy making during the formulation of the NHS and Medicare acts. The apparatus transformed politicians' traditional interest in identifying and responding to the public from an irregular, ad hoc process to a regular organizational routine; and this transformation had a direct impact on health policy. For instance, it helped to persuade Kennedy and Johnson to select the Medicare issue as one of the few they campaigned for. This state apparatus also had an important indirect role: its development had an inward "recoil effect," sensitizing government officials to the importance of responding to, rather than simply manipulating, public opinion. By the period of health policy formulation, politicians and civil servants recognized that government decisions must incorporate not only rigorous technical research but also the concerns of the "man in the street": as a British civil servant explained, "officers must not merely keep their noses hard down to the administrative grindstone."[16]

Political developments created a second link between the mass public and government elites, affecting policymakers' timing and motivation for pursuing reform. Politicians and civil servants decide to respond to public sentiment based on calculations that their behavior can advance their power and position. The making of the NHS and Medicare acts was shaped by the struggle of real, breathing politicians and civil servants to maintain (and, if possible, improve) their respective positions.

The political calculations of policymakers are made within a strategic universe, defined in this book in terms of two factors: public opinion toward reform and specific policy directions, and political struggles inside and outside government. Major political events, such as historic electoral landslides and the extraordinary popular demand for enacting the Beveridge Report, are especially effective in recasting political calculations and in linking public sentiment and policy making. These major political events provide an indisputable and highly visible signal concerning public opinion: they mobilize policymakers in fragmented political institutions (such as Congress) to re-

15. Elections and political parties supply two additional means by which public sentiment might be transmited to policymakers; I examine these in subsequent chapters in the context of other institutional and political developments.
16. Ministry of Health (MH) 78/147, Memo from S. H. Wood, "Intelligence and Public Relations," 7/2/35.

evaluate and respond to public preferences. Electoral competition, then, creates strong incentives for politicians to identify potentially popular goals, which less visible policy experts specify alternative means for achieving.

A major similarity in the formulation of the NHS and Medicare acts is that political struggles created three parallel stages in the policymaking process. Political developments during Britain's early war years and Eisenhower's last presidential term transformed the topic of major health reform from an issue considered impractical to one accorded a prominent position on governmental agendas. The intensification of political struggles within Britain's coalition government and within the Democratic administrations between the 1960 and 1964 elections prompted policymakers to pursue reform. Political deadlock, though, pressured them into pursuing a risk-averse consensus approach, which outlined the basic features of future legislation but failed to build sufficient agreement to win passage. During the third stage of the process, electoral landslides created a new political environment favoring a bold approach to policy making and the pursuit of major innovations believed inconceivable even a few years earlier.

Incorporating both culture as well as political and institutional processes is necessary to avoid two common extremes, treating public opinion as simply irrelevant to detailed policy making or assuming that public opinion is merely ratified into government decisions. Analyzing the mass public's influence on policy making requires an investigation of both public sentiment and the behavior of elites. The mass public's influence on health legislation was neither automatic nor coincidental but stemmed from the institutional development of a public opinion apparatus and from state actors' attempts to advance their power and position.

Diverse traditions of empirical research on liberal democracies have agreed that the mass public's role in policy making is and ought to be sharply limited. Weberians illustrate this research orientation by claiming that specialists and elected politicians have relatively free rein in determining detailed policies, and that their decisions are primarily the product of state actors' assessment of administrative capacity. Clearly, Weberians have helped shift the study of politics from the system's "required" functions toward the evolution of specific institutional change and the potential of state actors to design and pursue distinctive policies.

On the basis, though, of the Medicare and NHS cases, I argue that the Weberians' causal argument for institutional change is misspecified and contradicted by important developments. The state's "objective" administrative capacity is the primary focus and determinant in Weberian analysis: state autonomy from interest groups is presented as a function of capacity, and existing administrative resources are expected to prefigure new institutional changes. American and British health policy suggests, however, that state actors' perceptions of public preferences and understandings account for the variations in state autonomy; even with administrative resources uniform in a single policy area, state capacity still cannot account for the alternating weakness and strength of medical interest groups.

In addition, the dramatic differences in the language and decisions of American and British policymakers as they considered detailed changes in state capacity stemmed from important variations in the public's understanding and preferences concerning the state and different forms of health care delivery. Constrained by their public's comparative unfamiliarity with state provisions of social welfare and by preferences for merely extending the established Social Security system, American policymakers were reticent state builders. For instance, even as a major new role for the government was forged, American politicians and officials repeatedly compromised Medicare's hierarchical organization in order to minimize direct state control. As a result, the American state was strictly limited to relying on the established insurance approach to supplement nonstate arrangements for providing and financing health care. In Britain, in contrast, officials were able to draw on the public's familiarity with hospital and community-based care as well as on its acceptance of a state-run medical service. The American practice of ceding important administrative functions to nonstate bodies was inconceivable in Britain, where it was assumed that the state would play a major role in financing *and* providing health care. Public opinion (rather than administrative capacity) "loaded the dice," making certain institutional changes conceivable in Britain (e.g., a massive state role in the actual provision of hospital and general care for the entire population) while barring them in the United States.

Evidence that Weberians misspecify the causal argument for institutional change could be interpreted as ambiguous in certain respects: findings of the American government's concessions to interest groups and its decisions to establish weak hierarchical control could reasonably be interpreted as consistent with Weberian accounts. I argue, though, that health policy making offers significant counterevidence. During the formulation of specific policy issues, American state actors relied on moderately weak administrative capacity, but they persistently exercised a high degree of independence from interest groups; even risk-averse policymakers, who were intent on building consensus, dismissed particularistic claims.

Moreover, contrary to Weberian expectations, senior administrators in the United States did have strong confidence in their own capacity, and they aggressively lobbied President Kennedy for direct federal administration. Policymakers, then, did not turn away from establishing hierarchical control because it was "too much for the government machinery." Rather, capacity-enhancing arguments were not seriously considered because the White House and members of Congress primarily focused on, and were influenced by, Americans' enduring ambivalence toward the state and public preferences for medical reform, which built on the Social Security approach. Finally, after identifying a reform approach consistent with public preferences and understandings, American policymakers (despite their comparatively weak institutions) significantly expanded the scope of government responsibility for, and financial commitment to, health care.

I conclude that public preferences and socially shared understandings have a critical influence on the process of detailed policy making and on selecting the means for implementing policy goals. It is not tenable, then, to argue that the public's role is limited to identifying broad policy goals while elite experts have free rein to fashion the means to achieve those goals. In both the United States and Britain, public sentiment was critical in shaping the administrative means.

2 | Policymakers' Sensitivity toward Public Opinion

In our own time, policymakers openly rely on pollsters to get a direct, immediate sense of public concerns. Over the course of American and British history, governmental officials' relationship with the mass public has not always been characterized by this kind of sensitivity. Earlier policymakers were more preoccupied with manipulating public sentiment; elite norms discouraged prominent political leaders such as American presidents from establishing a direct, responsive relationship with the mass public (Tulis 1987). As a result of political struggles during the twentieth century, however, American and British policymakers' perceptions of the mass public qualitatively changed: by the time the NHS and Medicare began to be formulated, government elites were acutely sensitive to public opinion. The evolution of this disposition and behavior toward the public was tied to the institutional development during the twentieth century of a public opinion apparatus within the executive branch of the American and British governments.

The public opinion apparatus developed the state's capacity in two areas, manipulation of and responsiveness to public opinion. The aspect developed first and most extensively was the capacity to conduct public relations campaigns aimed at shaping popular preferences. The second capacity involved gathering intelligence on public opinion; in particular, polling became a central aspect of government efforts to gain a regular and reliable grip on public opinion. Policymakers' capacity to influence and track public opinion directly affected the motivations and behavior of state actors as they formulated American and British health policy.

More than creating new organizational capacity, though, the public opinion apparatus had a profound effect on policymakers' perception of the mass public. During the evolution of the apparatus, its "recoil effect [was] greater than the blast" (Ogilvy-Webb 1965, 196). As well as an outward effect on public opinion, this apparatus had an inward effect: it educated politicians and bureaucrats to be sensitive to public opinion. The consequent new outlook among politicians and civil servants involved a shift from a preoccupation with secrecy and seclusion to a recognition of public opinion as a critical influence on government decision making.

In this chapter I examine historic developments within the executive branch's apex (the presidency and the prime minister's No. 10 Downing Street office) and within each country's national agency responsible for health (in America, HEW; in Britain, Ministry of Health). Despite important differences in American and British institutional development, the public opinion apparatus that emerged in the two countries evinced remarkably similar features. Moreover, in both countries the apparatus's development was tied to the struggle for political power and institutional position: the apparatus became integrated into the policymaking process when policymakers in the executive branch recognized that it presented opportunities to offset advantages possessed by others, the legislature as well as nongovernmental groups and individuals.

The analysis of the public opinion apparatus is divided into two main sections.[1] In the first I consider initial developments in the period up to the 1930s. Elements of what would become a public opinion apparatus often emerged on a piecemeal, ad hoc basis and were either isolated in far reaches of the government or abandoned, leaving only precedents for later developments. In the second section I trace developments through the period when the Medicare and NHS acts were formulated; I examine the institutionalization of the public opinion apparatus as an enduring, routine component of government operations. In part because of limited data, this institutionalization is not primarily analyzed in terms of organizational resources such as personnel and budgets.[2] Instead, I focus on the changing meaning of the apparatus to government officials—the routinization of new patterns of thought and behavior regarding the mass public.

HISTORIC ROOTS OF THE PUBLIC OPINION APPARATUS

The government's public relations capacity was developed earlier and more extensively than each country's capacity to track public opinion. His-

---

1. This chapter merely outlines the institutional development of the public opinion apparatus. For a more detailed analysis see Jacobs, 1990.

2. The political risk of appearing to snoop for partisan advantage led government officials, at critical junctures, to deliberately refrain from assembling relevant information.

torically, politicians and bureaucrats have attempted to influence public opinion by media coverage: state actors used their words and initiatives to manipulate the media and, through it, public opinion. The public opinion apparatus originated, then, in policymakers' attempt to have an outward effect in manipulating the public.

Britain

The development of the British government's public relations structures was conditioned by the evolution of news organizations, in particular, the rise and fall of the political press. In his two-volume study (1981, 1984), Stephen Koss argues that by the mid-1800s "ownership by a political tendency" dominated the British press; as a result, politicians could rely on a group of newspapers to transcribe and endorse their positions. The political press, however, rapidly began to disappear after World War I: with the commercial tendency superseding the earlier political tendency, newspapers became less explicitly party political and more geared to providing what was thought of as independent and nonpartisan coverage.

With the erosion of ironclad bonds between politicians and newspapers, policymakers in the executive branch felt compelled to look for alternative ways to manage the media. In particular, state actors introduced government institutions to perform four public relations tasks. First, new state structures organized the media's daily routines as it covered the executive branch (providing necessary services to allow news organizations to file their stories before their deadlines). In addition, these structures channeled information to the media: they determined what information to release, the form in which such information should appear, and the appropriate forum. Third, they arranged contacts with policymakers. Finally, politicians and bureaucrats developed state structures to promote government policies and actions by appealing directly (and not through the media) to the public.

In Britain, World War I was a watershed event, prompting the gradual emergence of new government structures to perform three public relations activities—organizing the media's daily routines, arranging contacts with policymakers, and channeling information.[3] Wartime developments set important precedents and introduced the idea that public relations was a critical feature of modern administration. The postwar government, however, dismantled the new structures because of real and potential controversy associated with government attempts to manage the press and to produce propaganda.

---

3. Unless otherwise noted, the discussion of the British public opinion apparatus is based on Ogilvy-Webb 1965 and 1970.

Nonetheless, during the period between the wars important institutional developments led to the establishment of public relations offices within individual departments. Thus, within the Ministry of Health, officials reached a consensus by 1935 that, because a "great deal of publicity is being lost," the ministry faced unnecessary difficulties fending off political attacks and implementing its policies. These officials concluded that it was necessary to revamp the department's public relations apparatus significantly: they became committed to an active type of public relations whereby information was funneled into the press "on the initiative of the Ministry rather than at the request of the public."[4] Accordingly, the department changed its internal administrative arrangements and appointed an appropriately trained individual to manage the press by performing the various public relations tasks. The prime minister's involvement in public relations was limited. Although a press spokesman at No. 10 Downing Street was appointed in 1931 to distribute information from the prime minister and to coordinate ministerial relations with the press, even this new position was severely constrained.[5]

By the 1930s, then, the prime minister and especially the departments attempted both to manage (although not in a coordinated, systematic way) the increasingly independent press and to appeal directly to the public through the preparation and distribution of posters, photographs, films, and exhibitions. The departments and specifically the Ministry of Health were discouraged, though, from developing this direct capacity to manipulate public opinion by the political reaction to government-sponsored propaganda.

Intelligence gathering. Politicians and bureaucrats not only discussed government public relations in the executive branch but also contemplated ways to improve the government's capacity to collect intelligence on the general public. As a result, during the interwar period survey techniques were occasionally used to measure "habits of everyday life," such as family budget patterns (Ogilvy-Webb 1965, 56). But with formal opinion polling not introduced in Britain until the late 1930s and not regularly used until the latter half of the 1940s, much of the intelligence work was directed at systematizing traditional methods such as monitoring political events (e.g., by-elections) as well as collecting "factual" information issued by important groups, Parliament, or newspapers. Thus, throughout the executive branch

4. MH 78/147, MH 78/147, Memo from G. H. Shakespeare to secretary and minister, 6/26/35; MH 78/147, Minute from W. A. Robinson to minister, 7/5/35. Also see Memo from W. A. Robinson to J. Rucker, 2/11/35; MH 78/147, Memo, "Intelligence and Publicity Work," 1/18/35, by H. Leggett. For an early discussion of departmental public relations, see MH 78/147, "Memo," undated but probably written between 10/33 and 3/34.

5. In particular, the prime minister's spokesman did not have a full-time position and was unable to overcome the department's continued control over the flow of information to the press.

policymakers attended to revamping public relations arrangements and took a few measures on the intelligence front as well.

Mirroring this pattern, the revamping of the Ministry of Health's public relations arrangements in the early months of 1935 was accompanied by attempts to gain intelligence on lay and medical opinion. Thus, the department's new public relations director was supposed to contribute to the anticipation of future problems by studying the trend of "social and political opinion." But civil servants, anxious not to give the impression of snooping, were reluctant to conduct surveys of public opinion; they concentrated instead on collecting factual information from internal documents and external periodicals and reports.[6] Thus, despite the ministry's repeatedly stated intention, its intelligence gathering failed to develop significantly during this period.

Perhaps most important, the evolution of government arrangements to outwardly influence public opinion had an inward recoil effect: policymakers throughout the executive branch were increasingly preoccupied with what the mass public was thinking. In contrast to the prewar period, the eve of World War II found general acceptance of the "need to take positive and considered steps to publicize departmental policies" (Ogilvy-Webb 1965, 55). As Crossman observed, politicians realized during the interwar years that their influence was tied to their ability to educate or stimulate public opinion (1981, 105–6).

Echoing a similar sentiment, officials in the Ministry of Health repeatedly stressed that their new "watertight machinery" would be worthless without a significant change in the department's perception of the mass public. To "make the work of the Ministry a matter of legitimate interest to ordinary men and women," one official argued, "officers of the Ministry [had to accept] the labor involved as a necessary and legitimate part of their duties. ... This means that officers ... must in fact be 'publicity minded' and not merely keep their noses hard down to the administrative grindstone."[7] A senior civil servant acknowledged that he was not too old to depart radically from old civil service traditions: he accepted the new administrative norm that "the public has a right to be told what we are doing."[8]

United States

The evolution in the United States of the public opinion apparatus followed the same general path as that in Britain: public relations structures

---

6. MH 78/147, memo by H. Leggett, 1/18/35; MH 78/147, handwritten comments by W. A. Robinson on note from S. H. Wood, 7/2/35.
7. MH 78/147, Memo from S. H. Wood, "Intelligence and Public Relations" 7/2/35.
8. MH 78/147, Minute from W. A. Robinson to minister, 7/5/35.

were gradually developed throughout the executive branch, with intelligence gathering left comparatively less developed.

As in Britain, the government's major explicit channel of communication with the public was the media. The relatively less politicized nature of the American press was a major factor in the comparatively greater development of the American public relations apparatus. In the absence of the partisan bonds found in Britain, presidents were forced at a much earlier date and to a far greater extent than policymakers in Britain's executive branch to establish regular, institutional ties with the media.

Elected officeholders had recognized the political importance of newspaper coverage well before the twentieth century. But the first major institutional development in the executive branch's public relations apparatus occurred at the turn of the century in response to a presidential "desire for control and centralization of information."[9] Prompted by foreign policy developments that heightened the importance of controlling public opinion, President William McKinley initiated a series of innovative practices to manipulate the press as a public relations instrument.[10]

Staffed with more personnel specializing in press relations than any of its predecessors, the McKinley administration shaped the press's daily routine: it set the practice of providing regular press briefings, press releases, and copies of speeches in advance and provided accommodations that allowed the press to set up shop near the presidential offices. Moreover, the McKinley White House took a systematic interest in producing a timely supply of information that would keep the administration and its activities constantly before the public. It managed the media in order to focus journalistic attention on issues of its own choosing and to present its interpretation of those issues.

The two subsequent presidents accepted McKinley's new approach to the media: Theodore Roosevelt did so willingly; William Taft was politically forced to acknowledge the new practices as a regular part of the presidency. Woodrow Wilson, however, significantly strengthened McKinley's public relations apparatus: he further systematized relations with the media and centralized control over it in the White House.[11]

To enhance the president's control over the information the press received

9. Hilderbrand 1981, 164. Unless otherwise noted, this section on the United States is based on Hilderbrand 1981.

10. McKinley was specifically motivated by his political need for public support of a greatly expanded role in world politics, one that involved American military actions against Spain, China, and the Philippines.

11. Although Tulis (1987) identifies Wilson as the transitional figure in ushering in presidential leadership based on appeals to the public, my research on the public opinion apparatus emphasizes institutional developments and Wilson's place as one among several presidents who redefined the presidency.

and the interpretation it offered, the Wilson administration expanded the White House's involvement in structuring the media's routines, contacts, and information sources. As in Britain, World War I prompted major changes. Both before and during the war, when the Committee on Public Information was created, Wilson developed the means to communicate directly with the public through promotional campaigns and to centralize control further over press relations. As in Britain, though, political concerns within the legislative branch over government propaganda convinced policymakers in the executive branch to dismantle these public relations structures at the end of the war.

Whereas in Britain the evolution of the public relations apparatus largely occurred in the departments, in the United States this development was primarily generated in the White House. Initial forays into the field of public relations occurred in the State Department near the turn of the century; the departments of Agriculture and Commerce also became active in government public relations.

Intelligence gathering. As in Britain, the development of an intelligence-gathering capacity remained limited before the 1930s. Like their British counterparts, American politicians traditionally relied on a variety of techniques for assessing public opinion (e.g., newspaper coverage and election results). Indeed, one of the McKinley administration's innovations included systematic assessment of press coverage in order to inform White House strategy on managing press and public relations.

Since the 1700s, however, American policymakers had also turned to a range of polling techniques, such as straw polls and canvasing (Jensen 1980). Routine presidential use of modern statistical survey techniques, though, did not emerge until the 1960s.

Overall, the development of new government institutions that were focused outwardly on public opinion had an inward impact on state actors, forging a new outlook among policymakers. Twentieth-century White House preoccupation with public relations was unimaginable in the nineteenth century. By the 1930s, however, a publicity-mindedness encouraged policymakers in the executive branch to track and try to mold public opinion.

INSTITUTIONALIZATION OF THE PUBLIC OPINION APPARATUS

Beginning in the 1930s, attempts to influence and track public opinion escalated, prompting new institutions and intensifying policymakers' sensitivity to popular preferences. Public relations structures were expanded and institutionalized in both countries as a routine part of the government's administrative structure; an intelligence gathering capacity was introduced during wartime Britain but was not firmly institutionalized as a routine part of government operations as it was in the United States. This development of institutions and a receptiveness to public opinion stemmed from the political pressures of adversarial debate and competition: the typical pressures were exacerbated in the United States by the emphasis after the late 1950s on presidential primaries and in Britain by World War II and the virtual collapse of the political press.

Britain

In Britain, World War II began a period in which public relations arrangements were integrated into the decision-making process. Recognizing that a successful war effort required the public's active cooperation, state actors introduced at the onset of the war an extensive centralized public opinion apparatus—the Ministry of Information. To accomplish its primary objective of maintaining morale, this new ministry expanded the four public relations tasks that had begun to emerge during the interwar period. As the government's publicity agent for maintaining morale, it structured the media's routines, contacts, and information sources. Moreover, the state's capacity to influence public opinion directly also greatly expanded during the war. The ministry created the machinery to enable the government to produce and conduct direct public relations campaigns instead of relying on the transmission of publicity through the media.

Although the Ministry of Information did increase centralized control over the government's press and public relations, the departments continued to dominate. With many ministries having evolved their own public relations offices during the interwar period, even the prime minister's intervention failed to ensure the Ministry of Information's control over government public relations. Reflecting the continued control of departments, the Ministry of Health did not allow the Ministry of Information to conduct its publicity; rather, it relied on its own public relations office.[12]

Moreover, during the war, state actors created the first administrative structures to track public opinion systematically. The purpose of building an intelligence-gathering capacity was "to provide...[an] effective link between the people of the country and the government...convey[ing] the thoughts, opinions, and feelings of the public...[so that they were] con-

---

12. MH 80/27, Minute from Fife Clark to S. F. Wilkinson, 1/4/44; MH 77/28, Memo from Clark to Wilkinson, "National Health Service," 1/13/44.

stantly in the minds of administrators."[13] In particular, the Ministry of Information produced two distinct types of data on public opinion, a qualitative survey conducted by the ministry's Home Intelligence Division and a statistical report by its Social Survey Division. During the course of the war, the focus of intelligence gathering shifted from assessing the effectiveness of government publicity efforts and measuring general morale to studying public preferences toward particular government policies, especially as they related to postwar reconstruction.[14]

Within the Ministry of Health, interest in public opinion data was dramatically heightened. Thus, in June 1942 officials discussed using the Ministry of Information's intelligence service to measure both "how the ordinary citizen fares when he needs hospital treatment... [and] the untreated disabilities... that for financial reasons... [citizens] do not bring to the hospital."[15] Moreover, beginning in this period, the Ministry of Health commissioned the Ministry of Information's Social Survey Division to conduct several quantitative studies of the effectiveness of the ministry's publicity campaigns and to gauge public attitudes toward personal health.[16]

Even with this new interest in opinion surveys, policymakers did not systematically integrate polling data with decision making. Within the Ministry of Health, officials found the new opinion data only occasionally useful, providing merely "a sort of atmosphere... [or] picture of the feeling of the country."[17] In terms of the cabinet, divisions between the coalition's Labour and Conservative members prevented the government from using data of strong public support for major postwar reform. The failure to use this data left the government unprepared for the outpouring of public support for the Beveridge Report during the winter of 1942; the government's miscalculation irreparably damaged its credibility and contributed to the coalition's collapse in 1945.

Although the wartime government expanded the public opinion apparatus, it was still not accepted as a regular aspect of decision making. The reluctance to institutionalize the capacity to conduct public relations and

13. Ministry of Information (INF) 1/290, "Public Opinion in the U.K.: A Comprehensive Report on the History, Functions, and Administration of the Home Intelligence Division."

14. For instance, a survey was conducted on the public's reaction to the wartime government's published proposal for health care reform, see INF 1/293, "Home Intelligence Special Report: Public Reaction to the White Paper on a National Health Service," by Ministry of Information, 3/14/44.

15. MH 77/19, Letter from N. McNicoll to W. Jameson, 6/9/42.

16. Ministry of Information, Social Survey: Reports and Papers (RG) 23/24, Wartime Social Survey, "Public Attitudes to Health and to the Autumn Health Campaign," Report no. 21, Summer 1942; RG 23/38, Wartime Social Survey, "The Campaign against V.D.," new series, G. 5, Spring 1943.

17. INF 1/285, Letter from H. E. Magee to Ministry of Information, 9/43.

intelligence gathering led the coalition government to announce that the opinion apparatus and specifically the Ministry of Information would be dismantled at the end of the war to prevent the use of government facilities for political objectives.

Nevertheless, when the coalition government collapsed in May 1945 and the Labour government came to power in July, the new cabinet institutionalized the public opinion apparatus. Although senior ministers recognized the political risk in reversing the coalition government's decision, Labour transformed the apparatus from an ad hoc, extraordinary, wartime operation into an accepted peacetime routine of government. In the absence of the demands created by wartime pressures, Labour did decide to scale back the apparatus it incorporated into the postwar administrative structure. In the period following World War II, then, the public opinion apparatus was characterized by continuation and not by the termination and dismantling that followed World War I.

As the press's ties with political parties continued to unravel, politicians and bureaucrats believed that government public relations presented significant political advantages for pursuing their central policy objectives. Although senior policymakers repeatedly justified these arrangements as fulfilling the government's "duty to keep the public adequately informed," the public relations activities were a deliberate attempt to manage public preferences for political benefit.[18] In particular, the Labour government replaced the Ministry of Information with the Central Office of Information, and Prime Minister Clement Attlee appointed the first full-time public relations adviser, who enjoyed significant responsibilities as a press liaison.[19] These postwar arrangements further systematized the government's capacity to reach the public directly and to manage the media's routines, information, and contacts. The point was to "present to the public the facts necessary for an understanding of the Government's activities."[20] While the ministries continued to hold ultimate responsibility for keeping the public informed, the Labour government preserved the war's centralization: it encouraged the departments to see their individual efforts as part of a coherent whole.[21]

18. MH 77/577, Minutes of an informal meeting of Herbert Morrison, Francis Williams, and departmental and civil servants from the Central Office of Information, 10/3/46. Also see Cabinet file (CAB) 78/37, Memo by Morrison, "Postwar Organization of Government Publicity," 9/14/45; CAB 78/37, Minutes of meeting on the "Postwar Organization of Government Publicity," 9/18/45.

19. Continuing the Ministry of Information's role, the Central Office of Information's specialized staff and equipment provided a central agency for supplying publicity material, services, and advice to departments on request.

20. CAB 78/37, Minutes of meeting on the "Postwar Organization of Government Publicity," 9/18/45.

21. Centralization of public relations activities was encouraged by the establishment of both

In addition to public relations, Labour maintained the capacity to assess public opinion; the Social Survey office was preserved as a division within the new Central Office of Information. During the government's deliberations over the public opinion apparatus, ministers and civil servants repeatedly stressed—as one cabinet paper did—the importance of "interpret[ing] . . . public feeling to the Department, both in advance of and after decisions on policy."[22] In general, though, politicians and bureaucrats in the Labour government (as in previous governments) avoided surveys of public opinion, instead collecting "facts" from departmental and outside reports.[23] Even when opinion surveys were conducted during the immediate postwar period, they were not integrated as a critical piece of evidence into the deliberations of the cabinet and the Ministry of Health.[24] This failure to integrate opinion data stemmed from policymakers' distrust of survey techniques and their concern about the political risk of being attacked for snooping.

In short, by the time the NHS was enacted, the public opinion apparatus had become institutionalized. In spite of the personal disinterest or outright opposition of such central leaders as Attlee and Churchill, politicians and bureaucrats came to accept the public opinion apparatus as a routine part of British government that should be preserved and expanded. As Herbert Morrison, the Labour government's second-in-command, explained in the late 1940s, the apparatus's structures were an "indispensable" and "essential part of the administrative machinery . . . [that] have come to stay."[25]

Although the apparatus was initially created to have an outward effect in manipulating the public, its development—by the postwar period—created an inward recoil effect: politicians and bureaucrats became more sensitive to what the public thought. This recoil effect stemmed at least in part from policymakers' recognition of the limitations of an outward effect: they were forced to acknowledge that the public was not simply a passive receptacle to be manipulated but rather possessed a "good deal of power to frustrate the intentions of its elected representatives by peaceful means" (Ogilvy-Webb 1965, 72).

---

the prime minister's public relations adviser and government-wide coordinating committees, which were supervised by a senior minister (Herbert Morrison).

22. CAB 129/5, Annex to CP (45) 316, "Report by the Lord President."

23. CAB 128/5, Minutes of cabinet meeting, 4/1/46; CAB 129/8, Paper presented to the cabinet by Morrison, "The Social Survey," 3/27/46; CAB 129/11, Paper presented to the cabinet by Morrison, "The Social Survey," 7/1/46; CAB 128/6, Minutes of cabinet meeting, 7/8/46.

24. Interview with Sir George Godber, by L. R. Jacobs, 12/13/86 (hereafter, Godber Interview); Interview with John Pater, by L. R. Jacobs, 12/15/86 (hereafter, Pater Interview).

25. Prime Minister's Office (PREM) 8/1064, "Statement on the French Report," by H. Morrison and approved by Attlee, 11/28/49. Also see MH 77/577, Minutes of an informal meeting of Morrison, Francis Williams, and departmental and civil servants from the Central Office of Information, 10/3/46.

Policymakers' sensitivity to public opinion was evident in policy debates during and after the war. Whether arguing for or against the coalition government's endorsement of major postwar reform, cabinet ministers and top civil servants based their cases on public opinion—either to respond to the public's preferences in order to bolster morale or to discourage the public from developing unrealistic expectations about postwar conditions. After the war, Morrison insisted that "there should be no return to the old timidity and reticence in the relations between Government Departments and the public."[26] Indeed, another senior Labour minister, Stafford Cripps, instructed his department that sensitivity to public opinion was a fundamental part of policy making, requiring both a "striptease performance" in distributing information and a receptiveness to public opinion (quoted in Ogilvy-Webb 1965, 71).

United States

As in Britain, the 1930s began a period of major expansion of the public opinion apparatus. Although the Roosevelt administration set important precedents regarding public relations and intelligence gathering, it was during the Kennedy and Johnson presidencies that the apparatus was institutionalized as a routine and regular component of the White House.

Motivated by the pressing political demands of the New Deal period, Roosevelt orchestrated a major development in the executive branch's public relations capacity. In this prewar period, his administration initiated fruitful ties with a new media form (radio), strengthened existing ties with others (newspapers and film), and centralized these efforts in the White House (Steele 1985a). Before and during the war, the White House took several steps to centralize public relations efforts in order to make the administration speak with one voice. Committed to institutionalizing the ad hoc White House roles that had been emerging since the turn of the century, Roosevelt designated a press secretary to systematically structure the press's routines, contacts, and information sources. The White House also revived the centralized type of organization Wilson had established in the Committee on Public Information: it created the National Emergency Council before the war and a new series of institutions, a "publicity trust," during the war.[27] Facing political pressure to build popular support for the New Deal and later for the war effort, the White House used the press secretary and the

---

26. CAB 78/37, Memo by Morrison, "Postwar Organization of Government Publicity," 9/14/45.

27. This publicity trust involved the establishment of the Office of Government Reports within the Executive Office of the President and later the Office of War Information (Steele 1985 and 1978; Winfield 1984).

new centralized organizations to oversee the Departments and to insist that they move beyond their narrow circle of clients (Winfield 1984; Cohen 1968; Hess 1984).

The Roosevelt administration also launched the first systematic attempt to develop an intelligence gathering capacity in the executive branch. Determined to capitalize on the discovery of modern survey methods, Roosevelt initiated a relationship with modern pollsters (especially Hadley Cantril) and encouraged the development of government polling. The emergence of polls as the president's most important gauge of public opinion influenced his administration's policies during the New Deal and the war.[28] Nevertheless, Roosevelt and subsequent presidents supplemented polling data with other sources of information, such as White House mail and the personal judgment of their aides.

In spite of the importance the Roosevelt administration attached to the public opinion apparatus, many of its arrangements (including both the relationship with pollsters and the government's own polling operations) were abandoned under presidents Truman and Eisenhower.[29] The establishment of a presidential relationship with pollsters as a regular, routine part of the operations of the White House—one that would be maintained and expanded by subsequent presidents—was delayed until the arrival of John F. Kennedy. The seeds of this institutionalization of intelligence gathering in the presidency lay in Senator Kennedy's campaign to win the 1960 Democratic presidential nomination.

Documents in the Kennedy Presidential Library reveal that Kennedy and his aides sought out several nongovernmental pollsters in 1959 as they weighed the prospects of running in state primary elections. Acknowledging their importance on the American scene, Kennedy sought to hone polls into a tool that would provide him and his aides the critical insights to conduct a long-shot candidacy—one that required them to try to sweep the primaries.[30] Attracted in part by Louis Harris's repeated reassurance that he could not "separate . . . polling from the other problems of strategy," Kennedy established by August 1959 a formal relationship with the pollster that would last through the general election and stretch into his presidency.[31]

28. Public opinion data had isolated influence on the government's military policy as well as on its public relations efforts (Cantril 1967; Steele 1974, 1978, 1985a, 1985b; Winfield 1984).

29. Sudman 1982; Letter from Benedict K. Zobrist (Director, Harry S. Truman Library) to L. R. Jacobs, 8/24/87; and Letter from Martin M. Teasley (Dwight D. Eisenhower Library) to L. R. Jacobs, 8/21/87.

30. John F. Kennedy Presidential Library files (JFK Library), Sorensen Papers, Box 24, Letter to George Gallup from J. F. Kennedy, 7/24/59, and Letter to J. F. Kennedy from Louis Harris, 7/23/59.

31. JFK Library, Sorensen Papers, Box 24, Letter to J. F. Kennedy from L. Harris, 7/23/59;

Harris conducted at least sixty-seven polls during the primary and general election campaigns, twenty-seven of them between September and November 1960. During the 1960 contest, Harris's polls influenced the Kennedy campaign's itineraries and advertising as well as its campaign speeches and strategies.[32] The polls were an important factor, for example, in prompting Kennedy to advocate Medicare during a relatively issue-free campaign in which party identification and candidate image predominated (see Chapter 5).

Kennedy's inauguration as president in January 1961 marks the institutionalization of public relations and intelligence gathering as part of the White House's normal peacetime routines. The political needs of Kennedy and then Johnson made them especially sensitive to the potential advantage of expanding the apparatus. Because of his precarious political position after the close 1960 general election, Kennedy and his senior aides viewed the apparatus as an opportunity to "marshal public support for our legislative proposals," which would offset the political advantages of other groups and individuals.[33] The Johnson White House also came to appreciate the political usefulness of polls as it designed its strategy for the 1964 election campaign and sought to capitalize on its landslide victory. Although each president's political needs varied, both Kennedy and Johnson were pressed by the growing emphasis on direct primaries to campaign throughout their terms.

Public relations was a central presidential concern. As a close aide recalled, Kennedy was preoccupied with "public communication—educating, persuading, and mobilizing . . . [public] opinion." (Sorensen 1965, 310). Johnson similarly came to accept, despite initial doubts, the importance of "maintain[ing] press concentration on the White House as the vital center of news and interpretation"; the danger was that "reporters will move to other places in Washington—to the departments and to Capitol Hill—where others seek to inject their own prejudices and priorities into the news."[34]

Clearly very important, public relations consumed a growing portion of

Robert F. Kennedy Papers, Pre-Administration, Political, Box 39, Memo to J. F. Kennedy from Louis Harris, 7/5/60.

32. JFK Library, Sorensen Papers, Box 24, "Comments on Louis Harris' Proposed Program," undated but probably late summer 1959; Robert F. Kennedy Papers, Pre-Administration, Political, Box 36, "Media Campaign: Wisconsin Primary, 1/21/60–4/5/60"; for the general election, see R. F. Kennedy Papers, Pre-Administration, Political, Box 36, Memo to campaign coordinator from Steve Smith, "TV Spot Campaign," 10/19/60, and Box 38, "Priority States—Spot T.V."

33. JFK Library, Presidential Office Files (POF), Box 63, Memos from Dutton to president, 2/28/61 and 3/5/61. Also see Ex FG1, Box 108, Memo from Dutton to president, 3/23/61; Salinger Papers, Box 11, Memo from Salinger to Sorensen, 4/17/61.

34. Lyndon B. Johnson Presidential Library Files (LBJ Library), Ex PR18, Box 356, Memo from Cater to Johnson, 12/26/64.

executive branch officials' time and prompted further efforts to manage the media's routines, information, and contacts in the dawning of an age of television and daily briefings. Moreover, the Kennedy and Johnson administrations expanded White House capability to bring the president's message directly to the public through the use of writers and advance teams for travel (Grossman and Kunar 1981). In particular, they structured the cabinet into a public relations mechanism to launch direct promotional activities that would rally public support for pending legislative programs. Finally, both administrations attempted to enhance coordination by maintaining the position of the White House press secretary and his institutional base, the Press Office, as the central focus of media relations. Central control over information released by the departments was strengthened to prevent conflicting stories and to ensure that the White House released news items that would attract favorable publicity.[35]

The White House made changes in public relations arrangements that were aimed not only at its own operations but also at those throughout the executive departments. Concerned that "too often citizen experiences in direct contact are embittering memories [and are] detrimental to public support of their Government," the White House insisted that the departments become more sensitive to public opinion.[36] The increased departmental concern with public relations was evident in HEW, where public relations became accepted as an integral part of operations (Cohen 1968, 43).

In addition to changing the government's public relations apparatus, the Kennedy and Johnson administrations also revamped the White House's intelligence-gathering capacity. Following his election, Kennedy's relationship with private pollsters became a regular, routine part of the process of making decisions in the White House.

After 1961, then, the White House became a veritable warehouse stocked with the latest public opinion data. In addition to receiving polls that were published or conducted for others, the Kennedy and Johnson White Houses received private surveys by Harris, and later by Oliver Quayle, of public opinion in states and cities across the country. The regular flow of these private opinion surveys into the White House provided data on the president's pop-

35. JFK Library, POF, Box 63, Memo from Dutton to president, 2/24/61; POF, Box 92, Memo from Frederick Dutton, 1/28/61; POF, Box 92, Memo from Dutton to all cabinet members, 2/1/61; LBJ Library, Ex FG100, Box 130, Memo for the 1/17/64 cabinet meeting, initialed "LBJ"; Ex PR18, Box 356, Memo from Johnson to department and agency heads, 1/9/65; LBJ Library interview with George Christian by J. Frantz, 12/4/69; Salinger 1966, 135–37.

36. LBJ Library, FG100/M, Box 130, Letter from Johnson to John Macy. Also see Ex FG1, Box 11, Memo to all personnel handling correspondence, 3/26/65; Ex FG100, Box 130, Memo from Busby to Johnson, 2/20/65.

ularity as well as on public preferences for policy issues and for candidates in congressional and gubernatorial electoral races. Thus, although Kennedy and Johnson used other sources of information on public opinion and did not share the same level of enthusiasm for them, polls were consumed under both presidents at the highest levels in the White House. Reflecting the Kennedy White House's interest in polls as a reliable measure of public opinion, Harris conducted a survey only a few months after Kennedy's inauguration to identify the key policy issues that represented the "central pivots" for bolstering the president's popular following.[37]

The Johnson White House enhanced the new role of opinion surveys by directly commissioning polls to a much greater extent and by instituting organizational changes in the White House. In July 1964 the White House private pollster noted that an opinion survey in Maryland was "geared specifically to provide information on the race for President in the upcoming election and to assist in the development of a campaign strategy."[38] Conducted for the most part by Quayle, private polls for the White House continued into the 1964 general election and throughout Johnson's term in office. No longer restricted to the development of campaign strategy, polls were regularly conducted after the 1964 election to monitor the political climate in states and cities across the country. Moreover, Johnson initiated such organizational changes as introducing more and better specialized White House staff members to regularly analyze the polling data.[39]

This vast expansion in the White House demand for polling directly affected presidential decision making. Polls influenced the Kennedy White House's choice of Medicare as one of the few issues it was willing to "go to the people" with in 1962. Similarly, Johnson's campaign selected Medicare as a salient and popular issue after it had been tracked in a series of Quayle's surveys. In addition to affecting the presidents' agendas, polls had an impact on the formulation of major legislation; they persuaded politicians to adopt reformers' proposal to piggyback Medicare onto the Social Security system.

Most significant of all, the Kennedy and Johnson presidencies institutionalized the public opinion apparatus. In contrast to the abandonment of polling after Roosevelt's presidency, the legacy of Kennedy and Johnson

37. JFK Library, POF, Box 105, "Public Reaction to the President during the First Sixty Days," by Harris, 3/22/61.

38. LBJ Library, Confidential File (CF), PR16, Box 80, "A Survey of the Presidential Race in Maryland," by Quayle, 7/64.

39. LBJ Library, CF, PR16, Boxes 80, 81, 82. Under the Kennedy administration, the only major political figure (other than the President himself) who seems to have come into regular contact with the polling data was Robert Kennedy. Under the Johnson administration, polls were analyzed and then directly forwarded to the president: these analyses were conducted by Hayes Redman, Richard Nelson, and Fred Panzer.

was that public opinion data became an institutional part of presidential decision making. Nonetheless, the White House recognized the constraints on its attempts to track and influence public opinion. White House public relations efforts, when they became public, could ignite a storm of controversy in Congress and the media, as illustrated by criticism of the Kennedy administration's operations. Moreover, policymakers were concerned about the political risk of conducting opinion surveys, and of seeming to snoop on the public.

The Kennedy and Johnson administrations' institutionalization of the public opinion apparatus ushered in a new level of sensitivity to public opinion. To those working within the government, the change from the previous administration was dramatic: as a Kennedy aide proclaimed, "the President is no longer a mysterious figure operating behind closed doors."[40] The White House persistently struggled to instill a greater sensitivity in the "Government's attitude toward and treatment of the people in direct contact at all levels."[41] Reflecting this new outlook during the Kennedy and Johnson administrations, the executive branch dedicated almost the same amount of time to preparing public relations material as it spent preparing documents for presentation to Congress (Cohen 1968).

In the postwar period, the public opinion apparatus became established in the American and British executive branches: regardless of their personal predilections, politicians and bureaucrats demonstrated a permanent shift in their inward dispositions and behavior. Initially, policymakers were narrowly interested in public relations in order to gain greater control over their political environments; they introduced extensive developments to manage media coverage and to enable direct appeals to the people. Following the development of institutional arrangements to manipulate public opinion, policymakers then also began to create an intelligence-gathering capacity.

The development of this apparatus had a recoil effect: although it initially emerged as an attempt to outwardly affect and manage public opinion, the creation of a substantial apparatus had an inward effect on the dispositions of American and British policymakers. In attempting, then, to manipulate public opinion, policymakers became more sensitive to popular preferences. The shift from an emphasis on manipulation to an emphasis on responsiveness grew from policymakers' recognition that there were major institutional restrictions on the apparatus's capacity to manipulate the public. Institutional and partisan competition within and between the executive and legislative branches repeatedly frustrated efforts to create a cohesive, cen-

---

40. JFK Library, Salinger Papers, Box 11, Memo from Salinger to Sorensen, 4/17/61.
41. LBJ Library, Ex FG100, Box 130, Memo from Busby to Johnson, 2/20/65.

tralized public opinion apparatus. Both state actors and nongovernmental observers recognized that only a fine line separated the use of the apparatus for administrative tasks from its use for political purposes (e.g., pressuring the legislature or attracting voters). In particular, legislators and the media persistently criticized executive branch expenditures on public relations because they would create a partisan political advantage or pose a threat to individual privacy.

In spite of the significant budgetary cost and political risks associated with building the public opinion apparatus, the political pressure on presidents and British cabinet ministers to secure and maintain popular support provided a powerful rationale for its development. Thus, whereas previous policymakers repeatedly abandoned aspects of the apparatus because they did not recognize them as important, by the period of health policy formulation a new outlook on public opinion had emerged; the apparatus seemed vital to the task of modern policy making.

3 | Public Understandings of the State and Health Care

If state actors' greater sensitivity to public opinion opened the gate for American and British citizens to influence health policy, then the content of this influence lies in socially shared meanings; these meanings evolve over time from the interaction of ordinary people and become embedded in institutions. In this chapter I outline the cultural context in which the NHS and Medicare acts were designed—the mass public's enduring understandings of health care and the state. In effect, the enduring aspects of American and British culture loaded the dice during the formulation of the NHS and Medicare acts, making certain institutional changes seem conceivable while barring others. The basic terms on which elites and the public would understand and discuss these two acts were gradually constructed as part of the historic formation of cultural patterns.

Traditionally, the study of American and British culture emphasizes the two countries' common antistate national character. Here, I challenge the conventional wisdom about the shared Anglo-American liberal tradition, arguing that the historic evolution of American and British culture produced patterns of understandings that exhibit neither statelessness nor a fixed, uniform rejection of state involvement in social welfare provisions. I reinterpret existing histories of political and medical developments in the United States and Britain by arguing that the liberal tradition has been significantly reformulated: the enduring legacy of public uneasiness with state provisions has over time become interlaced with American and British acceptance (to differing degrees) of the state's role in social welfare. I suggest that the public's changing understandings of the state both influenced the organization of health care and was itself affected by changes in medical practice and in public perception of orthodox medicine.[1]

My treatment of culture modifies the two conventional approaches, which rely on survey research and intellectual histories. The "political culture" tradition equates culture with an individual's preferences as measured in opinion surveys. Although polling data capture the public's more explicit (often transitory) preferences, treating culture as isolated attributes of individuals neglects to incorporate the shared meanings that are produced from the interaction of ordinary people. Enduring understandings, which are widely shared and transmitted down generations, pattern individual preferences; they offer individuals a slim but important cue in organizing their immediate preferences.

A second conventional approach to culture focuses precisely on the development of enduring meanings. But these meanings are identified not by examining the mass public but by studying elites—politicians, policy experts, and scholars (e.g., Hartz 1955; Fox 1986). Intellectual histories of American and British elites traditionally emphasize the persistence of liberal ideals, the commitment to individualism and a fundamental aversion to state interference (Hartz 1955; Rimlinger 1971). Continuing this liberal, antistate tradition, researchers have minimized the variation between the United States and Britain and emphasized the countries' "ideological similarities" (Hollingsworth 1986, xiii). The meaning of the state is assumed not only to be relatively constant across the two countries but also to be a fairly fixed, unchanging characteristic within each country (Hartz 1955; Pelling 1968). Thus, Morone argues that the "fear of public power has been a [dominant] fixture on the American political scene since [the country's colonial beginning]" (1990, 3).[2]

In this chapter I also seek to trace enduring meanings, but I return to the practice of using evidence about the mass public. I rely on social historical studies of ordinary Americans and Britons in order to identify each country's often divergent understandings of major institutions, which helped to form and organize socially shared meanings (Thompson 1966, 1978a, and 1978b; Gutman 1975; Starr 1982; Rosenberg 1987; Smith 1979; Abel-Smith 1964).[3]

1. I do not intend the term "orthodox" to convey any particular moral connotation about the value of medical science.

2. It should be added, though, that Morone's interpretation of America's liberal tradition emphasizes the impact of democratic ideology in temporarily lifting the "dread of government" and allowing state development.

3. Social historians study the perceptions of the ordinary man or woman regarding health, medical care, and the state through a range of primary sources: their analyse focus on national and local newspapers and magazines; hearings and reports of government bodies and medical facilities (like hospitals); socioeconomic characteristics and behavior of ordinary people who

INITIAL FORMATION OF PUBLIC UNDERSTANDINGS

Britain

Public perceptions of the state and health care, have their roots in the seventeenth and eighteenth centuries. Although political rights were historically restricted in the United States and Britain, this did not stop a wide spectrum of American and Britons from embracing representative democracy and particularly the franchise as the appropriate mechanism for ensuring popular participation in government decision making. American and British understandings of the state diverged, however, in important respects: whereas Americans' perception of the state centered on its democratic procedures, British attitudes extended to an acceptance of state involvement in social welfare. The British acceptance of state benefits was borne from the public's comparatively greater familiarity with poor-law relief.

In spite of important differences, the American and British poor-law systems did share one basic characteristic: the development of each was closely related to public perceptions. The American and British poor laws were both deliberately designed to be negatively perceived to deter all those who were not truly destitute. The combination of demeaning income tests and loathsome benefits led the public to detest the two central components of the poor laws—"indoor" relief in poorhouses and "outdoor" assistance (outside poor-law facilities). The public's uniformly negative perception of poor law provisions served as a self-regulating mechanism for distinguishing the poor from the truly indigent: the stigma of poor relief led the poor to choose starvation over the surrender of their respectability, thereby putting a brake on the number of requests for assistance.

Despite this similarity, the British state was far more involved in distributing both general and medical relief. The national government initiated the poor-law system with Parliament's enactment of the Elizabethan or Old Poor Law of 1601; subnational governments and specifically local municipalities administered indoor and outdoor relief.

In health care, Britain developed during the eighteenth century both non-hospital, community-based treatment and two types of hospital care: private, voluntary hospitals, which relied on the charity of the rich, and a haphazard government system of workhouse infirmaries and poor law hospitals. The limited development of therapeutics (the methods of treating

---

participate in the political system and enter medical facilities; and diverse sources of everyday life (e.g., diaries and advertisements for cures). For a discussion of social history's sources of data and its relevance for social science, see Jacobs 1990, chap. 3, and Jacobs and Shapiro 1989. For useful reviews of relevant historical studies of American and British health care, see Fox 1986, Smith 1979, Woodward and Richards 1977, Rosenberg 1977and 1979e, and Reverby and Rosner 1979.

sickness) meant that hospital care was characterized by long periods of confinement rather than a definitive course of medical treatment (Abel-Smith 1964, 10–11). Indeed, given their limited abilities and the high risk of infection, hospitals actually posed a threat to patient health, and eighteenth-century hospitals refused admittance to patients who were acutely sick or had contagious diseases. Because hospitals presented the unattractive offer of custodial care and the risk of infection, the public dreaded them: both private and government facilities were negatively perceived as a form of care intended for the sick poor, who required free treatment.

Community-based care developed as an outgrowth of British medicine's early organization of medical professionals into specialists (surgeons and physicians) and generalists (apothecaries) who typically treated patients outside hospitals.[4] Because hospital treatment was considered neither safe nor respectable, nonpaupers from all classes preferred by 1800 to be treated in a doctor's office, or in their own home by family members and (if they could afford it) private practitioners. Moreover, the sick poor in urban areas also received drugs from community-based dispensaries, which emerged as a less expensive alternative to hospitals. Thus, although poor relief was viewed in uniformly unfavorable terms, it began to familiarize the British public with state involvement in social welfare.

United States

Despite similarities, Americans' understandings of the state and health care before 1800 diverged from those in Britain. Although the public in both countries was strongly attracted to the democratic procedures associated with a representative state, most Americans found government involvement in social welfare provision inconceivable. Moreover, the absence in the United States of an organized and cohesive medical profession opened the way for unorthodox medical sects to dominate the healing arts and prevented hospital- and community-based care from developing as they did in Britain.

Americans tended to understand the state in terms of its procedural mechanisms. Early American state builders deliberately drew upon the tradition of representative democracy, which was established during the settlement of colonial communities (Wood 1969; Lockridge 1970). The comparatively wide issuance of suffrage rights convinced many Americans that state in-

4. Physicians and surgeons organized royal colleges (in 1518 and 1800, respectively) and treated the wealthy, whereas apothecaries originated as dispensers of drugs and provided the same general practice services as physicians but for the nonwealthy. Apothecaries were little more than tradesmen who charged for drug sales until they were granted the right to charge for advice in the mid-1800s (Homigsbaum 1979).

stitutions were impersonal and enduring mechanisms for impartially representing the popular will; thus, the notion of a machine or instrument is perhaps the oldest popular image of the Constitution (Kammen 1986). Whereas British access to institutions was contested, Americans believed that access transcended conflict: with the vote and other democratic rights widely granted during the initial phase of state building (and not conceded in the face of popular unrest), American state institutions and procedures came to be viewed as morally significant in themselves rather than as contested objects or instruments used to press for popular demands.

In comparison to the strong, favorable meaning associated with the state's democratic procedures, government involvement in social welfare was alien to most Americans. In Britain the central state established a broad framework for poor relief, and local governments developed complex administrative networks for providing that relief; but in the United States the enactment of a national poor law was inconceivable, and the limited poor relief that did exist was ad hoc and piecemeal.

The public's understandings of health care and in particular hospital- and community-based care was affected by the exceptional history of American orthodox medicine. The American medical profession could not organize itself into distinct branches along the lines of the British categories—physicians, surgeons, and apothecaries. Not only were American doctors unable to impose demarcations within their own ranks, but they could not even separate themselves from other unorthodox practices and establish who was and was not a doctor.

In the absence of a medical profession that could establish itself as the dominant form of medical treatment, Americans failed to become accustomed to either hospital treatment or orthodox care outside hospitals. In colonial America, hospital care was both comparatively rare and based on ad hoc medical arrangements (e.g., occasional visits by local doctors to government poorhouses). The comparative absence of hospitals, however, did not translate into public use of orthodox care outside hospitals. Rather than surrender their judgment to medical "experts," the nonpoor looked to unorthodox medical treatment—namely, to domestic medicine and lay practitioners.[5] For most colonial Americans, then, the meaning of health care was associated not with the principles of organized, orthodox medicine but instead with oral traditions or self-help guides (Starr 1982, 32–37).

In short, by 1800 the meaning of the state and health care differed in important respects in the United States and Britain. Whereas Americans

5. The challenge of lay medicine to the medical profession's therapeutic tenets seems to have been less severe in Britain. Unorthodox medicine was practiced in Britain, especially for diseases orthodox medicine could not cure, but Americans of various different classes used unorthodox treatments more extensively than did Britons (Smith 1979, 109, 340).

tended to understand the state in terms of its procedural mechanisms, the British were beginning to accept state provision of social welfare as legitimate—even though its particular form (poor relief) was universally detested. Moreover, with orthodox medicine more firmly established, the British (unlike Americans) began to associate medical treatment with hospital- and community-based care.

The Period of Gestation, 1800–1875

Britain

During the first three-quarters of the nineteenth century, American and British understandings of the state and health care continued to develop within the already established patterns. In Britain, the New Poor Law of 1834 maintained the local government's control of everyday administration and expanded the central state's coordination of poor relief through the creation of a national board. To ensure that relief would be less than the lowest wages, the 1834 act deliberately and successfully reinforced the public's negative perception of poor-law provisions; the image, in particular, of workhouses as harsh prisons for grinding the poor down was used to deter all but the truly indigent from requesting relief. Nonetheless, the New Poor Law's reform of administration and expansion of relief (especially the enlargement of workhouses) embedded and helped to widen public acceptance of state involvement in social welfare. Although the relief was not attractive to members of society as a whole, the poor laws did enhance the legitimation of a centralized mechanism of administration and make large-scale economic aid conceivable (Quadagno 1982, 137–38).

The emergence during the nineteenth century of working-class organizations known as Friendly Societies affected the development of public perceptions of social welfare. Through a vast network of local and national branches that stretched across Britain, Friendly Societies came to encompass 4.5 million of the most respected portion of the working class by the organization's peak in the late 1800s. The societies relied on the favorably perceived mechanism of insurance: their members earned the right to emergency financial security by making voluntary contributions to an insurance fund. The growth of these voluntary associations instilled among a significant portion of the working class a relatively widespread familiarity with, and an expectation of, social welfare provisions from large institutions.

Moreover, medical advances within hospitals, together with the evolving organization of the medical profession, continued to encourage two separate spheres of health care—hospital- and community-based treatment. During the nineteenth century, hospitals began to become the focus of medical research and training: to serve the needs of medical students and their teachers (rather than those of the sick poor), patients began to be admitted based not on their degree of poverty but according to medical criteria. Improvements in medical knowledge and procedures led hospitals to accept significantly more patients during the first half of the nineteenth century and to spread rapidly after mid-century. Medical advances also helped to create a system of government hospitals: government workhouses were gradually transformed from refuges for the truly destitute into curative institutions in which admission was increasingly limited to sick paupers; other workhouse inmates were evicted in order to make room. As part of the evolution of medical practice and organization, specialists (surgeons and physicians) assumed control over the admission and care of patients in hospitals; apothecaries (and what became general practitioners) were excluded from hospitals and left to provide general community-based care for dispensaries and Friendly Societies (Abel-Smith 1964).

By the 1860s, public perception of improved health care, combined with widening acceptance of state and nonstate provision of social welfare, increased the attractiveness of hospital treatment and community-based care in dispensaries and especially the Friendly Societies. Capitalizing on the widening attraction of drugs and general practitioner (GP) services, the societies attempted to recruit new members by expanding the general medical services available in their club practices. Although club practices encouraged a sizable portion of the working class to expect such services, the stigma associated with poor relief deterred the public from seeking general medical care from state facilities. Indeed, poor-law authorities, who wanted to encourage general community care as a less expensive alternative to hospital treatment, used the more favorably perceived non state dispensaries to attract and treat the sick poor (Hodgkinson 1967).

During the nineteenth century, important changes also occurred in perceptions of hospitals. The uniformly negative meaning that had become associated with government and voluntary hospitals gradually weakened, and the public increasingly identified these facilities with treatment of the sick and not simply refuges for paupers; this change induced increasing numbers to flock to the hospitals by 1870. This perception of hospital medical improvement prompted a surge in the number of both inpatients and outpatients seeking the hospitals' advice (Smith 1979, 278–80).

The gradual emergence of a new understanding of hospitals' benefits intermingled with the public's changing perception of the state. The public's widening acceptance of state involvement in hospital care was embodied in the Metropolitan Poor Act of 1867, which contained the first explicit acknowledgment that the state had a duty to provide hospitals for the poor and that the sick poor had the right to institutional care (Abel-Smith 1964,

82,65). After 1867, the definition of those eligible for care was widened and government hospitals were expanded until they were more extensive than voluntary hospitals. Reflecting the widening public interest in hospital care, growing numbers of nonpaupers requested and received treatment in government and voluntary facilities.

Even though hospitals gradually became relatively more attractive, the general public continued to fear them. This fear stemmed in part from objective circumstances: up to the last third of the nineteenth century, British hospitals continued to be more a threat than a benefit to inpatients. The emergence of surgery introduced "hospital disease": hospital patients often died in outbreaks of epidemics that were not evident outside the hospital (Woodward 1974, 122–23). Wealthy patients were more safely treated in their homes; those who felt they had no choice entered hospitals, but only with trepidation. Thus, even after improvements in health care began to change the character of poor-law medical services, the pauper stigma and uneasiness about medical treatment continued to dampen demand for the government's services, discouraging even many deserving sick from entering hospitals.

United States

American understanding of the state and health care continued to evolve in ways that were strikingly different from the pattern in Britain. Clearly, the state's democratic procedures were meaningful to the British, motivating the Chartists during the 1830s and the social movements of the 1860s and later (Thompson 1984). What distinguished the United States, though, was the overarching preoccupation with the impersonal guarantees of political institutions and procedures. De Tocqueville referred to this preoccupation as a type of "paternal love" (1969, 241) and Ostrogorski called it a "constitutional fetish-worship" (1902, 46–47). During the Civil War, the public's understanding of the state in terms of democratic procedures led both northerners and southerners to portray themselves as fighting to protect the Constitution and the impersonal mechanisms it had established (Kammen 1986; Foner 1970). America, then, was founded on and continued to be influenced by the fact that "government is valued more for its moral than for its material benefits" (Wood 1984, 19).

In contrast to the British public during the nineteenth century, Americans remained largely unaccustomed to central state involvement in social welfare provisions; up to the late 1800s "the central government did not exist as a social welfare entity" (Berkowitz and McQuaid 1980, x, 2–3). With people thinking of society and government in terms of the locality in which they lived, Americans' contact with government social welfare was largely limited to the state and local levels (Leiby 1978, 35); it was these subnational governments that were responsible for the increased expenditures on poor relief and the expansion of poorhouses (Katz 1986, 3–16, 85–86, 91–109; Axinn and Levin 1975, 43–45; Leiby 1978, 45). As in Britain, public perception of government benefits was strongly negative; poorhouses served as the "heavy artillery in an assault on popular culture"; they were aimed at deterring requests for assistance (Katz 1986). Even with the expansion of poor relief by subnational governments, neither the number of facilities nor the administrative arrangements matched British developments.

An important element in the distinctive evolution of American understanding of social welfare provisions was that working class organizations in the United States did not develop to the extent they did in Britain. Although a nationwide movement of Charity Organization Societies and settlement houses did form, these middle- and upper-class organizations concentrated on rationalizing the provisions of poor relief (Leiby 1978, 90–91, 179–91; Axinn and Levin 1975, 91–99, 124–43). Private, nonstate institutions did not encourage (as Friendly Societies did in Britain) the widespread expectation of social welfare provisions.

In health care, the organization and practice of medicine in the United States continued to depart from patterns emerging in Britain and continental Europe. During much of the nineteenth century, American doctors placed comparatively little faith in medical science; they resisted improvements in medical knowledge and procedures in the belief that environment rather than universal scientific principles determined the appropriate treatment. Moreover, the American medical profession remained weakly organized: American doctors could neither create distinctions within the medical profession nor prevent the growing practice of unorthodox medical sects.

By 1870, American hospitals for the civilian population were also comparatively unaffected by advances in diagnostic tools and knowledge. Hospital trustees and administrators (even at the advanced Massachusetts General Hospital) imposed limits on the normal practices of medical science, obstructing the development of their facilities into centers that would specialize in curative treatment. As a result, hospitals continued to be operated on religious and moral criteria and to provide custodial care not unlike that found in convalescent homes.[6] By 1875, American health care was distinished by comparatively inferior quality of hospital treatment and relatively fewer private hospitals and separate facilities for the indigent. The number of American government hospitals never expanded to the levels reached in Britain (Rosenberg 1987; Vogel 1976; Shonick 1984; Katz 1986).

6. A notable exception to American hospitals' general imperviousness to medical advances involved the hospitals constructed by the Union for the injured during the Civil War.

In the absence of breakthroughs in medicine and professional organization, by 1875 Americans were—compared to the British—unfamiliar with organized orthodox care; instead, significant numbers of Americans continued to be attracted to self-treatment and medical sects. The public's unease with orthodox scientific medicine was reflected in the successful movement during the 1830s and 1840s to revoke state licensing regulations and to encourage such unorthodox treatments as homeopathy and botanic medicine (Starr 1982, 30–31; Numbers 1985, 187; Young 1977; Rosenkrantz 1985, 222; Rosenberg 1979b, 44–46). Voluntary hospitals found that suspicion of orthodox medicine depressed public support and charitable contributions for their efforts to treat the sick poor (Rosenberg 1977; Vogel 1976; Starr 1982, 152–55). In Britain, the public's long-standing negative perception of hospitals was gradually blunted by a growing appreciation of their curative benefits; in the United States, hospitals continued to be uniformly dreaded and to serve as a last resort for those who were isolated and had no family (Starr 1982, 72, 152). Americans associated hospital residency with infection, experimentation, and the stigma of failure and misery (Rosenberg 1977 and 1979).

General medical care in community-based facilities sidestepped the dread of hospitalization and developed into an attractive alternative to hospital treatment (Vogel 1976, 289–91; Rosenberg 1977, 428–41). In contrast to health care provision in Britain, American dispensaries provided by 1870 far more urban health care than did hospitals (Rosenberg 1977, 434–43, and 1974). Despite the attractiveness of dispensaries, widespread public interest in general medical care did not form. Thus, the few health insurance plans that did develop primarily provided protection from lost income rather than coverage of medical expenses (Numbers 1979; Starr 1982, 206–7, 240–42, 294–95). The combination of the public's disinterest in orthodox medical care and the absence of private, nonstate institutions comparable to the Friendly Societies meant that large numbers of Americans did not become accustomed to receiving community-based care.

Overall, by 1875 important differences had begun to emerge in American and British understanding of health care and the state. In the United States, with orthodox medicine still facing significant challenges, the public did not come to expect hospital and general medical care. Americans' unfamiliarity with orthodox health care was reinforced by the comparative detachment of the state from social welfare. In Britain, hospital and especially community care was increasingly attractive by the late nineteenth century, and the state's involvement in its provision and financing was becoming accepted. Indeed, by the 1870s growing familiarity with both state provisions and health care meant that nonpaupers were on the verge of demanding the hospital- and community-based care that had originally been intended for the indigent.

HISTORIC CONTEXT OF THE NHS AND MEDICARE ACTS

By the period during which the NHS and Medicare acts were formulated, the American and British public were coming to expect (with important variations) both scientific medicine and state involvement in the provision of health care. Encouraged by dramatic advances in therapeutics, especially surgery, all British classes were attracted to community- and hospital-based care; Americans largely associated health care with hospitals. In addition, whatever fundamental aversion to state intervention might have once existed was altered by the gradual emergence (following the British reforms of the early 1900s and the American New Deal) of genuine public support for state involvement in health care. Nevertheless, the new meanings of health care and the state, which members of American and British society began to articulate, drew on and therefore were structured by established patterns of understandings.

Britain

In Britain, public understanding of state provision of social welfare was reformulated by the early twentieth century: government benefits, which had been dreaded because of the poor laws' means tests and stigma, were now seen in a new, more positive way. In an effort to widen their electoral following, David Lloyd George and the Liberal party designed the Old Age Pension (OAP) and National Health Insurance (NHI) acts to embody and help encourage the growing attraction of state benefits. For instance, the Liberals hoped to reap the political rewards of enacting the NHI, which provided general medical care to wage earners; it would appeal to the general public and avoid the stigma associated with targeting programs to the indigent. To be sure, the public's negative perception of the state did not simply disappear. But, for the first time in the provision of institutional and financial benefits, most members of British society in the 1930s shared a favorable understanding of central state programs like OAP and NHI (Emy 1973; Morgan 1971; Collins 1965; Gilbert 1966).[7]

7. Henry Pelling (1968) claims that the British working class was in general hostile to the new social welfare measures, which were proposed at the turn of the century. I argue here,

After the 1870s, hospitals were also fully transformed into centers of curative treatment that strictly concentrated on the acutely sick. Although infectious disease and, for example, radium treatments continued to represent a danger, the combination of fundamental improvements in surgery and the acceptance of germ theory and antiseptic principles made hospitals significantly safer and more beneficial. By the early 1910s, advances in medical knowledge and procedures spread (though unevenly in rural areas) from the more advanced, private, voluntary hospitals to government hospitals and infirmaries. Government hospitals selected patients according to their level of sickness, and not indigence: medical considerations replaced the poor laws' preoccupation with financial status as the criterion for admission. By the 1910s, specialists fully dominated hospital care; GPs were excluded, especially in big city hospitals, but were firmly established—after a compromise within the medical profession—as the point of entry into the health care system (Honigsbaum 1979).

In the context of medical changes after the late nineteenth century, the public came to perceive orthodox health care positively. With concern over the country's military capability heightening the Victorian interest in health, the public became fixated with the curative benefits of health care "as though there were some magic in it" (Mackintosh 1953, 122; Smith 1979, 258; Gilbert 1966; Searle 1971 and 1979). As a major consequence of the public's increasing awareness of medicine's curative benefits, the strong negative perceptions of state and nonstate provisions for the poor weakened, opening the way for nonpaupers to use facilities that had previously deterred all but the destitute.

By the early twentieth century, the home lost its attraction as a treatment center and the working and middle classes favorably perceived hospitals as the center for the most advanced medical treatment: the number of requests for admission to state and voluntary hospitals increased, and the number of beds in hospitals also rose.[8] In the context of the public's new favorable understanding of hospitals, the state extended free hospital care to nonpaupers; it encouraged the development of general hospitals (through the Local Government Act of 1929) for those outside the poor-law ambit (Abel-Smith 1964, 127–29, 152–54).[9]

---

though, that this era was an important transitional period in which state involvement in social welfare became sufficiently attractive for significant numbers of the nonpoor to do what was unthinkable to an earlier generation—accept government benefits.

8. In the two decades after 1891, the total number of hospital beds increased at a higher rate than did the population of England and Wales (Abel-Smith 1964, 200–201). Moreover, World War I prompted the rapid development of hospitals for the middle and upper classes.

9. Despite its intentions, the 1929 act was implemented in a way that continued the poor-law system; local authorities controlled hospital care and used means tests (Digby 1982, 37; Crowther 1986; Abel-Smith 1964, 383).

Nevertheless, the meaning associated with government hospitals and private, voluntary hospitals did differ: whereas the public favorably associated voluntary hospitals with spectacular cures and sensational surgery, government hospitals continued to be tainted by the shadow of the poor law. Thus, even though government facilities continued to provide the majority of hospital treatment, by the 1920s and 1930s a growing proportion of patients were willing to wait months to be treated in voluntary hospitals (Smith 1979, 153–54; Meacham 1977, 153–54; Abel-Smith 1964, 356).[10] Voluntary hospitals increasingly abandoned their original devotion to the sick poor and instead responded to the general public's growing attraction to their facilities: they improved the comfort of private patients and increased the proportion of costs that were collected by charging patients (from approximately 10 per cent before World War I to 40 percent in 1931).[11]

Whereas the state's hospital system continued to be tainted by the poor-law stigma, local government infirmaries were increasingly understood by the public as medical rather than poor-law facilities. As the distinction between the infirmary and the workhouse grew, patients far above the pauper class were attracted to local government infirmaries (Abel-Smith 1964, 130–32, 236–38; Hodgkinson 1967, 520–49, 602). The growing public expectation of general medical services from local governments was reflected in the decision of poor-law authorities after 1918 to welcome greater use of government dispensaries by both the nonpoor and, in particular, the dependents of those insured under NHI (Honigsbaum 1979, 128–29; Abel-Smith 1964, 255–57).

The public was becoming accustomed to general medical care not only through the services of local governments but also because of the provisions of Friendly Societies. Thus, the NHI Act of 1911 reflected and helped form new socially shared meanings about GP care and state provisions (Honigsbaum 1979; Gilbert 1964; Briggs 1961; Meacham 1977). In particular, the act both established a panel system along the lines of the societies' club practice and broke with the poor laws' local government structure: the central state coordinated administration and financed the program through social insurance. In the decades before World War II, however, even this nationale panel system failed to satisfy public expectations for GP services:

---

10. The proportion of patients treated in state-provided beds declined from 75 percent to 64 percent between 1921 and 1938, while the proportion in voluntary hospitals increased from 25 percent to 36 percent. Moreover, the nonpoor's attraction to voluntary hospitals was reflected in the fact that by 1920 half of voluntary hospitals' patients were persons insured under NHI.

11. Voluntary hospitals in the 1930s found that raising their fees to levels that seemed more appropriate to the middle class actually attracted more affluent patients who would not have attended general hospitals (Abel-Smith 1964, 24–37, 294–98, 398).

it did not cover the middle class and dependents of wage earners, and its care was perceived to be of poor quality.

United States

In contrast to the British, Americans did not become familiar with state provisions or GP care. By the end of the nineteenth century, the state was associated with democratic procedures; the state's widespread distribution of social welfare to the general population remained a foreign idea to most Americans. Although special programs for such discrete groups as Native Americans and especially Civil War veterans grew to significant proportions (Skocpol 1992; Orloff and Skocpol 1984; Quadagno 1988), the absence of widespread public acceptance of state social welfare presented a stubborn barrier to generalizing these arrangements to the entire country.

Amid the reformism of the Progressive Era, American preoccupation with the "moral stratosphere" of the state's democratic procedures served to divert attention from the state's provision of social welfare (Kemler 1947, 166). The benefits the government did widely distribute through a decentralized patronage system were attacked as the corrupt payoffs of a spoils system. Popular interest in the type of social welfare legislation passed in Britain was overshadowed in the United States by a spree of institutional tinkering with democratic procedures: while old age pensions and national health insurance were being enacted in Britain, most state governments, from New York and Mississippi to California, found a groundswell of support for laws that required political parties to conduct direct primaries to select their candidates.

By the 1920s, the state's provision of social welfare remained largely restricted to poor relief, and even those benefits, which continued to be harshly administered by subnational governments, were comparatively quite limited. The programs for Civil War veterans faded, and new programs such as workmen's compensation continued to minimize the state's involvement by relying on the action of private employers. In the context, then, of Americans' enduring perception that substantial state involvement in social welfare was inappropriate, even poor relief could not be expanded or even defended as a legitimate end (Lubove 1968, 106–11).

The New Deal and especially the passage of the Social Security Act of 1935 represented an important shift in the meaning of the state. The Roosevelt administration designed national social welfare programs such as old age pensions (or Social Security) to be widely perceived, for the first time, as attractive and untainted by the stigma of the dole (Schlesinger 1960; Leuchtenberg 1963). Commenting in 1947 on the "ethical revolution" in

Americans' perception of the state, Edgar Kemler observed that the passage of the 1935 act reflected a shift from "inflated ideas" about democratic procedures and moral uplift to a more sober acceptance of concrete "material objectives" (1947, 71,122). But, even as the state's meaning was being rearticulated, the public's uneasiness toward government provisions continued, albeit in a modified form. The result was a deep ambivalence: Americans simultaneously harbored concerns about the state's role and accepted state involvement based on Social Security's insurance system. Thus, research on public opinion has persistently found that Americans' enduring unease regarding state interference awkwardly coexists with an acceptance of state involvement in specific social welfare programs (Page and Shapiro 1992; Marmor et al. 1990; Feldman and Zaller 1992).

After the late nineteenth century, American medicine also developed rapidly: it embraced the principles of scientific medicine and advanced medical knowledge to the point that the United States supplanted Europe by 1920 as the dominant research center (Stevens 1976; Rosenkrantz 1985). The acceptance of germ theory and antiseptic principles, combined with improvements in surgical operations, transformed hospitals from refuges providing custodial care into centers for curative treatment (Rosenberg 1979a).

In comparison with British developments, though, American medical advances were more narrowly confined to hospitals, making them the hub of health care. Unorthodox care outside hospitals was replaced by hospital-centered scientific medicine; licensing statutes and university medical schools established orthodox medicine's control over the medical labor market. With the waning of unorthodox medicine, general care outside hospitals (such as in Friendly Society club practice or company programs) remained comparatively insignificant; hospitals encouraged their own growing centrality by allowing virtually all doctors (including GPs) access to their facilities (Rosner 1982; Starr 1982; Stevens 1976 and 1989).

In the context of major medical changes after the late 1800s, the public's understanding of health care also shifted. Health became synonymous with orthodox medicine and the diagnostic and curative procedures of modern hospitals; the previous attraction of lay practitioners and self-treatment faded, and hospitals supplanted the home as the preferred setting for treatment (Starr 1982).

The reformulation of health care's meaning was constrained by American unfamiliarity with either widespread state provisions or general medical care. Thus the expansion of poor relief after the 1930s to include general medical services did not attract strong public interest as it did in Britain. Moreover, the depressed level of public interest in GP care led to relatively low levels of health insurance coverage for general medical or doctor services; it also contributed to the collapse of dispensaries and neighborhood health centers, which could not emulate their British counterparts by attracting the general public (Rosenberg 1974; Starr 1982; Rosen 1971).

Voluntary and other private hospitals attracted a wide spectrum of Americans, from the "respectable" working class to the middle and upper classes. As patients inside private hospitals began to reflect the occupational distribution of the population as a whole, hospital construction soared, first during the last quarter of the nineteenth century and then after the 1920s (Stevens 1976 and 1989; Starr 1982, 158–60; Sicherman 1979, 104).[12] Moreover, American voluntary hospitals responded to the growing attraction of their facilities just as their British counterparts did: they increasingly relied on charging patients and improved the accommodations and services of paying patients (Stevens 1989; Rosenberg 1979a and 1977, 438–40; Starr 1982, 74–78, 159; Rosner 1982, 2–8).

The new meaning of health care did not become associated (as it did in Britain) with a direct, visible state role. Indeed, the public's resistance to state provisions created a major barrier to the enactment of government health insurance during the Roosevelt and Truman administrations. Roosevelt appreciated what Truman did not—the political significance of a public that was found in social histories and opinion surveys to be "uninformed and largely apathetic concerning government reform of the medical care system"; indeed, national health insurance proposals suffered deteriorating support during Truman's term (Hirshfield 1970, 43; Schiltz 1970, 138, 180).[13] The public's enduring uneasiness with state provisions led Roosevelt and his administration to omit health insurance from their draft of the Social Security Act; Truman's insensitivity to public understandings contributed to congressional defeat of his proposals for compulsory insurance for the entire country (Poen 1979; Hirshfield 1970; Schlesinger 1960).

The American state did become significantly involved in health care after the 1920s, but in an indirect, nonsalient way: it encouraged nonstate institutions to organize and finance the country's health care. In particular, the state promoted private health insurance schemes such as Blue Cross by granting them special tax-exempt status, and it funded most of the boom

12. Hospitals expanded from 178 in 1873 to 4,359 in 1909 and nearly 7,000 by the 1920s; the period after World War I saw another burst of construction. Between 1925 and 1945, the number of hospital beds jumped 80 percent, with 60 percent of this increase occurring before the onset of World War II.

13. Schiltz (1970) and Payne (1946) suggest that interpreting polling data to indicate support for national health insurance during the Roosevelt and Truman terms conflates preferences toward the means and the ends of health policy. These polls, it is argued, actually capture the public's preferences for the objective of financing health care; when it comes to the means for achieving this the public is "as much for *any* type of prepayment plan as it is for government medicine" (Payne 1946, 95).

in the construction of nonstate hospitals; by 1939, government financing surpassed private support by a 4-to-1 ratio (Fox 1986, 74–79, 115–31). As a result, the number of private hospitals skyrocketed and private health insurance rapidly developed; by 1960, private nonprofit insurers (namely, Blue Cross) and the increasingly dominant private commercial insurers were an accepted part of society, covering 81 percent of the civilian population for some kind of hospital benefits.

In contrast to the development of nonstate insurers and hospitals, the number of government hospitals in the United States never approached the level of those in Britain, where they constituted the country's largest system of medical care (Rosenberg 1977; Starr 1982, 149–51, 178–80; Shonick 1984). Agreement about the appropriate role of public hospitals simply never developed in the United States (Shonick 1984, 54; Fox 1986, 74–77).

In short, government health insurance and other forms of state activity failed to attract the necessary backing not because they were "socialized medicine"—as the American Medical Association was to repeatedly charge—but because "socialism" symbolized for many Americans their own sense that direct, salient state involvement in social welfare was unfamiliar and foreign. The public was gradually coming to accept a direct state responsibility for social welfare based on the Social Security system, but this was a slow process, one just beginning when Truman declared comprehensive national health insurance his top domestic priority. Without the formation of widespread support for a major direct state role, nonstate institutions came to dominate America's hospital-centered health care system.

Public understandings of the state and health care prefigured the formulations of the NHS and Medicare acts. Gradually emerging from an interaction with medical and professional developments, the meaning of health care became associated in the United States with hospitals and in Britain with both hospital treatment and community-based GP care. Without an established tradition of general medical care along the lines of Britain's club and panel practices, Americans did not develop a comparable understanding of (and attachment to) community-based care.

American and British understanding of health care was closely related to the meaning associated with the state. Long-standing British experiences with government provisions created the basis for the public's acceptance of direct state involvement in providing and financing health care. Americans, in contrast, historically identified the state with democratic procedures and did not come to understand (and ultimately accept) direct state involvement in hospital and general medical care as an emanation of the poor law system. Instead, the American public became accustomed to nonstate institutions financing and providing health care. But the public's widening acceptance of Social Security's massive and direct provision of benefits gradually modified Americans' enduring uneasiness with state provisions. What was conceivable in Britain—direct government operation of hospital and general care—was unfathomable in the United States.

The historic development of American and British culture created multiple social meanings—elements of which overlapped and at times contradicted each other. The state, then, never meant just one thing, even though important tendencies did emerge. In Britain, for example, the public historically tended to enunciate its prevailing repertoire of understandings in terms of greater state involvement; but this pattern contained a lingering (and generally subordinate) element of fear—that state interference would become excessive.

In short, enduring cultural patterns prefigured (but in a general, indeterminate manner) the terms on which policymakers and the public would understand and discuss health policy reform. The details of the NHS and Medicare acts were not preordained, but each act was designed within specific cultural parameters: state provision of hospital- and community-based care for the entire population in Britain, and narrow, hospital-centered care in the United States, which drew on public acceptance of Social Security. In the United States, them, extensive state involvement in health care failed to attract the necessary backing not because it represented socialized medicine but because socialism articulated for many Americans their own sense that a massive government-operated social welfare system was alien to their repertoire of understandings.

PART II

The Health Care Debate Moves to the Mainstream

4 | Britain, 1930s–1942:
Reform Becomes Practical Politics

By 1942 in Britain and 1960 in the United States, proposals to reform health care were attracting the serious attention of both elites and the general public; only shortly before, the issue had been relegated to the margins of governmental deliberations. Before authoritative decisions on the NHS and Medicare acts were reached, policymakers made critical choices regarding what issues were placed on the agenda. More than simply the pressure of real-world problems, it was the political dynamics of agenda setting that moved the health reform issue from the margins of policy debate to the top of the governmental agenda (Kingdon 1984; Cobb and Elder 1972; Nelson 1984; Light 1991).

Policymakers' discussions of reform emerged from policy networks of specialists outside the government as well as bureaucrats and elected politicians in the executive and legislative branches. By transcending political and formal divisions, these networks made it possible to accumulate and distribute information as well as to organize bargaining. In general, visible political figures (the U. S. president or prominent members of Congress or the British cabinet) are attracted by the publicity associated with setting the general direction of policy and use this national attention to dominate the selection of agenda items; the hidden clusters of experts from the bureaucracy and professional communities concentrate on specifying alternatives (Kingdon 1984). During the first phase of health policy formulation, politicians were especially instrumental in determining the subject of governmental debate, while specialists began to generate the content and details of possible reforms.

The placement of the reform issue on the governmental agenda raises the following central question: what determined policymakers' definition of the problem, their selection of the issue, and their specification of alternative arrangements? For Weberians, an institution's existing administrative capacity is the primary focus and determinant of elite decisions in agenda setting. According to Skowronek (1982), for instance, elites' perception at the turn of the century that existing institutions were incapable of meeting the country's "developmental imperatives" led them to define this problem in terms of organizational weakness and to devote sustained attention to the development of state hierarchy and specialization. The culturalists' explanation differs from that offered by Weberians (and by other analysts of agenda setting):[1] they expect policymakers' perceptions of public preferences and understandings to affect significantly the definition and selection of an issue, as well as the specification of policy alternatives.

INITIAL POLICY DISCUSSIONS

The 1930s in England was a formative period in the emergence of major health care reform.[2] Problems in health care had been an ongoing concern of the Ministry of Health and policy community professionals; but in the period just before World War II, policymakers' alarm over the limitations in the prevailing health care system prompted them to address these problems systematically and with renewed vigor.

Ministry of Health files, which recorded the deliberations of senior and middle-level civil servants as well as nongovernmental experts, indicate that these policy discussions produced two significant developments, both tied to public preferences and understandings: first, policymakers came to agree that there was a major crisis in health care; then, they responded to this new demand by discussing incremental adjustments to expand and coordinate the existing health care system.

The Problem

Although the old arrangements for health care delivery did not attract the same attention as the dire economic and foreign crises of the 1930s,

1. Agenda-setting research has emphasized the "severe limits on the ability of general public opinion to affect policy formulation" (Kingdon 1984, 69; Light 1991).
2. The group of senior ministry officials who were most intimately involved in health policy formulation included the permanent secretary, the deputy secretaries, and the chief medical officer. The middle-level officials were assistant secretaries and principals, who were less senior. During the period up through the fall of 1942, the critical senior officials included W. A. Robinson, E. J. Maude, A. S. MacNalty, G. Chrystal, A. N. Rucker, and W. Jameson. The relevant middle-level officials included H. A. de Montmorency, A. W. Neville, J. C. Wrigley, T. H. Sheepshanks, J. Hawton, S. F. Wilkinson, and John Pater.

policymakers and experts agreed by September 1939 that these arrangements were increasingly incapable of meeting the public's new level of demand. A series of Ministry of Health memoranda concentrated on the widening gap between changing public opinion and old administrative arrangements for hospital care. In considering "the future development of the hospital system," a ministry official contrasted the long-standing public beliefs that had previously undergirded administrative arrangements with the new sentiment: "Formerly the Public interested in hospitals represented a very small proportion of the community. Today the hospital public and the population of the country are synonymous terms. Formerly the hospital public was interested in the cure of others. Today it is interested also in the cure of itself."[3]

By the latter half of the 1930s, the shift in the public's understanding of hospital care—from one of fear to one of attraction—created major problems for the existing municipal and voluntary hospitals. The public's negative perception of municipal hospitals, which originally deterred all but a narrow section of the population, was now becoming increasingly ineffective in discouraging requests from the more hospital-minded public. With acceptance of the hospital spreading up the social strata, public hospitals attracted working- and middle-class patients; although originally created for the destitute, by the 1930s only 18 percent of London's municipal hospital patients were paupers (Abel-Smith 1964, 368–404; Fox 1986, 62–64). The demand for municipal hospitals reflected the development of public expectations toward the state provision of hospital care; this trend was echoed in a March 1939 Gallup poll, which reported that 71 percent of respondents preferred making "hospitals a public service supported by public funds."[4] As a result of changing public understandings and preferences, the larger local authorities were now competing with voluntary hospitals for paying patients.

Nevertheless, because the organization of municipal hospitals was premised on providing care to a limited audience, these facilities found it impossible to meet the new demands, even after significant expansions. One of the leaders of the London County Council recalled that by the late 1930s the "change of public opinion" toward municipal hospitals had increased demand beyond the capacity of their facilities: "The old stigma attaching to the poor law Infirmaries and Institutions had absolutely and entirely

3. MH 80/24, Memo, "The Future Development of the Hospital System," undated, probably written in 1938.
4. The poll question was the following: "1,092 hospitals in Great Britain are dependent upon charity for their support. Do you favor continuing this system, or should hospitals be a public service supported by public funds?" Twenty-two percent favored the present system, while 7 percent had no opinion (Gallup 1976, 14).

disappeared and it was becoming more and more difficult to cope with the enormous demand made by the public for Hospital accommodation."[5]

The pressure facing municipal facilities was even more severe for voluntary hospitals, in part because they were more desirable. A Ministry of Health official noted that the state's municipal hospitals "do not arouse the same feelings of enthusiasm" as the voluntary hospitals, which attract a strong "patriotism" among the middle class because they "possess features that are in consonance with [the public's] own outlook."[6] As a result of the particularly strong public demand for treatment in voluntary hospitals, a broad range of voluntary insurance schemes (such as the Hospital Savings Associations) emerged during the 1930s to make treatment in voluntary facilities affordable to both the working and upper classes (Abel-Smith 1964, 384–404). Voluntary hospitals expanded their capacity but were simply unable to satisfy the demand for care; large numbers of sick were either left waiting for long periods or simply denied admission.

By the late 1930s, it was clear that new public attitudes toward hospitals had created a level of demand that threatened to overwhelm the capacity of the prevailing system. Even as local authorities and voluntary bodies expanded their services to meet increasing demand, Ministry of Health officials reported that "all the general hospitals, voluntary and municipal are severely taxed."[7]

Policymakers were especially concerned with the difficulties facing hospitals, but they were also aware of the growing problems in the area of community-based GP care. With the growing division between hospital- and community-based practitioners, by the late 1930s GPs were excluded from hospitals, especially in big cities; they came to dominate general medical care and its largest system for delivery—the NHI's panel practice. The combination of this widening division and growing popular expectations created two problems. First, a growing portion of the country came to expect community-based GP care: despite expansions, the demand to enlarge further the coverage of the existing GP provisions (especially, the panel practice) grew. Moreover (and somewhat ironically), the quality of care provided by GPs and in particular the NHI's panel doctors came under increasing attack. Excluded from hospital practice, these doctors failed to keep abreast of the medical advances the public came to expect from modern medicine (Honigsbaum 1979, 135–70).

5. MH 77/25, Memo, "Hospital Policy in London," 8/41, by Frederich Menzies (medical officer of health for the London County Council).

6. MH 80/24, Memo, "The Future Development of the Hospital System," undated, probably written in 1938.

7. MH 80/24, Memo, "The Future Development of the Hospital System," by A. S. MacNalty, 5/24/38. This remark was made in specific reference to Glasgow hospitals, but it reflects the general thinking within the ministry.

Policymakers' understanding of the problem facing health care, contradicts Weberian expectations. The problem was believed to originate not in the inherent organizational weakness of existing institutions but in changing public understandings and preferences. Officials became convinced that the increasing public demand for more and better health care could not be satisfied by existing arrangements for providing hospital and community care; reforming existing arrangements would ultimately involve addressing the source of the problem—the changing social meanings of health care and the state.

Incrementalism Considered

The recognition of serious problems in Britain's health care system prompted Ministry of Health officials during the 1930s to begin discussing health reform, though not the major sort of change involved with creating the NHS. Concern with health care developed as part of the society-wide "middle opinion" in favor of economic and social reforms (Marwick 1964). Reflecting the formation of this broad reform-oriented consensus, a former Ministry of Health official recalled deliberately joining the Department in 1933 "because I was sure there was going to be an NHS and I wanted to be in on the organization of it and I [was] not unique in that."[8]

Nevertheless, with the economy and foreign policy the dominant concerns of governments and political parties, major health care reform was a relatively marginal issue in government deliberations during the 1930s. Certainly, the cabinet did not identify its vital political interests with this issue, nor did it press the Ministry of Health to formulate new policies. Thus, although ministry officials began to consider policy reforms systematically, the issue of a national health service was limited to the margins of policy debate; an important participant in health policy discussions recalled that "in 1939, an NHS was scarcely discussed" (Taylor 1979a, 173). Instead, policy discussions during the 1930s were largely limited to proposals for incremental adjustments to the existing system.

In particular, during the latter half of the 1930s Ministry of Health officials considered two incremental reforms: expanding existing services and rationalizing their provision (but without imposing hierarchical control by the state). Both reforms were aimed at preserving the old arrangements: the discussions before September 1939, one civil servant recalled, centered on improving the present system and not on proposals of a comprehensive new health service. In February 1938, officials broached the topic of gradually expanding access to both GP care (i.e., by including the dependents of those

---

8. Godber Interview.

insured under NHI) and intrahospital treatment by the specialists.[9] Officials came to agree that these extensions should be achieved through incremental adjustments in the administrative framework of local authorities; expanding the scope of reform to provide comprehensive services and universal coverage was assumed to be impractical.

To rationalize the existing hospital and GP care, existing providers were encouraged to coordinate their services voluntarily; strengthening the national government's hierarchical control was not seriously considered. Like the proposals for extending health services, the discussions of voluntary coordination were aimed at prompting incremental changes to prolong the prevailing arrangements, especially the role of nonstate bodies. As one Ministry of Health official noted, "there is no desire to see [voluntary efforts] disappear. The desire is that they should take steps to save themselves." Although the organization of GP care was discussed, policymakers' attention was on hospitals. Ministry of Health officials generally agreed that coordination and rationalization of all hospitals would provide the solution for preserving the existing system. By coordinating hospitals within regions that were larger than a single local authority, officials argued (with some agreement from leading interest groups) that it would become possible to build cooperation between the local authorities and the voluntary hospitals. The network of departmental and nongovernmental policy experts discussed this regional scheme as a strategy to encourage voluntary and municipal hospitals to behave—through their own voluntary actions—less as independent units and more as partners in a general scheme.[10]

The discussion of these two incremental reforms did not, however, produce a new policy: with interest groups opposed to encroachments on their prerogatives and the public seemingly apathetic, officials in the Ministry of Health concluded that it was "impractical" to press for even incremental changes. Mistakenly convinced that local authorities had escaped the taint of the poor law and had developed because of the "force of opinion," administrators of these municipal governments opposed all policy changes that threatened to diminish their role in health care. Moreover, ministry officials recognized that the medical profession opposed any changes that introduced "restrictions" by the state.[11]

9. Pater Interview; MH 80/24, Minutes and memos, Office conference on the development of the health services, 2/7/38, 4/6/38, 5/31/38, 6/27/38.

10. MH 80/24, Memo, "The Future Development of the Hospital System," undated, probably written in 1938; MH 80/24, Memo, "The Future Development of the Hospital System," by A. S. MacNalty, 5/24/38; MH 80/24, Notes on the fourth office conference, 6/27/38; MH 80/24, Minutes, "Conference at the Ministry of Health . . . on the Question of Financial Assistance to Voluntary Hospitals," 1/27/39. Between 1936 and 1939, ministry officials regularly met with representatives of doctors, voluntary hospitals, and local authorities: MH 71/51 and 71/52, Minutes, memos, and newspaper clippings relating to Medical Advisory Committee meetings.

11. MH 80/24, Memo, "The Future Development of the Hospital System," undated, prob-

The opposition of the medical profession and local authorities was reinforced by national policymakers' inaccurate perception of an apathetic public. Stressing that "there was precious little" public opinion on reforming health care during the 1930s, one administrator in the national government recalled feeling that "the great mass of the public were not really conscious of the need for an improved health service."[12] In addition to deciding that the reforms would not "command great popularity," officials in the Ministry of Health accurately recognized that local authorities were still tainted by the poor laws: challenging the assumptions of municipal hospitals, administrators thought it "doubtful if public opinion ... [would] approve" of an expansion of local authorities. The "attitude of the public mind [in preferring voluntary over local authority hospitals]," a ministry official stressed, "must be taken into account."[13]

These unfavorable conditions for health reform were compounded by what ministry officials saw as the practical difficulties presented by the general political climate. Between the two world wars, the Conservative party became associated with economic recovery and prudence, and the Labour party was discredited by its ineptitude in responding to the economic decline of the 1920s and the financial crisis of 1931. The Conservatives' status-quo-oriented policies, then, seemed certain to win them reelection on the eve of World War II.

The combination before the war of an unfavorable political environment, interest group opposition, and the perception of an apathetic public convinced the health policy community that pursuing even mild reform was "impolitic." Ministry of Health officials and interest groups acknowledged that extending and rationalizing existing services was desirable but agreed that "no such simple solution was possible"; "a revolution was necessary to achieve the desired end."[14]

In short, even before World War II policymakers had come to recognize that health care arrangements were faced with a serious problem: changing public opinion created a demand for hospital and GP care that was increas-

---

ably written during 1938; MH 80/24, Minutes, "Conference at the Ministry of Health," 1/27/39. Also see Memo, "Conference with the Voluntary Hospitals and the LCC," 2/1/39, by T. S. McIntosh; MH 71/51 and 71/52, Minutes and memos associated with the Medical Advisory Committee between 1936 and 1939; MH 80/24, Memo, "The Proposals for Subvention of the London Voluntary Hospitals 5/24/38"; MH 77/25, Memo, "Hospital Policy in London," 8/41, Frederick Menzies; MH 71/52, "Statement by Sir Frederick Menzies," 12/7/37, and Minutes, Medical Advisory Committee, 12/31/37.

12. Pater Interview.

13. MH 80/24, Memo, "The Future Development of the Hospital System," undated, probably written during 1938; MH 80/24, Notes of the third office conference, 5/31/38; MH 80/24 Notes of the first office conference, 2/7/38; MH 80/24, Memo, "Provision of Specialist Services," 3/15/37, by A. S. MacNalty.

14. MH 71/51 and 71/52, Minutes, memos, and newspaper clippings relating to Medical Advisory Committee meetings held between 3/5/36 and late 1939.

ingly straining the existing delivery system. In response, policymakers began by September 1939 to consider modifying the health care system. Their initial policy discussions focused on incremental reforms and preservation of the status quo. But with policymakers not perceiving strong public backing for major reform, even these proposals were found to be revolutionary and impractical.

THE SHIFTING STRATEGIC UNIVERSE, 1939–1942

From the outbreak of war in September 1939 until the eve of the Beveridge Report's publication, the issue of major health care reform was propelled onto the governmental agenda by political disputes involving rival parties, politicians, civil servants, and interest groups. As political calculations changed, politicians and bureaucrats assumed by October 1942 that major reform was no longer impolitic and that they could begin to move beyond incremental changes. As a result, policymakers became both more sensitive to changing public opinion and more concerned with incorporating shifting public expectations into the formulation of new health policy.

The war went through three general phases. In the initial phase before March 1940, it created little direct disruption of normal domestic and political life; the eerie calm of this period became referred to as the "phony" war. But, in April 1940 with the German invasions of Scandinavia and France and the attempted evacuations from Dunkirk, the war entered a new period; during the next eighteen months, Britain experienced significant social and political disruption as it struggled to defend itself. Finally, the war took a favorable turn in October 1942 with the victory at El Alamein; no longer struggling to fend off a German invasion, Britain and its allies spent the next three years on a long march to defeat Germany. During the first two of these phases, health care became a central focus of public opinion and political struggles.

Public Opinion

Although the war contributed to the evolution of public opinion, the development of public understandings and preferences should not merely be reduced to the war. The public's enduring understanding of state involvement in health care was echoed in a range of evidence about public preferences during the war—quantitative surveys by Gallup and the government as well as qualitative studies by the government, including one

William Beveridge commissioned.[15] Although the representativeness of the qualitative studies is far from clear, they are nonetheless informative given the limited availability of opinion data; their reliability is strengthened when they are examined in conjunction with quantitative polls and evidence on enduring understandings.

Before November 1942 and the completion of the Beveridge Report, two trends in public opinion had emerged: the quality of existing health care arrangements and state provisions had become a salient issue (attracting widespread dissatisfaction), and a new policy direction that would introduce major new initiatives was demanded.

Existing social welfare benefits aroused strong public interest, because the public found them very unsatisfactory. The hostility toward social welfare provisions was directed both at the continuing use of a means test and at the perceived inadequacies of the benefits. In November 1942, the government used the Ministry of Information's system of regional investigators to finish a qualitative study of "public feeling on postwar reconstruction." The study reported that the "continuance of anything in the nature of a Means Test is generally condemned"; this hostility carried over to health care, where there was "very strong and in some cases unanimous" feeling that care be provided "without the stigma of charity."[16] The government study echoed the public's long-standing hostility toward arrangements that differentiated beneficiaries according to their financial means.

Polls and qualitative studies during the war also found that the public was anxious about deteriorating health, and that the existing arrangements for hospital and community care attracted widespread attention and criticism.[17] Explaining the public's dissatisfaction with hospital care, Eckstein noted that "many upper- and middle-class patients were compelled, for the first time in their lives, to enter public hospitals.... They got first hand experience of workhouse-turned-hospital and their response generally was furious" (1958, 98). The public not only resented municipal hospitals be-

15. Beveridge commissioned a group of academicians at Oxford's Nuffield College (led by G. D. H. Cole) to interview "responsible people" across the country during the first half of 1942. The goal was to use "numerous local inquiries" to identify the country's "consensus" or "general opinion and views about the existing [health care] schemes." CAB 87/78, Minutes, Interdepartmental Committee on Social Insurance and Allied Services (SIC) (42) 20th, 6/24/42; CAB 87/80, Memo, SIC (42) 85, "Report for Sir William Beveridge's Interdepartmental Committee," 6/23/42; CAB 87/80, SIC (42) 114, Memo, "Nuffield College," by Miss M. Ritson, 7/20/42. For a more detailed discussion of the Nuffield survey see Harris 1977, and 1983.

16. CAB 117/209, Memo, "Public Feeling on Post-War Reconstruction," by Ministry of Information, Home Intelligence Division.

17. RG 23/24, Wartime Social Survey, "Public Attitudes to Health and to the Autumn Health Campaign," Report no. 21, conducted July-August 1942; CAB 117/209, Memo, "Public Feeling," 1942; Gallup 1976, 42.

cause of their connection to the poor laws but also disliked voluntary hospitals. In particular, the public widely criticized voluntary hospitals for their unsatisfactory treatment and their financial reliance on charity, as epitomized by "flag days" to raise contributions.[18]

Perhaps the harshest criticism was directed against community-based GP care, especially the NHI panel treatment. Both the 1942 government poll and the Nuffield College Survey which Beveridge commissioned reported that panel treatment was strongly and widely disliked. In particular, both found public resentment against inferior, "second-class" treatment and inadequate coverage.[19] As a result of the NHI system's exclusion of both dependents and intrahospital specialist services, many of the nonpoor turned to local authorities, but only with great resentment: the Nuffield survey reported that "there is a strong feeling of resentment against an Insurance system which so inadequately provides for sickness . . . [that it] forces people of independent spirit . . . to seek assistance through the same channels as the unemployables [and] the destitute."[20]

The selection of the health care issue for the general, nongovernmental agenda is indicated not only by studies of the mass public but also, to a lesser extent, by examination of the mass media. A review of articles published in the *London Times*, in particular, indicates that the health issue attracted relatively more coverage than other prominent domestic policies.[21] Although this evidence on media coverage is not compelling by itself, it does provide some additional indication of the relative concern over health care.

As the inadequacy of health care and government provisions became quite salient, the public also came to prefer that future policy move in the direction of major innovation; this would expand the state's social welfare provisions and make its benefits universally available. With the war accelerating change in the patterns of public understandings, the 1942 government survey reported broad agreement that the state (especially at the national level) play a greater role in administering and financing social services in general. Echoing this finding in terms of health care, the Nuffield survey reported fairly widespread demand that medical services become a state matter: "The state is looked to more and more as the [public's] best guardian." In particular,

18. CAB 117/209, Memo, "Public Feeling," 1942.
19. CAB 87/78, Minutes, SIC (42) 20th, 6/24/42; CAB 87/80, SIC (42) 64, Memo, "National Health Insurance," by Nuffield College, 6/5/42, pp. 4–10; CAB 117/209, Memo, "Public Feeling," 1942.
20. CAB 87/80, SIC (42) 64, Memo, "National Health Insurance," by Nuffield College, 6/5/42, pp. 27–28 (quotation from a Nuffield investigator in Aberdeen).
21. During 1942, the *Times* published five articles on health care, only one on housing, and two on social insurance and unemployment. The low number of articles published on these issues probably reflects Britain's preoccupation (particularly during 1942) with the war front.

there existed widespread support for the central state to finance medical services directly rather than to rely on insurance. Moreover, the 1942 government survey reported that, although a small body of opinion favored the retention of a voluntary hospital system, the majority were for state ownership and control of hospitals.[22] The public support for greater state involvement in health care provisions is confirmed by an April 1941 Gallup survey of public preferences for three alternative approaches for delivering hospital and doctor services: 55 percent favored state control in order to provide free services, while 30 percent supported extending the panel system and 15 percent preferred making private arrangements.[23]

In addition to favoring expanded state involvement, the public supported the egalitarian aim of making state benefits universally available. The feeling that the war had created a single community may have helped crystallize support for universalism. The combination of wartime experiences and the development of a new social understanding of the state produced strong support for making government benefits a right of citizenship and removing the detested means tests (Addison 1977, 128–63). Articulating the emerging expectation that state social welfare provisions should attract rather than repulse recipients, Beveridge's committee assumed that "the general population of this country favor a scheme … which enables … benefits to be obtained as a right and without a means test."[24] In the area of health care, this widespread expectation was identified by the Nuffield College report and the 1942 government survey; both reported "very strong and in some cases unanimous" feeling that "in the future, the best possible medical, surgical, and hospital treatment should be available to everyone."[25]

The public's hostility toward existing health care arrangements and support for new policies was expressed in the widespread demand for a particular policy direction: it supported innovative reconstruction after the war of the economy and domestic affairs. A November 1940 Gallup poll reported that 42 percent felt that "the government should draw up and publish our war aims"; a differently worded question in April 1942 found that one-third of the British civilian population felt that the government

22. CAB 117/209, Memo, "Public Feeling," 1942; CAB 87/80, SIC (42) 64, Memo, "National Health Insurance," by Nuffield College, 6/5/42, p. 66; CAB 87/78, Minutes, SIC (42) 20th, 6/24/42.

23. The Gallup poll asked: "Which would you prefer of the following: all doctors and hospitals under state control with their services free as education is now; an extension of the panel system to include everybody; having a private doctor whom you pay for his visits and medicine?" (Gallup 1976, 43–44).

24. Official Committee on the Beveridge Report (PIN) 8/86, Memo by subcommittee of Beveridge committee, 2/42.

25. CAB 117/209, Memo, "Public Feeling," 1942; CAB 87/80, SIC (42) 64, Memo, "National Health Insurance," by Nuffield College, 6/5/42.

"should...start thinking now about the kind of peace we want."[26] The strong public support for major domestic reform after the war was reflected in the popularity of Beveridge's social security scheme seven months *before* its official publication in December 1942.[27] By fall, the 1942 government survey reported an important change in the public's policy concerns: "Three years ago, the term social security was almost unknown to the public as a whole. It now appears to be generally accepted as an urgent post-war need."[28] Evidence of the increasing salience of the social security issue was accompanied by public support for governmental insurance; a Gallup poll reported in October 1942 that 70 percent favored a government insurance scheme, that would provide sickness and unemployment benefits "even if it would mean...paying more insurance than you are paying now" (Gallup 1976, 67).

Thus, even before the Beveridge Report was published in December 1942, there was a widespread expectation that after the war a major reform of prewar policies would occur. In terms of health care, the strong dissatisfaction with existing arrangements had aroused public interest and placed the health issue high on the general public's policy-making agenda. The growing salience of this issue was accompanied by strong public preference for major policy innovation, which would expand the state's involvement in health care and establish universal coverage.

Political Struggles

Political struggles were an important link between public support for a major change in health care arrangements and senior policy-makers' selection of this issue for serious attention. As public opinion was solidifying behind what was referred to as domestic "reconstruction," changes in British politics altered the calculations of politicians and bureaucrats and increased the strategic importance of major domestic reform.

The war significantly disrupted British politics, which the Conservative party had largely dominated since World War I. During the interwar period, the Liberal party continued its slide into obscurity, and the governments formed by Labour in 1924 and 1929–31 were political disasters, discrediting that Party and throwing the entire organized labor movement into retreat. With the onset of significant wartime hostilities in May 1940,

26. Gallup 1976, 37. The latter question was, "Should we win the war first and then think about the peace, or should we start thinking now about the kind of peace we want?" As a government memo noted, the question's wording probably depressed support for the second alternative because it did not mention victory; CAB 117/209, Memo, "Public Opinion on 'After the War'," Ministry of Information, Home Intelligence Special Report, no. 21, 6/4/42.
   27. CAB 117/209, Memo, "Public Opinion on 'After the War,'" 6/4/42.
   28. CAB 117/209, Memo, "Public Feeling," 1942.

however, the Conservatives replaced Neville Chamberlain with Winston Churchill as prime minister and struck a political bargain with its opposition, especially the Labour party. In exchange for supporting Churchill's conduct of the war and refraining from overt electoral politics, Labour was brought into the government as a virtual equal partner and made "the chief though not the sole animating force in civilian affairs" (Addison 1977, 75). In the wartime coalition, political struggle for personal and party advantage was not suppressed for the national interest but rather inundated the government; this was especially true on homefront issues in which the Labour party's representation and influence were greatest. The coalition's domestic policies, then, did not merely echo cross-party consensus; they resulted, in part, from significant political conflict (Morgan 1984; Webster 1987).

The political struggle within the coalition quickly coalesced in a dispute over public opinion. The shock of Dunkirk and the fall of France in June 1940 prompted policymakers to focus on public morale to sustain what would have to be a people's war: morale and public willingness to contribute to the war effort were recognized as having decisive military importance (McLaine 1979, 2; Calder 1968). Indeed, the government's public opinion apparatus was built precisely because of this growing sensitivity to the man in the street. Reflecting this interest in incorporating public concerns, the Ministry of Health requested opinion surveys to "examine statistically the public mind in connection with health problems."[29]

The interest in public opinion became directed at domestic policy making and especially reconstruction policy for postwar Britain. Only a day after France sued for peace, coalition members began to discuss the importance of establishing their war aims. Political struggles within the coalition, however, quickly enveloped the discussion of public opinion and reconstruction issues. Liberal and especially Labour politicians vigorously argued (with the often unspoken agreement of senior bureaucrats) that responding to public opinion by announcing government support for postwar social reform was necessary to bolster civilian morale and prevent panic. They directly linked the war effort to reconstruction planning; in the face of intense German bombing, a government pledge for the popular issue of reform would maintain public morale and give the nation something to fight for (McLaine 1979, 50–52, 59, 100–101). But the Conservatives (especially Churchill) opposed a government commitment, emphasizing its dangerous impact on public sentiment. Instead of stressing the benefits of responding to public opinion, the Conservatives warned that making reconstruction a war aim

29. RG 23/24, Wartime Social Survey, "Public Attitudes to Health and to the Autumn Health Campaign," Report no. 21, conducted July-August 1942.

would distract attention from conducting the war and create (as the previous war had) unrealistic expectations.

To prevent these political tensions from dividing the coalition, a political compromise was quickly reached: the government would investigate policies for postwar reform but would strictly avoid committing the postwar government. The contentious issue of reconstruction policy, then, was funneled into a policy-making process centered on committee investigation. Although the Conservatives viewed this process as a means for limiting policy discussion and restraining public expectations, it ultimately encouraged policymakers and the public to expect major postwar reforms.

The process of committee investigation into postwar policy began in the summer of 1940, when the cabinet established a committee to study the reconstruction issue. Although its membership and title changed, a cabinet committee on reconstruction existed until the coalition disbanded in May 1945. Churchill instructed the coalition that "provision must now be made for the study of postwar problems," and by early January 1941 the committee investigation was widely referred to within and outside the Government.[30] It was this process for defusing the divisive issue of postwar reconstruction that ironically gave rise to Beveridge's committee, charged with exploring possible reforms. The government committed itself in May 1941 to a comprehensive review of Britain's social services; by December, Beveridge circulated a memoranda to his committee that outlined the three fundamental aims—national health service, universal children's allowances, and maintenance of employment—which would be publicly announced a year later.

The process of policy investigation, which led to the Beveridge and cabinet committees, had a tremendous impact on government officials. It transformed the atmosphere of policy making, recasting common assumptions of what was practical. In this new atmosphere, bureaucrats tried to follow the apparent shift in official thinking and the perception that "public interest in [reconstruction] questions is increasing."[31] The sense of a new atmosphere was evident in remarks made by Beveridge a year before completing his report: assuring members of a private conference on reconstruction that he was "not concerned at the nonemergence of a 'slogan'," he stressed the importance of a "common . . . consciousness that we were at a revolutionary

30. CAB 117/1, Memo, "PM's Minute: Study of Postwar Problems," by W. Churchill, 12/30/40.
31. CAB 87/1, Committee on Reconstruction Problems (RP) (41) 4, "Provisional Plan of Work To Be Done under the Auspices of the Committee on Reconstruction Problems," by A. Greenwood, 2/27/41.

period in world history."[32] Beveridge's sense of the new climate was apparent in the growing feeling among civil servants that "further nibbling would seem to be a waste of time"; it is necessary, one official remarked, not to be "afraid of being too revolutionary."[33]

The new atmosphere emerging in the government was felt in the Ministry of Health through two types of pressure. First, the cabinet and its committees broadly supervised the department through its ministers, especially Ernest Brown. Because of his membership on the reconstruction and other policy committees, Brown became a conduit; he relayed to the department the desire of cabinet committees (and especially their Labour members) that postwar health policy embody the government's "general aim . . . to secure freedom and security to every human being." With the cabinet and its committees overseeing the ministry's activities, Brown instructed his administrators to begin designing major changes in the prewar arrangements for health care delivery, especially hospital care.[34]

Second, the ministry's perception of the Beveridge committee as a threat to its domain and institutional position motivated the department to consider major health care reform. Almost immediately after the committee's formation, word leaked out that "something large was afoot," and officials widely assumed that Parliament and the public would strongly press the government to state what action it proposed to take when the committee's report was completed.[35] Ministry officials reacted by unsuccessfully arguing with Beveridge that his focus should be narrowed because it was unnecessary and overlapped with the ministry's work.[36] But Beveridge insisted on recommending a broad framework for postwar reconstruction that would include a national health service for comprehensive treatment available to all members of the community.[37] By passing up "mere administrative tidying" in favor of setting the broad governmental agenda, he put the ministry in a threatening position: the forthcoming release of his report could catch it unprepared to respond to cabinet requests for information and proposals. Pushing aside objections within the ministry, a senior official acknowledged: "I feel pretty sure that we must here work out some sort of a scheme for a general medical service, if only for the reason that in its absence Beveridge,

32. CAB 117/164, Copies of the minutes of private conference, 6/4–5/41.
33. CAB 117/177, Memo from C. V. Davidge to secretary (George Chrystal), 2/27/41, and Letter from C. V. Davidge to A. Owen, 3/22/41.
34. CAB 87/1, RP (41) 1st, 3/6/41; CAB 117/2, Memo to George Chrystal, 2/17/41.
35. CAB 123/43, Memo to lord president, 7/15/42.
36. CAB 87/76, Minutes, SIC (41) 1st, 7/8/41; MH 80/31, Minutes of a meeting between William Beveridge and members of the Ministry of Health, 2/17/42.
37. CAB 87/76, SIC (41) 20, Memo, "Basic Problems of Social Security with Heads of a Scheme," by William Beveridge, 12/11/41.

who is thirsting to do the job himself, will probably induce [the minister responsible for reconstruction] to invite him to make a report on the subject."[38]

This twofold pressure on the Ministry of Health to consider major policy changes was reinforced by medical profession reports. In particular, the profession generally favored comprehensive service for everyone—a position, according to a ministry official, "which only a few years ago they would have regarded as dangerously heterodox."[39]

As a result of this pressure, a new policy-making atmosphere emerged: ministry officials perceived a major shift in public expectation toward fundamental reform. Brown argued in 1942 that wartime developments had "no equal as a method of presenting facts to us in a new light, and of stimulating us to think in new ways."[40] Concerned that "all opinion is in a state of flux," ministry officials sensed that the public was expecting the postwar government to "take all possible measures to safeguard the health of the people": even in the event of a postwar economic decline, "the question is sure to be asked, with insistence, if [state involvement in hospital care] can be done in time of War why cannot it be done in the difficult times of peace?"[41] This atmosphere of receptivity to new ideas prompted ministry officials to reject their previous assumption that major health care reform was an impractical, revolutionary change. Now they agreed with the Nuffield study of prewar health care arrangements that "no half measures or tinkering with the present chaotically constructed machine would be considered at all adequate."[42] By January 1941 it was "practical" politics, as one administrator explained, to "thin[k] whether we can't take the whole business at one gulp."[43]

Political struggles within the coalition had become an important link between public opinion and the emergence of a new policy-making atmosphere: political conflict altered the calculations of officeholders and bureaucrats, enhancing the importance they attached to responding to strong public interest in, and demand for, innovative reform. In particular, the process for defusing the political struggle over the reconstruction issue pro-

38. MH 80/31, Letter from J. Maude to H. A. de Montmorency, 2/9/42.
39. MH 80/31, Letter from H. A. de Montmorency to J. Maude, 2/23/42; Hill 1964, 82–83. Two especially important medical profession reports were by the BMA's Medical Planning Commission in May 1942 and by the Medical Planning Research group in November.
40. MH 80/24, Notes on Ernest Brown's speech to a conference at the Royal College of Nursing, 6/11/42.
41. MH 80/24, Memo, "Notes on Postwar Hospital Policy," from E. R. Forber to G. Chrystal, 5/40; MH 77/19, Memo, "Hospital Survey: Personal Impressions Gained at the Outset of a Survey," by E. R. C, 9/22/42.
42. CAB 87/80, SIC (42) 64, Memo, "National Health Insurance," by Nuffield College, 6/5/42, pp. 68–70 (quotation from an Aberdeen investigator).
43. MH 77/22, Memo to J. Maude, 1/23/41.

duced a new receptivity within the government: policymakers became sensitive to public opinion and were willing to prepare "definitive and authoritative" plans for reconstruction.[44]

POLICY DISCUSSIONS, 1939–1942

The changing political context fundamentally altered the course of policy discussions within the cabinet and among health care experts. In particular, changes in Britain's political atmosphere increased the sensivity of politicians and Ministry of Health officials to public opinion and led them to perceive a significant change in public sentiment. The shift in elite perceptions had two major impacts on policy discussions. First, it recast policymakers' assumptions regarding what was practical and propelled the issue of comprehensive and universally available health care to the top of the governmental agenda. Second, policymakers' perception of public preferences and understandings became an integral part of the initial discussion of major health care reform, policy professionals' specification of alternative arrangements for providing hospital and GP care.

Reform as the Policy Objective

With the coalition's formation altering civilian politics, the discussion of health policy underwent a major shift. As indicated by official responses in the cabinet, Parliament, and the Ministry of Health, major health care reform was selected from a large set of conceivable subjects and given a high priority on the governmental agenda. In particular, by October 1942 governmental attention was on reform proposals that significantly widened the coverage of services and population from that previously envisioned. A critical factor in the decision to discuss major reform seriously was the perception of a high level of public interest in and support for extending hospital and GP care to the entire population.

Immediately before and after the war's outset, the scope of policy discussions remained limited, with hospital care the primary focus of attention. The Ministry of Health concentrated on creating the Emergency Hospital Scheme (EHS) to ensure that voluntary and municipal hospitals set aside the necessary beds for air-raid casualties. Wartime events like the establishment of the EHS and the German bombing raids led policymakers to assume that future reform should begin with hospital rather than GP care. The idea of a comprehensive health service was recognized early in the war as a

44. CAB 75/13, HPC (42) 28th, Minutes, 9/22/42.

general (albeit distant) aim, but not as a practical matter for current discussion. Summarizing the ministry's thinking, an official observed: "Ideally, a thorough revision of... the hospital service and the domiciliary medical service should be undertaken simultaneously. It is fairly certain that this will not be practicable and that the hospital service must be tackled first [even though GP care was probably in more "urgent need" of reform]."[45] While wartime events made the formulation of a new hospital policy seem urgent, it was felt that "the GP system,... as regards panel and private practice, will not be radically altered by the time the new hospital policy must operate."[46]

In the immediate period of the war's beginning, policymakers seldom explicitly discussed expanding coverage of the population. In the planning before the war, officials in the Ministry of Health (and Treasury) designed the EHS to be strictly limited to treating air-raid casualties. But with the war's onset, access to EHS was significantly expanded to encompass the entire civilian population. As a ministry official noted only several weeks into the war, "patients are being admitted to [the emergency casualty hospitals]... whose treatment in peace time would be paid for by the rates or by the patients themselves. The Government, therefore, is being made directly responsible for the hospital treatment of the community as a whole."[47] The expanded EHS coverage, though, did not initially influence discussions of future health policy.

Nevertheless, the new policy-making atmosphere, which emerged as the coalition's political infighting intensified, profoundly affected discussions within the Ministry of Health: by October 1942 the issue of comprehensive health reform was accepted by the minister of health and his senior administrators (with some significant support within the cabinet) as the government's policy objective. Increasingly sensitive to public expectations, politicians and bureaucrats accepted the establishment of adequate hospital facilities as a central assumption: "The object of the new policy," Brown explained to a supportive cabinet committee in the fall of 1941, "was to carry through into the peace the standards of hospital service which had been achieved for war purposes."[48] Moreover, as the Beveridge committee

45. MH 77/22, Memo, "Suggestions for a Postwar Hospital Policy," 8/41. Also see MH 80/24, Memo, "Hospital Policy and Regionalization," by J. C. Wrigley, 12/18/40; MH 77/22, Memo, Office committee on postwar hospital policy, by A. Rucker, 2/6/41.

46. MH 77/22, "Suggestions for a Postwar Hospital Policy: Conditions under Which a Policy Must Be Framed," 8/41.

47. MH 80/24, Memo, "Proposed National Hospital Service," from A. S. MacNalty to secretary (G. Chrystal), 9/21/39. Also see MH 80/24, Memo from Alford to secretary (G. Chrystal), 9/29/39; MH 79/311, Memo prepared in the Treasury Department, "Savings and the Means Test," 1/27/40.

48. MH 80/34, Minutes, Lord President's Committee, LP (41) 48th, 10/41.

began its deliberations, ministry officials became concerned with the possibility of considerable public concern about GP care. In early 1942 officials began stressing that the likely "demand for some large-scale alterations" made it "imperative" that "the Government should be prepared with proposals . . . for domiciliary medical services." Indeed, by March 1942 the ministry had already prepared a comprehensive memorandum on the GP service.[49]

In addition to encompassing both hospital and GP care, ministry discussions of future health policy also came to accept 100 percent population coverage as a central principle. The principle of universal coverage was first accepted in connection with postwar hospital policy. By August 1941, ministry officials acknowledged that "public opinion will not . . . be satisfied with less than a scheme under which hospital treatment . . . is available to anyone who needs it."[50] As an outgrowth of this type of concern with public expectations, the cabinet decided—as Brown announced to Parliament—that postwar hospital policy would "ensure that . . . appropriate treatment shall be readily available to every person in need of it."[51]

In contrast to support for expanding access to hospitals, there was strong opposition within the Ministry of Health and the medical profession to making GP care universally available. Even after Beveridge's work became known, ministry officials objected: as one official noted, "I don't believe that either the medical profession or the community want the . . . institution of a free domiciliary service open to all."[52] Instead, officials emphasized lingering public unease with excessive state interference and mistakenly argued that the public would be more receptive to a GP program that encompassed 70–85 percent of the population since "the idea of switching over to a State doctor would be very unpalatable to many people." Within the ministry, objections to universal coverage were reinforced by the BMA's insistence that 10–15 percent of the population be excluded from the GP service to "keep the more lucrative side of the private practice in being."[53]

Nevertheless, as policy discussions and political struggles intensified, by March 1942 senior ministry administrators were increasingly concerned with the strong public support Beveridge's call for a national GP service

49. Government's Actuary (ACT) 1/708, Memo, "Postwar Medical Policy: General Practitioner Service," by J. Maude, 3/42.

50. MH 77/22, "Suggestions for a Postwar Hospital Policy: Conditions under Which a Policy Must Be framed," 8/41.

51. Hansard, Brown's statement in the House of Commons, 10/9/41.

52. MH 80/31, Letter from H. A. de Montmorency to J. Maude, 2/6/42.

53. MH 80/31, Letter from J. Maude to H. A. de Montmorency, 2/9/42; MH 80/31, Letter from H. A. de Montmorency to J. Maude, 2/23/42; MH 80/31, Letter from J. Maude to W. Beveridge, 3/4/42.

seemed likely to enjoy. Officials now began to perceive a shift in public opinion and to assume that the new GP service "must cover the whole population." They concluded that it was no longer appropriate to allow means tests to act as a deterrent; senior administrators began to concede readily that the use of a means test to exclude the 10 percent or so of the population "seems scarcely defensible" and "certainly unpopular."[54] With officials convinced of public support for a universal GP service, the BMA's opposition seemed less significant; by September, administrators declared that "there is no justification for excluding any section of the population from sharing in the proposed [GP] service."[55]

New Administrative Arrangements

Because the government began to accept the objective of GP and hospital care for the entire population, bureaucrats began (under the minister's supervision) to specify alternative administrative arrangements for organizing the state's involvement in and hierarchical control over the new health care system.

Before the coalition's formation, the dscussion of administrative arrangements was limited. At the war's outset, a range of ministry officials agreed that the repercussions on the postwar problems must be taken into account; the EHS was the starting point for future developments.[56] The idea, though, that wartime experiences should precipitate a radical change in the policy of the ministry was rejected by both senior and middle-level administrators because "this was not the moment for so far-reaching a change."[57] Even the prewar discussion of altering administrative arrangements to rationalize and coordinate health services was dismissed: as a former senior official explained, the "theoretical advantages" of unifying municipal and voluntary hospital care did not "outweigh the disadvantages of the difficulties, friction, and expense of working on an untried machine in the time of war." Instead, top civil servants anticipated that administrative arrangements would evolve through the "inevitability of gradualness." Agreeing that "no precipitate action [should] be taken," they discussed incremental adjustments that

54. MH 80/24, Memo, "Beveridge Scheme and Health Services," 3/42; ACT 1/708, Memo, "Postwar Medical Policy: General Practitioner Service," by J. Maude, 3/42.
55. ACT 1/708, Memo, "Medical Practitioner Service," approximately 9/42; MH 80/31, Memo regarding the BMA's Medical Planning Commission, 5/20/42.
56. MH 77/25, Memo, "The EMS as a Starting Point for Future Developments," by A. W. Neville, 1940–41; MH 80/24, Memo from S. F. Wilkinson to George Chrystal, 10/16/39; MH 80/24, Notes of an office meeting, 10/19/39.
57. MH 80/24, Notes of meeting of ministry civil servants, 9/27/39; MH 80/24, Letter from E. R. Forber to George Chrystal, 9/17/39; Memo from S. F. Wilkinson to George Chrystal, 10/16/39.

would achieve "a cautious and safe movement in the direction of normality."[58]

After the coalition's formation, however, and the placement of a comprehensive health service on the governmental agenda, officials began to consider major changes in administrative arrangements; assumptions based on gradual change became increasingly anachronistic. In response to the altered political environment and the minister of health's call for radical reorganization of hospital arrangements, administrators began meeting regularly after December 1940 "to evolve as soon as possible a . . . fairly detailed blue-print" for significant administrative changes.[59]

Initial policy discussions of such changes occurred in a central state whose actual hierarchical organization is often portrayed as weak in comparison to that of continental European countries. But the British state's capacity and, in particular, specialization—which had been enhanced even before the war because of the NHI's development and the Ministry of Health's expert and committed administrative staff—was if anything further strengthened after 1939. In wartime Britain, the state's coordination and funding of the country's economy and social services bolstered its administrative experience and capabilities (Titmuss 1950). This strengthening of the British state's administrative capacity has particular significance for Weberians: future institutional changes should enhance the state's capacity and hierarchical control.

Policymakers began to specify new arrangements for both GP and hospital care. In response to their perception that public opinion had significantly changed, Ministry of Health officials decided by early 1942 to abandon long-held assumptions and to eliminate altogether the NHI's panel system. They no longer viewed this system as a suitable basis for building a new GP service and doubted that the country would stand for its continuation.[60] Policymakers stressed the public's understanding of existing GP care. As one critical policy document explained, "a mere extension of 'panel treatment' would not appeal to the middle classes": its reputation for inferior quality would be resented and "the existence of two classes of patients, panel and private, in itself creates a distinction which tends . . . to lower the repute of the panel service."[61]

58. MH 80/24, Letter from E. R. Forber to George Chrystal, 9/17/39; MH 80/24, Memo, "EHS: Finance"; MH 80/24, Notes of meeting of ministry civil servants, 9/27/39; Memo, "Proposed National Hospital Service," from A. S. MacNalty to secretary (G. Chrystal), 9/21/39.

59. MH 80/24, Notes of meeting among civil servants, 12/7/40; MH 80/24, Memo, "Notes on Hospital Policy," J. Pater, 12/18/40.

60. MH 77/22, Memo to J. Maude, 1/20/41.

61. ACT 1/708, Memo, "Postwar Medical Policy: General Practitioner Service," by J. Maude, March 1942.

To replace the panel system, the ministry's senior officials began specifying new administrative arrangements for GP care. Sensing quite accurately that "public opinion demands more and not less State interference," officials suggested that designing a virtually universal salaried service, and a high quality general medical service in health centers, would command considerable popular appeal. Officials concluded that there would be substantial support for placing the new service under the ultimate control of a minister. Moreover, given public expectations that had evolved from the poor laws, Friendly Societies, and the NHI, top administrators contemplated that GP care would be a free service.[62]

Strong opposition within the health policy network did not deter ministry officials from attempting to create a new GP service. Convinced of public support for the new arrangements, officials simply assumed that "encroachment on the sphere of private practice must invariably increase" and bring with it outcries by doctors over restriction of their private practice.[63] Suggesting in January 1941 what would later become a conviction, an official noted that "it may be that vested interests are too powerful, but I think the kite should be flown."[64] Although the ministry specified new administrative arrangements that would introduce a strong professional element through the formation of a doctor-controlled central board, administrators remained committed to a universal GP service. Concerned, however, that suddenly introducing a new service would create "startling and sometime unwelcome changes in the habits of the great bulk of the population," a senior official suggested that "transitional arrangements" involving "more gradual change would be more practicable."[65] It would take additional changes in the country's political environment before policymakers perceived public demand for the immediate establishment of new administrative arrangements for GP care.

While they discussed significant reorganization of GP care, officials also sought—as the ministry's senior civil servant explained—to "make a com-

62. MH 77/22, "Office Committee on Postwar Hospital Policy: Salaried Medical Service," by J. Pater, approximately 4/41; ACT 1/708, Memo, "Postwar Medical Policy: General Practitioner Service," 9/42; Godber Interview; ACT 1/708, Memo, "Postwar Medical Policy: General Practitioner Service," by J. Maude, 3/42.

63. ACT 1/708, Memo, "Postwar Medical Policy: General Practitioner Service," by J. Maude, 3/42; Act 1/708, Memo, "Postwar Medical Policy: General Practitioner Service," 9/42.

64. MH 77/22, Memo to J. Maude, 1/20/41; MH 77/22, "Office Committee on Postwar Hospital Policy: Salaried Medical Service," by J. Pater, approximately 4/41; MH 77/22, Memo, "Hospital Policy and Regionalization," by J. C. Wrigley, 12/18/40.

65. MH 77/22, "Office Committee on Postwar Hospital Policy: Salaried Medical Service," by J. Pater, approximately 4/41; ACT 1/708, Memo, "Postwar Medical Policy: General Practitioner Service," by J. Maude, 3/42. Also see MH 80/31, Letter from J. Maude to H. A. de Montmorency, 3/4/42; ACT 1/708, Memo, "Postwar Medical Policy: General Practitioner Service," 9/42.

prehensive hospital service available while making all possible use of existing machinery"; authority would continue to be dispersed to private operators and local governments.[66] Officials realized, though, that to provide adequate facilities they had to overcome the public's long-standing attitudes about the difference between voluntary hospitals and local authority (albeit poor-law) hospitals. To challenge the public's perception of these hospitals as representing a two-class system, administrators sought to equalize the treatment and status of all facilities: in the new hospital service "all patients should be on the same footing and ... no distinction [should] be made on the ground of the patient contributing to a savings association, or on any other ground."[67] The critical question, addressed only later, was whether existing administrative arrangements could be used to create a hospital service which the public would understand as a new single-class system.

Policymakers, then, attempted to use the administrative machinery of both voluntary bodies and local authorities: discussions centered on "find[ing] the right relation between the local authorities ... and the voluntary hospitals" without significantly altering either.[68] Based on their (outdated) perception of public attachment to voluntary hospitals, officials decided to use voluntary hospitals, even though they were clearly on the brink of collapse. Emphasizing that the public's attraction to voluntary hospitals would continue to sustain them, a ministry administrator observed that their "roots [go] so deep in the national life that I should not expect [their] immediate break-up even under the pressure of postwar financial conditions."[69] Officials argued that to preserve voluntary hospitals it was necessary to avoid state interference, which would divert public charity to other objects and prompt voluntary contributions to fall off entirely.[70]

Policymakers were also committed to using the existing administrative machinery of local authorities. The discussion of the state's involvement in the new hospital service centered on achieving prewar aims: eliminating inefficiency and coordinating state and nonstate providers. In contrast to

66. MH 80/34, Memorandum regarding a discussion with J. Maude, approximately 5/42.
67. MH 77/22, "Suggestions for a Postwar Hospital Policy: Conditions under Which a Policy Must Be framed," 8/41.
68. Letter from Malcolm MacDonald (minister of health) to W. Goodenough (chair of Nuffield Provincial Hospitals Trust), 1/6/41, quoted in MH 77/22, Memo to Lord President's Committee, LP (41) 167, "Postwar Hospital Policy," 10/14/41.
69. MH 77/22, Memo, Office committee on postwar hospital policy, by H. A. de Montmorency, 2/12/41.
70. MH 80/24, Memo, "Public Medical Service," sent to the Beveridge committee, 8/13/42; MH 77/22, "Suggestions for a Postwar Hospital Policy: Conditions under Which a Policy Must Be Framed," 8/41; MH 80/24, Letter from E. J. Maude to E. R. Forber, 10/26/39; MH 80/24, Notes of a meeting of ministry civil servants, 9/27/39; MH 80/24, Memo, "Proposed National Hospital Service," from A. S. MacNalty to secretary (G. Chrystal), 9/21/39; MH 77/22, Memo, "Hospital Policy and Regionalization," by J. C. Wrigley, 12/18/40.

prewar deliberations, however, wartime discussions sought significant administrative changes, that would expand the state's role and strengthen its hierarchical control over hospital care: the previous "informal and unorganized partnership between local authorities and voluntary hospitals should be ... put on a more regular footing."[71] Thus, from the war's outset, officials were attracted to the organizational advantage of strengthening the central ministry's role to create a more firmly ordered system of authority. As one official explained, "it is only in a national service that the fullest coordination is possible."[72]

But policymakers submerged their interest in enhancing the state's hierarchical capacity because of their perception of public attitudes: the public's unfamiliarity with central control led officials to "assume reluctantly that this solution must be ruled out."[73] Instead, it was agreed within the ministry that the only practical alternative for state involvement in hospital care was through highly decentralized local authorities, which were seen as the objects of strong public attachment. Committed to "preserv[ing] a wide popular interest in the running of these services," one official insisted that "*it is more important that the general body of people should be interested in these services ... than they should be provided from above with a mechanically perfect organization ... in which they can take no interest.*"[74] Hospitals, then, would be administered by local authorities in collaboration with voluntary hospitals.

During the 1930s and 1940s, the upheaval and destruction of war created problems in all aspects of British society; it was not possible for elites and the mass public to recognize and consider seriously each of the exceptionally large number of challenges. The issue of health care was privileged; it was recognized as an important problem not only by the general public but also by politicians and specialists.

Weberians expect the capacity of existing British institutions to be the primary focus and determinant of elite decisions to select an issue and specify new alternatives. The emergence of the health issue in Britain, though, suggests that the Weberian argument for agenda setting is misspecified and contradicted by important developments. The primary focus and determinant of agenda setting was policymakers' perception of public opinion rather than administrative inability to meet developmental imperatives. Politicians

71. MH 77/22, "Suggestions for a Postwar Hospital Policy: Conditions under Which a Policy Must Be Framed," 8/41.

72. MH 80/24, Memo, "Postwar Hospital Policy: Papers A and B," approximately 7/20/42.

73. MH 80/24, Memo, "Postwar Hospital Policy: Papers A and B," approximately 7/20/42.

74. MH 77/22, Memo, "Hospital Policy and Regionalization," by J. C. Wrigley, 12/18/40.

and bureaucrats defined the health problem as originating in changing public views, and they selected it for serious attention because of strong public interest in and support for postwar reconstruction, specifically for major health reform. The selection of comprehensive and universally available health service was a response to popular hostility toward existing hospital and GP care, and the continued use of means tests to restrict coverage. Moreover, the decisions to abandon the panel system and expand state involvement in hospital care reflected popular dissatisfaction with existing arrangements. The government's agenda corresponded to the public's agenda: policymakers not only selected the popular health issue but also specified policy in a direction that was congruent, in important respects, with public preferences and understandings.

The temporal sequence of government decisions reinforces the argument that policymakers' perception of public opinion drove agenda setting: it was largely *after* this new perception that policy changed. Before the coalition's formation, major health reform was rejected as "impractical" in favor of tinkering with existing arrangements. But the political conflict that came with the coalition significantly altered policymakers' perception of public opinion; in the new political atmosphere, vote-seeking politicians and turf-conscious bureaucrats now found it now "practical politics" to propose "drastic reconstruction." Only after political struggles had changed policymakers' perception of public opinion did they select major health reform and begin specifying comprehensive alternatives. Contrary to Weberians expectations, policy change did not stem from a reassessment of existing administrative capacity; rather, decisions resulted from a new and more conclusive assessment of public preferences and enduring understandings.

In certain respects, the evidence that Weberians misspecify the causal argument for agenda setting could be interpreted as ambiguous. For instance, the British state's moderately strong administrative capacity could reasonably be interpreted as consistent with the coalition's decision to ultimately create greater hierarchical control over GP care. But policymakers put these plans on hold out of concern for the "habits of the great bulk of the population." Moreover, in the area of hospital care, the moderately strong capacity of existing institutions and policymakers' confidence in their capacity to create a national service coincided with decisions to continue low hierarchical control. Bureaucrats (under the watchful eye of politicians) pointed to what they perceived to be public attraction to local authorities and voluntary hospitals; they were simply more concerned with preserving a wide popular interest in health services than with providing a new program "from above with a mechanically perfect organization" in which the public would take no interest.

Government decisions, however, were not merely an epiphenomenon of public preferences and understandings; policymakers were unresponsive to several important trends in public opinion. Politicians and bureaucrats were unwilling to move beyond transitional arrangements to respond to the public's widespread hostility toward the panel system and its support for a greater state role in GP care. Moreover, officials did not seem to appreciate fully the strong popular interest in state ownership and control of all hospitals; instead, they favored retaining voluntary hospitals, at least in the short term. The unresponsiveness of Ministry of Health and cabinet to these public attitudes was reflected by Minister Brown's rejection in Parliament of the proposition that "the maintenance of voluntary hospitals . . . by public funds and flag-days is becoming increasingly repugnant to the conscience of the public."[75] It would take a further shift in the strategic calculations of policymakers before the specification of new administrative arrangements would become more responsive to public opinion.

75. Hansard, question by Aneurin Bevan following Brown's statement in the House of Commons, 10/9/41.

5 | United States, 1950s–1960: Medicare and Presidential Campaigning

Between the early 1950s and the conclusion of the 1960 presidential campaign, major health care reform moved from the margins of American policy discussions to the top of the governmental agenda. Although important policy innovations occurred before and outside legislative debates, congressional deliberations organized the bargaining among politicians, interest groups, and policy specialists. This policy network's organized discussions were affected by Congress's emphasis both on voting (in committee and on the floor) and on committee deliberations. In Medicare's case, these deliberations involved finance committees in the Senate and, especially, the House and its Ways and Means Committee. Whether inside or outside Congress, politicians' and specialists' perceptions of public opinion were the primary focus and determinant of government decisions to address the health issue and to begin specifying new arrangements.

As the Eisenhower presidency wound down, policymakers began to recognize the problem in health care, arguing that it originated in the culmination of historic changes in public understandings and preferences. Although a small group of policy specialists began specifying the new Medicare approach to health reform in the early 1950s, prominent politicians neglected or altogether ignored the issue for much of the decade. The 1960 presidential campaign, though, altered the country's political environment: John Kennedy's sensitivity to public opinion and use of Louis Harris polls to select health care reform for his campaign recast the calculations of policy professionals and other politicians. By November 1960, a new atmosphere emerged in which policymakers became more sensitive to public attitudes and more willing to pursue health care reform.

INITIAL POLICY DISCUSSIONS

Problems in American health care had been a prominent concern since at least the turn of the century. But in the period between the early 1950s and the Ways and Means Committee's hearings in 1958, the health policy network began to discuss formally whether the aged could finance their hospital treatment.[1] Ways and Means' initial hearings on the Medicare approach, which had been proposed by committee member Aime Forand, represented the first official recognition of what many had been emphasizing since the early 1950s—the problem in health care for the elderly. The committee's initial hearings also represented the first formal consideration of the Medicare approach, which had begun to be specified in the early 1950s by a small group of specialists. This group of reformers significantly scaled back Truman's comprehensive national health insurance schemes and designed Medicare as an extension of Social Security's financing system. New evidence as well as existing research suggests that the beginning of formal recognition and discussion of health care was tied to policymakers' perception of public opinion (Marmor 1973; see also Harris 1966; David 1985).

The Problem

After the defeat of Truman's proposals, the health care issue quickly slid off the governmental agenda. With even the Democratic presidential candidate in 1952 describing the health insurance issue as obsolete, serious discussion of the topic quickly faded from governmental deliberations for much of the Eisenhower presidency (Poen 1979, 202–7). The first formal discussion of the issue occurred during Ways and Means' June 1958 hearings, which directed the policy network's attention to the problem facing the sick elderly. Even though disagreement and conflict were the most visible features of the hearings, the collection and diffusion of information on the elderly's health care predicament helped build agreement among governmental and nongovernmental officials: a problem clearly existed, and it stemmed from changing public attitudes.

By the 1950s, policymakers began to become aware of a disjuncture between existing administrative arrangements and changing public understandings of health care. Although Americans historically had feared and resented orthodox medicine, by the late 1930s growing segments of the

1. My analysis of Medicare emphasizes the Ways and Means Committee because of its institutional authority in matters of taxation and its overall political influence. The Senate and its Finance Committee were not as central. For a detailed discussion of the Senate's constraints and occasional interference with the Ways and Means deliberations, see David 1985 and Harris 1966.

mass public became attracted to it, especially to its sophisticated hospital treatment. Summarizing for Ways and Means the trend of rising demand for hospitalization, an AHA representative pointed to the "tendency not only for persons to seek more hospital service, but for them to seek more complicated hospital services."[2]

The existing arrangements for financing hospital treatment were inadequate to meet the expectations of those entering retirement and old age. Since the 1930s, the rapid growth of nonstate insurance schemes to finance the greater demand for hospital treatment had been oriented to the employed. After retirement, however, many elderly who had previously enjoyed middle-class incomes began to find that nonstate arrangements for financing their care either had lapsed or were too expensive.[3] Stressing the limits of voluntary insurance in meeting the elderly's expectations of sophisticated treatment for their illnesses, the AHA representative found the existing financing arrangements inadequate: "the aged need more care than any other group in the population and are largely less able to finance it."[4] Precisely in order to address this disjuncture between existing administrative arrangements and public opinion, Forand targeted his bill to the bulk of the elderly who were neither wealthy nor indigent and eligible for charity.[5]

Summarizing their analyses over the previous decade, policy specialists identified two significant problems, which had resulted from the inadequacy of existing financial arrangements for meeting the elderly's expectations of hospital care. First, many retired people, who had earned middle-class incomes during their working years, were being forced into indigence, having to rely on the dreaded poor-law arrangements. Public welfare and hospital officials from around the country testified that, although most elderly were covered by health insurance during their working years, their retirement and the onset of sickness forced many to rely on public assistance: the AHA representative found that ill-health had become a major cause of destitution among the aged. Several witnesses reported that the elderly often forestalled needed medical treatment as they struggled to "cling to their waning independence on near-starvation incomes and refuse to apply for public assistance."[6]

2. Testimony by Dr. James Dixon (Commissioner's Department of Public Health, Philadelphia, and Chair of the AHA Committee on the Health Needs of the Aged), U.S. Congress, House, Ways and Means Committee, 1958, pp. 867.

3. Both nonprofit (e.g., Blue Cross) and for-profit insurers adjusted their rates downward to attract the low-risk groups and charged higher rates to the undesirable high-risk groups such as the aged.

4. Testimony by Dr. James Dixon, U.S. Congress, House, Ways and Means Committee, 1958, pp. 857–59.

5. Statement by Aime Forand, U.S. Congress, House, Ways and Means Committee, 1958, pp. 12–13, 573.

6. Quoted in Harris 1966, 80. Also see testimony by Raymond Hilliard (Director, Chi-

Second, and more pressing from policymakers' perspectives, the inadequacy of existing financing arrangements was creating a major problem for hospitals, which felt compelled to provide free treatment to the sick elderly. Typical of the difficulties faced by many hospitals, Massachusetts General reported that the major cause of its significant indebtedness was the treatment of social security recipients. As a result, the AHA representative argued that, even with the cooperation of voluntary insurance schemes during a period of prosperity, practically all hospitals were facing dire financial difficulties.[7]

In their testimony to Ways and Means, then, policy experts argued that the source of the health care problem, which had emerged by the 1950s, was changing public opinion: the existing financing arrangements were increasingly incapable of meeting the new level of demand for hospital care. Indeed, the bulwark of the resistance to government health insurance schemes, the AMA, felt compelled to abandon its previous position and acknowledge the inadequacies of existing arrangements; it was now "acutely aware of the existence of medical care problems among the aged."[8] Thus, even while the Ways and Means Committee overwhelmingly opposed the Medicare bill in June 1958 and witnesses questioned the extent of the elderly's difficulties, an influential group of politicians had joined policy professionals in recognizing that the gap between public expectations and medical financing arrangements had created a major problem.

The Birth of Incrementalism

The 1958 hearings constituted the first formal consideration of the new Medicare approach. Although the small group of reformers who had designed the new Medicare approach earlier in the decade could not control Congress, it did structure congressionel choices by generating a broad alternative framework. In designing the Medicare approach, reformers sought to circumvent the political firestorms that had consumed previous government health insurance proposals: they assumed that maximizing political support depended on incorporating public opinion into the formulation of policy.

---

cago's Public Welfare Department), U.S. Congress, House, Ways and Means Committee, 1958, pp. 333–34; Dr. Frank Furstenberg (Member, Board of Directors, Council of Jewish Federations), and Dr. James Dixon, U.S. Congress House, Ways and Means Committee, 1958, pp. 857, 1069;

7. Testimony by Dr. Allan Butler (Professor of Pediatrics, Harvard Medical School, and Vice Chair, Physicians Forum), U.S. Congress, House, Ways and Means Committee, 1958, p. 940; Testimony by Dr. James Dixon, U.S. Congress, House, Ways and Means Committee, 1958, pp. 857–65.

8. Testimony by Leonard Larson (Chair, Board of Trustees, AMA), U.S. Congress, House, Ways and Means Committee, 1958, p. 889.

Interviews with reformers themselves suggest that they traced the repeated failure of health insurance proposals since the early 1900s to a persistent insensitivity to public opinion.[9] Leading architects of the Medicare proposal such as Wilbur Cohen began with the assumption that in the past the positions of such interest groups as the AMA were influential because they drew on the public's enduring uneasiness with excessive state interference. The "overarching" factor, Cohen insisted, in the AMA's successful effort to "muster the negative" campaign against health insurance proposals was that it "buil[t] upon the innate frontier, capitalistic...local...atmosphere in which socialized anything was a big bogeyman."[10] The influence of interest groups, Cohen and others concluded, was not a monolithic barrier but varied according to how well it was rooted in public understandings and preferences. The key, then, to countering fierce opposition was to carefully redirect health reform to reflect the enduring meanings Americans associated with health care and the state.

Acknowledging the peculiar character of Americans' understanding of health care and the state's involvement in social welfare, the reformers' Medicare proposal scaled back Truman's comprehensive insurance scheme in two ways. First, health services covered by the new program would be largely limited to hospital care. The incentives to exclude the services of doctors were substantial: the AMA fiercely opposed interference with medical practitioners and the public lacked a strong expectation of GP provisions (as arose in Britain from the Friendly Societies and the panel system). Thus, Cohen publicly objected when Forand expanded the coverage of his bill to include the surgical procedures of doctors.[11] As Marmor convincingly argues, reformers chose to restrict the Medicare proposal to financing hospital care because such costs were "a 'problem' less disputable than the one to which the Truman plans had been addressed" (1973, 17).

Second, reformers decided to limit state involvement to existing arrangements that already enjoyed strong favorable public support. Cohen recalled that he was especially influenced by a February 1949 poll that indicated that the AMA's slogan for opposing any form of state involvement in health care—"socialized medicine"—was not widely understood by the public. For Cohen, *Americans' dread of government did not represent an unchanging and insurmountable obstacle to all forms of state involvement.* Rather, he explained, the reformer's task was to identify state arrangements that enjoyed

9. Interview with Wilbur Cohen by L. R. Jacobs, 4/1/87 (hereafter, Cohen Interview); LBJ Library, Interview with Wilbur Cohen by David McComb, 12/8/68; and Interview with Robert Ball by David McComb, 11/5/68; Poen 1979, 189–207.
10. Cohen Interview.
11. Testimony by Wilbur Cohen (representative of the American Public Welfare Association), U.S. Congress, House, Ways and Means Committee, 1959, pp. 343–45.

public support; once this was accomplished, "sooner or later we were going to win." Based on his sense of American culture and his review of existing polling data, Cohen concluded that, although the elderly tended to favor a smaller government role, they made an exception in the area of financing medical care costs.[12] Cohen and other reformers looked specifically to the Social Security system, which was widely recognized by the 1950s as enjoying universal support: as Cohen explained, "the reason we latched... Medicare [onto]... Social Security is because we knew people were very favorable to Social Security."[13] For the nonpoor, who were repulsed by poor-law arrangements, Social Security's reliance on contributions by beneficiaries during their working years was enormously appealing, giving its benefits "a different character [that]... separates it entirely from... [an] assistance or a welfare approach."[14]

Reformers' perception of American culture and their recognition of its political importance in deflecting opposition led them to restrict their Medicare proposal in two ways. First, they limited the central state's role to financing health care based on Social Security's insurance mechanism; the idea of significantly enhancing the state's specialization and hierarchical control was floated but not seriously considered. Second, they limited Medicare's coverage to Social Security beneficiaries; the British principle of 100 percent coverage did not seem to fit American understandings of social welfare. Reformers' preoccupation with the popularly accepted Social Security arrangements convinced them to "live with this gap between the problem posed and the remedy offered" (Marmor 1973, 20).

In Britain, policymakers also drew on widespread public understandings, which had gradually evolved from social interactions with poor-law institutions and with Friendly Societies and NHI; it seemed reasonable (if not always politic) to recommend state provision of comprehensive services to the entire population. In the United States, though, reformers designed proposals tailored to Americans' comparative unfamiliarity with either state involvement in social welfare or comprehensive medical treatment. The irony in America is that to mirror popularly accepted arrangements reformers often behaved as conservatives; the advocates of change persistently opposed efforts to liberalize the Medicare proposal to include more health services, wider coverage of the population, and a larger state role. In the hope of reversing the previous pattern of defeat, policymakers designed Medicare to be a cautious incremental reform: reformers identified a virtually indisputable problem—the inadequacy of existing financial arrange-

---

12. Cohen et al. 1960; Cohen Interview.
13. Cohen Interview.
14. LBJ Library, Interview with Robert Ball by David McComb, 11/5/68.

ments to pay for the elderly's hospital care—and proposed limited solutions rooted in public understandings and preferences.

Even though a small group of policy professionals had begun to outline a new approach to health care reform, by 1958 politicians were not prepared to either assign a top priority to the issue or devote serious attention to its details. With the health insurance issue slipping off the governmental agenda following Truman's departure, the Medicare proposal was met with indifference among most members of Congress, who assumed that it would share the same fate as previous schemes. This indifference toward the health insurance issue was reflected by Ways and Means chairman Wilbur Mills's reluctance in 1958 even to hold hearings.

In the absence of visible, strong public interest in the Medicare proposal, most members of Congress had little reason to challenge opposition claims that state involvement in financing hospital care for the aged was at odds with Americans' enduring beliefs. Basing their arguments on "ethical grounds," rather than on their financial or organizational interests, opponents of the Medicare plan argued in the 1958 hearings that the proposed expansion of the state was un-American and a harbinger of communism.[15] Thus, even after the 1958 hearings on Forand's Medicare proposal, when public interest did begin to awaken, health insurance remained a marginal issue in governmental deliberations; neither the executive branch nor legislature accorded importance to it. Forand himself agreed with Mills's assessment that the time was not right even to attempt to vote the bill out of committee.[16]

THE SHIFTING STRATEGIC UNIVERSE, 1959–1960

As in Britain following the coalition government's formation, American political struggles between 1959 and the 1960 presidential election prompted politicians and policy specialists to devote serious attention to health reform. Because of the exceptional prominence of American presidential candidates, Kennedy's decision to identify himself with what he perceived to be a popular issue—health reform for the aged—set off a political chain reaction, with Nixon and other political actors subsequently feeling compelled to devote significant attention to it. The result was a new policy-making atmosphere in which politicians and specialists became more

15. Testimony by Representative Walter Judd (appeared with the AMA delegation) and Frank Krusen (AMA representative), U.S. Congress, House, Ways and Means Committee, 1958, pp. 891, 905–6.

16. Interview with Wilbur Mills by L. R. Jacobs, 6/18/87 (herafter, Mills Interview); interview with Wilbur Mills by Charles T. Morrissey, 4/5/79, 6/7/79, Former Members of Congress, Inc.; Harris 1966, 73.

sensitive to public opinion and more willing to reform financing arrangements for the elderly's health care. By November 1960 major health reform no longer seemed impractical: a wide spectrum of policymakers agreed that it was necessary.

Public Opinion

Interpreted within the context of enduring public understandings, the Harris polls conducted for Kennedy's primary and general election campaigns provide new and better data for analyzing the effect of public preferences on policy making. Past research has presumed that public preferences found their way into the policy-making process (e.g., Page and Shapiro 1983); the Harris polls were actually assembled and used by a key politician. Moreover, the Harris poll results, which concentrated on twenty-four states (three-quarters of them surveyed at least twice), offer data for a period in which opinion surveys were infrequent (Schiltz 1970).[17] In particular, these polls measured voter preferences toward both candidates and issues, including medical care for the aged.[18]

The Harris data revealed that the general election campaign was very close. Over the course of the campaign, Kennedy had widened his initial lead or reversed early Nixon leads in the pivotal states of California and New York, as well as in Illinois, Ohio, Pennsylvania, and Texas. But it was clear from the outset of campaigning in August that it was going to be a close finish: in ten of the last surveys before election day, the candidates were reported to be within four percentage points of each other. Moreover, the Harris polls revealed that by November Nixon maintained leads in five of twenty-four races which the Kennedy campaign had targeted.[19]

The Harris polls indicated that in general old-age problems emerged as a salient issue. Of the approximately dozen major issue areas repeatedly explored, old-age problems were one of the five most frequently mentioned issues in 38 of 46 polls.[20] Moreover, the medical care issue was mentioned

17. For more detail on the Harris polls, see Jacobs 1990.

18. The public's policy preferences were elicited by the following type of open-ended question: "Now, what do you feel are the two or three biggest problems facing people like yourself that you feel the *national* government should do something about in the next four years? Any others?" Harris generally organized his reports on public preferences into seven major issue areas: war and peace, taxes and spending, economic bite, old-age problems, education, civil rights, and farm problems. Concerns about social security and medical care for the aged were listed as old-age problems.

19. The five states in which Kennedy trailed (Maine, Oregon, Virginia, South Carolina, and South Dakota) did not include any of the pivotal large states, although in a close race they were seen as important enough to warrant the commissioning of polls.

20. War and peace was listed as the top issue in the great majority of the 46 polls. Old-

as the top concern among old-age problems in a third of these polls and, overall, emerged in the Harris surveys as among the top eight most important issues.[21] Of the domestic and foreign policy issues that were consistently of concern to respondents during the entire campaign, only five other issues were ranked as high as medical care for the elderly.[22]

The selection of health care for the general, nongovernmental agenda is indicated not only by the evidence of public preferences but also by reports in the mass media. In particular, a review of articles published in the *New York Times* indicates that the health issue attracted more coverage than other prominent domestic policy matters.[23]

According to the Harris polls, the public not only cited the elderly's medical care as a salient issue but also backed Kennedy's position of supporting a change in policy to provide health insurance for the aged.[24] At times by wide margins, survey respondents preferred the policy direction advocated by Kennedy over Nixon's position of avoiding a major change: in seven polls, they preferred Kennedy's position on the direction of future policy to Nixon's by at least ten percentage points. In 18 of the remaining 39 polls, Kennedy's position on the medical care issue was favored by at least three percentage points; in 17 of the 39, the candidates were tied or the difference between them was two percentage points or less. Thus, in the 27 polls in which there was a difference of at least three points on the candidates' positions, Kennedy held leads in 25. Summarizing his polls in California and other states, Harris

age problems alternated with tax and spending, economic bite, and education as areas of top concern to voters. Of the eight polls in which old-age problems were not listed among the top five issues of concern, seven were conducted in the South, where civil rights and states' rights were especially salient.

21. Some of the research on Harris's polling data and Kennedy's policy positions discussed in this chapter is based on Jacobs and Shapiro's (1991) quantitative analysis. Evidence on the health issue's overall ranking was based on the percentage of respondents in each state poll that identified the issue as important; each issue's ranking was then averaged across the different state polls conducted during that month.

22. The five issues that were persistently ranked as high as medical care during the general election were rebuilding American prestige, the high cost of living, creating more and better schools, raising social security, and balancing the budget.

23. The index to the *New York Times* lists 275 references in articles and editorials to medical assistance or health insurance for the years 1959 and 1960. For the same period, there are 109 references to education and related federal policy and 106 references to federal aid for educational programs.

24. The Harris polls do not establish that respondents who supported "medical care for the aged" specifically favored Kennedy's proposed approach—financing the elderly's care through the Social Security insurance mechanism. But given Kennedy's highly visible identification with Medicare proposals and the Republican's opposition to a new approach, the public concern identified in these polls can reasonably be interpreted as reflecting support for a significant change in policy toward helping the aged. Indeed, Kennedy aides and Harris regularly interpreted respondents' support for "helping the aged" and providing "medical care for the aged" as backing for the Medicare approach of building on the Social Security system.

observed that medical care for the aged was an issue of prime importance across the country.[25] During the final two weeks of the campaign, the medical care issue received its highest average ranking in Harris surveys (Jacobs and Shapiro 1991). Even though the issue slipped slightly in some states, Harris reported in his last California poll that the candidate's position ranked high and was continuing to work for Kennedy.[26]

The public's preference for a new policy direction reflected a widening acceptance of state involvement in social welfare. A majority of respondents in a series of published opinion surveys between the mid-1930s and the 1960s favored maintaining or increasing government expenditures for poor relief (Schiltz 1970, 151–52). Survey results echoed the socially shared meanings that had become associated with government social welfare provisions: given the stigma associated with welfare, an extensive review of opinion surveys concluded that social insurance programs "are more warmly supported by the American public than programs that are or look like 'the dole'." The new meaning of state provisions, which was encouraged by Social Security's establishment, was confirmed by repeated poll findings that the American public was extraordinarily enthusiastic about social insurance programs (Schiltz 1970, 177–79).

In short, Harris's polling reports for the Kennedy campaign indicated that the race was very close and that problems associated with old age and in particular medical care were highly salient. Public support for a change in the current direction of health policy was bolstered by Americans' widening acceptance of the legitimacy of state provisions, especially when based on Social Security's insurance principles.

Political Struggles

As the focus of national public attention and media coverage, the presidential candidates for the Democratic and Republican parties can dominate agenda setting like no other single candidate for government office. The standard interpretation of the 1960 presidential campaign is that the close competition for independent "floating voters" produced an issue-free campaign centered on the public's image of the candidates' personalities and leadership qualities (Erikson and Luttbeg 1973; Page 1978). But, rather than emphasizing image to the exclusion of issues, the Kennedy camp in particular saw the two as interconnected: policy issues were viewed as a strategic campaign tool with which to influence the public's evaluation of

25. JFK Library, R. F. Kennedy Papers, Pre-Administration, Political, Box 43, "A Study of Presidential Election in California," by Louis Harris and Associates, Inc., 9/60.
26. JFK Library, R. F. Kennedy, Papers, Pre-Administration, Political, Box 43, "A Study of Presidential Election in California, Wave III," by Louis Harris and Associates, Inc., 10/31/60.

Kennedy's image. During its bid to win the nomination and then the general election, the Kennedy campaign faced a large pool of policy issues to choose from; it selected only a few issues based on public preferences. The campaign's responsiveness to public opinion in selecting issues, however, was used to mold an image of Kennedy that would be appealing to voters. The campaign, then, combined attempts to respond to and to direct public opinion; but its relation to voters was driven by public sentiment—popular issues were selected to "prime" or adjust the standards by which the public perceived and evaluated the candidate (Iyengar and Kinder 1987).

The Kennedy campaign's use of popular policy areas to widen the candidate's appeal became an important link between public support for a major change in health care policy and policymakers' selection of the health issue for sustained attention. Kennedy's selection of health care as one of the few domestic issues he repeatedly emphasized prompted other politicians—concerned to either bolster or neutralize Kennedy's strategy—to address the issue too.

Soon after the 1956 election, Kennedy faced the question, what am I going to be for? By the time the campaign gathered steam in 1959, his aides viewed Kennedy's identification with certain issues as a strategic campaign tool to adjust "the so-called Kennedy image."[27] Out of concern that the candidate was seen as too slick and lacking depth, an aide in 1959 suggested that a "Kennedy-identified program" should address in "clear and unmistakable terms" the "prevailing doubt . . . that Kennedy is a bonafide liberal" and "enable people to be for something [and someone] that excites their imagination."[28] Kennedy's aides also became concerned with his image immediately after the presidential conventions, when they agreed that the campaign had reached its low point. In response, the eminent historian and campaign adviser Arthur Schlesinger, Jr., suggested that "the present lethargy of the campaign" be reversed by "giv[ing] the enthusiasts something to believe in"; "once the issue-minded Democrats catch fire, then the campaign will gather steam."[29]

To charge the party faithful with "crusading urgency," campaign officials decided to mold a "move-ahead image" of a compassionate candidate who favored change—an image that would appeal to both the Democratic party's

27. JFK Library, R. F. Kennedy Papers, Pre-Administration, Political, Box 39, Memo, "Some Modest Realignments in the Kennedy Image," by J. Miller, 10/20/59. Also see Cohen Interview; LBJ Library, Interview with Cohen by David McComb, 12/8/68.

28. JFK Library, R. F. Kennedy Papers, Pre-Administration, Political, Box 39, Memo, "Some Modest Realignments in the Kennedy Image," by J. Miller, 10/20/59.

29. JFK Library, POF, Box 32, Special Correspondence, Letters to J. F. Kennedy from A. Schlesinger, 8/26/60 and 8/30/60. Also see R. F. Kennedy Papers, Pre-Administration, Political, Box 43, "Memorandum on the Last Nine Days of Campaigning," marked "Confidential" (undated).

liberal core and the general public. After eight years of a conservative president and Republican "do-nothingism," Kennedy aides suggested that backing popular issues could project an image of favoring new and dynamic approaches to the country's problems. Thus, in the final phase of the campaign, Harris pressed Kennedy to "go on the offensive" to press his "basic theme on all the issues: to get America on the move at home and abroad."[30]

Because they viewed issues as a campaign tool Kennedy officials carefully selected policy areas and proposals. Two criteria shaped these decisions, public preferences and the significance of these preferences for candidate image. The importance of strong, favorable public attitudes toward the campaign's selection of issues led Wilbur Cohen—the tireless reform advocate—to anchor his pitch to Kennedy for choosing Medicare in polling data. Cohen assembled recent poll results in order to tell "Kennedy and his people: this proves ... we've got public opinion."[31] Harris stressed in virtually every polling report during the general election campaign the strong public preference for the Kennedy medical care position, which he identified as one of the "sharpest cutting edge[s]" between the candidates. "There is no situation, no local or national speech," Harris argued, "in which the medical care issue should be ignored."[32] These poll findings of strong public preferences were confirmed by contacts with voters beginning in 1959: one campaign official recalled that Kennedy "would comment that of all the issues on which he campaigned ... the one that constantly provoked the most interest ... was the Forand bill."[33] Kennedy was reportedly impressed by this public interest and support in 1959 and 1960, and his advisers and campaign officials confirmed his reading of voter concerns.[34]

Indeed, quantitative analysis indicates an impressive and systematic relationship between the Harris survey results and Kennedy's policy stances (as evident in the four televised debates and the *New York Times* daily coverage). After allowing for a one-week or one-month lag between Harris poll reports and Kennedy's position taking on 124 issues raised during the

---

30. JFK Library, R. F. Kennedy Papers, Pre-Administration, Political, Box 45, "An Analysis of the Third Kennedy-Nixon Debate," by Louis Harris and Associates, Inc., 10/19/60.

31. Interview with Wilbur Cohen by LRJ, 4/1/87.

32. JFK Library, R. F. Kennedy Papers, Pre-Administration, Political, Box 43, "A Study of Presidential Election in California," by Louis Harris and Associates, Inc., 9/60, and Box 44, "A Report on the Presidential Election in Maine," by Louis Harris and Associates, Inc., 11/5/60.

33. The Oral History Collection, Columbia University, interview with Ivan Nestingen by Peter Corning, 1966 (hereafter, Nestingen Interview).

34. Nestingen Interview. Also see JFK Library, Interview with Akers, by William Moss, 7/17/71, and Interview with Love by William Young, 7/14/64; R. F. Kennedy Papers, Pre-Administration, Political, Box 25, Letter to R. F. Kennedy from Abraham Ribicoff, 10/15/60, and Box 43, "Memorandum on the Last Nine Days of Campaigning," marked "Confidential" (undated).

general election campaign, Jacobs and Shapiro (1991) found that Kennedy's stances were consistent not only with the issues identified by the public but also with the public's preferred direction for policy.

The Kennedy campaign viewed popular policy issues as a political resource for directing the public; Kennedy responded to the public's preferences in order to influence the standards by which voters evaluated candidates. The strong public support for Kennedy's position on the medical care issue was viewed as a means to project the candidate's "move-ahead image."[35] In particular, it was "through the issues" and especially by "hammer[ing] home" the medical care issue that the campaign attempted to contrast Kennedy's "caring" and willingness to offer new approaches to Nixon's cold "competence" and "drift and inaction."[36] Obviously, medical care would have special meaning for liberals and the aged (with whom, according to Harris, the Democrats stood poorly); but Kennedy aides also saw the issue as a way to shape Kennedy's image for many voters other than the elderly.[37]

Convinced of Medicare's strategic importance, the Kennedy campaign struggled to identify their candidate visibly with the health issue. Kennedy formally staked out his position favoring health insurance for the elderly by sponsoring legislation in the Senate during the spring and fall of 1960. The campaign attempted to publicize Kennedy's position through television advertisements as well as personal appearances including his debates with Nixon; it also used policy conferences by Kennedy's supporters to elaborate his position.[38] Of all the 124 domestic and foreign policy issues raised during the general election campaign, medical care for the elderly—according to the *New York Times* daily coverage of Kennedy's position—was in a select group of twelve policies that the candidate most frequently identified (Jacobs and Shapiro 1991).

Whereas the *Times* coverage may have picked up positions intended for specific audiences, the Nixon-Kennedy debates' national viewership pre-

35. JFK Library, R. F. Kennedy Papers, Pre-Administration, Political, Box 43, "Memorandum on the Last Nine Days of Campaigning," marked "Confidential" (undated).

36. JFK Library, R. F. Kennedy Papers, Pre-Administration, Political, Box 45, "A Study of Presidential Election in Ohio, Wave I," by Louis Harris and Associates, Inc., 9/6/60; Box 36, "Memorandum on the First Kennedy-Nixon Debate on Domestic Issues," 9/22/60; and Box 43, "A Study of Presidential Election in California, Wave III," by Louis Harris and Associates, Inc., 10/31/60.

37. JFK Library, R. F. Kennedy Papers, Pre-Administration, Political, Box 43, "A Study of Presidential Election in Florida," by Louis Harris and Associates, Inc., 9/13/60; Box 44, "A Study of Presidential Election in Maryland, Wave I," by Louis Harris and Associates, Inc., 9/23/60; Box 45, "A Survey of the Presidential Election in South Dakota," by Louis Harris and Associates, Inc., 9/19/60; and Box 48, Memo, "Simulatics, Report No. 2," 8/25/60.

38. JFK Library, R. F. Kennedy Papers, Pre-Administration, Politics, Box 39, Memo to R. F. Kennedy from Robert Wallace, August 1960, and Box 46, Memo to campaign coordinators from Steve Smith, 10/19/60.

sented the best medium for reaching a broad audience. Indeed, Kennedy and his advisers carefully prepared for the debates by identifying the most effective issues; Harris used his polls to select medical care as the first among ten leading domestic issues.[39] It was precisely during the televised debates that the health issue was elevated from one among a select group of a dozen policies to the top of Kennedy's domestic agenda. No domestic issue either received as much of Kennedy's time (with the exception of the recession) or was cited more frequently by the candidate (Jacobs and Shapiro 1991).

After the first debate, Harris reported to Kennedy that medical care had "become a major and enormously important question in this election."[40] The campaign's use of this popular issue raised an important strategic concern—protecting Kennedy's identification with a popular issue from Nixon's efforts (through his statements and Eisenhower's policies) to "fuzz up" the differences, as Clark Clifford (the prominent Democrate Party operative) put it.[41] Alarmed at Nixon's attempt to create the illusion of similarity between the candidates' positions, Kennedy aides repeatedly urged their candidate to emphasize the "documented" Republican record of "hav[ing] said 'no' to helping older citizens."[42] To resist Nixon's "fuzz up" effort as well as the Kennedy campaign's tendency to "move over to new issues" as election day approached, Harris frequently warned Kennedy to dramatize and press home the candidates' differences.[43] Accordingly, Kennedy reinforced his identification with medical care reform by pushing for a plank favoring Medicare at the Democratic national convention. And he pressed for support of Medicare during the special congressional session that met in August after the conventions. A Senate supporter of Medicare recalled that, even though Kennedy was under significant pressure to be out campaigning during the special session, "he thought it was more important that these principles be established... laying the blame on the Republicans for not adopting Medicare."[44]

---

39. Interview with Louis Harris by L. R. Jacobs and Robert Y. Shapiro, 6/17/91; JFK Library, RFK Papers, Pre-Administration, Political, Box 36, "Index to Topics Discussed and List of Topics Not Discussed by Senator Kennedy during the First Four Debates," and "Memorandum on the First Kennedy-Nixon Debate on Domestic Issues," 9/22/60; Second interview with Helen Lempart by N. Aldrich, 3/66.

40. JFK Library, R. F. Kennedy Papers, Pre-Administration, Political, Box 45, "An Analysis of the First Kennedy-Nixon Debate," by Louis Harris and Associates, Inc., 9/26/60.

41. JFK Library, R. F. Kennedy Papers, Pre-Administration, Political, Box 36, Memo to J. F. Kennedy from Clark Clifford, 9/27/60.

42. JFK Library, R. F. Kennedy Papers, Pre-Administration, Political, Box 43, "Memorandum on the Last Nine Days of Campaigning," marked "Confidential"; Box 45, Memo, "Most Americans Are Basically 'New Dealish,' " by George Belknap, 6–8/60; and Box 25, Letter to R. F. Kennedy from Abraham Ribicoff, 10/15/60.

43. JFK Library, R. F. Kennedy Papers, Pre-Administration, Political, Box 45, "A Study of Presidential Election in Ohio, Wave II," by Louis Harris and Associates, Inc., 10/19/60.

44. JFK Library, Interview with Clinton Anderson by John Stewart, 4/14/67.

The result of the Kennedy campaign's sensitivity to public opinion was a new policy-making atmosphere. As Mills stressed, "public opinion is a very important thing in legislation; there's always a time when...public opinion is right for action and that's when you have to enact a bill."[45] By the fall of 1960, policymakers began to perceive a change in public opinion and to recast their assumptions regarding the significance of the medical care issue; they began to believe that it was time to address the issue. With medical care reported in the media as the "most politically significant domestic issue of the election year," Nixon abandoned the Eisenhower administration's previous opposition to new legislation; he emphasized his agreement with Kennedy's aim of helping the aged but differed over the Democrat's particular solution.[46] Other politicians facing elections also became sensitive to the issue's popularity and political significance: as one member of Congress complained, "the heat is on full blast, and we are stewing" (quoted in Harris 1966, 103). Politicians' attention to the issue had a ripple effect on policy discussions among specialists in HEW and outside the government. Both politicians and specialists, then, sensed a new environment for policy making; they now calculated that it was in their interest to address the popular issue of health reform.

POLICY DISCUSSIONS, 1959–1960

As the 1960 presidential election approached and Kennedy used popular issues to press his "move-ahead image," policymakers' changing perception of public opinion became a primary focus of and influence on their decision to select the health issue and to begin serious deliberations about alternative arrangements.

Reform as the Policy Objective

Before the fall of 1958, health reform was seen as a marginal issue that hardly demanded congressional hearings. By November 1960, however, HEW, Eisenhower's White House, and Congress officially recognized the problem confronting the elderly and selected the issue of health reform from a large set of conceivable subjects for sustained attention.

Although policymakers had previously begun to recognize that existing financing arrangements were no longer meeting public expectations for medical care, by 1960 the typically acrimonious debate over health policy was characterized by virtually unanimous agreement that a problem did exist.

45. Mills Interview.
46. Edward Chase in the *Reporter*, quoted in Harris 1966, 102; David 1985.

The AMA now readily acknowledged that, although "there was a time when you almost had to drag the patient into the hospital...now it is rare you find anyone who wants to stay at home."[47] A 1959 congressional study similarly concluded that the "revolution of rising expectations" toward health care was undermining existing financing arrangements (Harris 1966, 98). By November 1959, HEW officials began to explore health insurance schemes for the aged based on the assumption that there was general agreement that a problem existed.[48] Reflecting the consensus that emerged, Forand was congratulated by an unlikely source—an AMA representative—for being "a catalyst in this whole problem of care of the aged... [and] dramatiz[ing] this problem before the American public."[49]

In the policy-making atmosphere that developed as the presidential campaign intensified, HEW began to discuss in its congressional reports and internal deliberations proposals for financing the treatment of the aged—independent of congressional requests for technical assistance. Department officials considered several financing schemes as a result of their judgment that "a satisfactory solution to the problem of paying for adequate medical care for the aged will become more...important."[50] Meeting the health care needs of the aged was not only on HEW's specialized agenda, it was also the subject of widespread concern in Congress (Harris 1966, 98). The Ways and Means Committee opened a new round of hearings in July 1959 to consider the elderly's problem. Although Mills preferred to avoid a committee vote on this politically sensitive issue, by March 1960 the public clamor forced him to consent to one (Harris 1966, 102–3). In spite of the 17–8 defeat of the Medicare proposal, Mills decided that it now made political sense to continue to consider possible policy responses to the elderly's health problem. By fall, the outcome of Mills's deliberations was a new program that proposed a major expansion in medical relief.

47. Testimony by Dr. Frederick Swartz (representative of the AMA), U.S. Congress, House, Ways and Means Committee, 1959, pp. 2304–5.
48. HEW Report, "Hospitalization Insurance for OASDI Beneficiaries," submitted to the Ways and Means Committee, 4/2/59, quoted by HEW Secretary A. Flemming, U.S. Congress, House, Ways and Means Committee, 1959, pp. 9–10; JFK Library, Dept. Healt, Education and Welfare (DHEW) Microfilm, Box 24, Memo from Ida Merriam to David Martin, Allen Pond, R. G. Conley, W. H. Stewart, and Agnes Brewster, 11/2/59, and Memo from W. H. Stewart to Agnes Brewster, R. G. Conley, David Martin, Ida Merriam, and Allen Pond, 11/5/59.
49. Testimony by Dr. Leonard Larson (Chair, Board of Trustees, AMA), U.S. Congress, House, Ways and Means Committee, 1959, pp. 294.
50. HEW Report, "Hospitalization Insurance for OASDI Beneficiaries," submitted to the Ways and Means Committee, 4/2/59, quoted by HEW Secretary A. Flemming, U.S. Congress, House, Ways and Means Committee, 1959, pp. 9–10. Also see JFK Library, DHEW Microfilm, Box 24, Memo from Ida Merriam to David Martin, Allen Pond, R. G. Conley, W. H. Stewart, and Agnes Brewster, 11/2/59, and Memo from W. H. Stewart to Agnes Brewster, R. G. Conley, David Martin, Ida Merriam, and Allen Pond, 11/5/59.

The placement of the health issue on the general governmental agenda was also evident in Eisenhower's decision, during his final months in office, to begin for the first time to actively consider health reform. With Kennedy and other Democrats drawing on strong public interest in the issue, Nixon and HEW secretary Arthur Flemming pressured Eisenhower to "agree to a bill that would at least take some of the pressure off of the Republican presidential candidate and the Republicans in Congress who were up for election" (Harris 1966, 102). Reversing his long-standing opposition to government involvement in health care, Eisenhower proposed by the summer of 1960 a government-subsidized but voluntary program for catastrophic care, which became the basis in Congress for several Republican proposals. It was a reflection of the new sensitivity to public opinion that Eisenhower and the Republicans concluded that they could no longer be seen as ignoring or opposing policy responses to the elderly's health care problems; by agreeing to put the issue up for active consideration, Republicans could argue that their differences with Democrats lay in their approach, not their objective. Both parties, then, now accepted the idea that the federal government had a responsibility to assist the aged who were sick and too poor to pay for medical care (Harris 1966, 106).

Initial Policy Formulation

With the financing of elderly health care gaining acceptance on the government agenda, the network of policy specialists began to publicly discuss new arrangements for organizing the state's involvement in new health policy. Beginning with the Ways and Means Committee's July 1959 hearings, formal policy discussions centered on the state's role. Should the elderly's expectations of treatment be met by nonstate health insurance schemes, or was it necessary for the state to intervene by financing care through Social Security's insurance mechanism? Medicare advocates based their argument on the public's changing understanding of government social welfare; the question, as they posed it, was how and not whether the central state should be involved in financing health care. Drawing on the new social understanding of the state that had been gradually evolving, reform-minded policy experts argued that when faced with sickness "more and more older people have . . . come to the public assistance authorities for medical care purposes." The result was a deepening of state involvement in health care to the point at which already "the Federal Government is taking care of the aged"; new social meanings were, in effect, overtaking existing arrangements. Given the elderly's expectation that the state would meet their health care needs, Cohen testified that "the basic problem of public policy is whether you wish to have people's economic and health needs met through public assistance or through social insurance."[51]

Cohen and others argued that the current health care provisions, which relied on means tests and other negatively perceived poor-law arrangements, should be replaced by a health insurance program that would use the widely accepted Social Security system. With many of the aged enjoying middle-class incomes and private health insurance coverage until retirement, Medicare advocates argued that the onset of sickness compelled them to face the "indignities of a means test for medical care": "public charity ... forces a [retired] worker to go through a means test, forces him into all kinds of embarrassments, loss of a sense of social status and worth and dignity, in order to get access to basic health care."[52] "We believe," Cohen testified, "that it is not the wish of the American people that substantial numbers of our aged citizens be required to turn to public welfare for help with their medical needs."[53] The central argument for the Medicare approach, then, was that it responded to Americans' belief that the aged "should not be forced by high medical bills to ... become medically indigent [and] ... to undergo the means test."[54] Instead, reformers publicly pressed for financing arrangements that would be favorably perceived, "provid[ing] medical care to the aged who need it, as a matter of right, with head up, with a sense of dignity."[55]

Members of the Ways and Means Committee, the AMA, and others repeatedly opposed the idea of reforming existing arrangements through the Medicare approach (Marmor 1973; David 1985). They emphasized "ethical" or "philosophic rather than administrative" or "financial" objections and offered a different interpretation of public opinion than that presented by reformers: stressing the public's uncompromising hostility toward the state, they could not "accept ... that there is need for the Federal Government to be involved."[56] Medicare's introduction of "Communism" and practices "foreign" to Americans' enduring cultural values would, they pre-

51. Testimony by Wilbur Cohen (representative of the American Public Welfare Association), U.S. Congress, House, Ways and Means Committee, 1959, pp. 321–22.

52. Testimony by Walter Reuther (President, United Auto Workers), U.S. Congress, House, Ways and Means Committee, 1959, pp. 410–411.

53. Written Testimony by Wilbur Cohen, U.S. Congress, House, Ways and Means Committee, 1959, 314.

54. Testimony by Nelson Cruikshank (representative of the AFL-CIO), U.S. Congress, House, Ways and Means Committee, 1959, pp. 88–89.

55. Testimony by Walter Reuther (President, United Auto Workers), U.S. Congress, House, Ways and Means Committee, 1959, pp. 410–411.

56. Testimony by committee member Bruce Alger, U.S. Congress, House, Ways and Means Committee, 1959, p. 345. Also see testimony by HEW Secretary Flemming, U.S. Congress, House, Ways and Means Committee, 1959, pp. 21–30.

dicted, "break up normal family obligations and responsibilities";[57] its infringement on nonstate arrangements meant that "individual responsibility is going to be taken away ... [until the citizen] will be finally dependent upon this great Central Government to take care of him."[58] But reflecting their sensitivity to the changes in public understanding of the state since the 1930s, opponents of Medicare repeatedly framed their objections in terms of the danger the program posed to "the acceptance and support of the [Social Security] program by the American public at large."[59]

Medicare was especially dangerous, it was argued, because its expansion of state involvement in social welfare would threaten the practice of American medicine. Even if Medicare duplicated nonstate financing arrangements, it would inevitably violate Americans' innate hostility to state interference.[60] In particular, opponents claimed that "a Governmental agency paying for so large a volume of care" would ultimately restrict both the public's ex- -pectation of a free choice of a provider and the medical profession's "independence and integrity that ... are essential to ... any practice."[61]

In addition to representing an immediate threat to accepted medical practices, the Medicare proposal was seemed to augur an unacceptable future. Attacking the incremental strategy that had guided reformers, Medicare's opponents charged that the attempt to achieve acceptance of compulsory health insurance for one group of the population was merely a "first step" in the development of a national health insurance program for the whole population.[62] By making people accustomed to state involvement in this area, Medicare would introduce "pressures to constantly improve the benefits and widen the scope of action."[63] Thus, while reformers were restricting policy discussions to arrangements familiar to the public, opponents were

57. Testimony by Herbert Berger (President-elect, New York State Society of Internal Medicine), U.S. Congress, House, Ways and Means Committee, 1959, pp. 40–44.

58. Testimony by Dr. R. R. Robbins (representative of the American Academy of General Practice, Arkansas), U.S. Congress, House, Ways and Means Committee, 1959, p. 549.

59. Testimony by Allen Marshall (representative of the U.S. Chamber of Commerce), U.S. Congress, House, Ways and Means Committee, 1959, pp. 122.

60. Testimony by Dr. Leonard Larson (Chair, Board of Trustees, AMA), U.S. Congress, House, Ways and Means Committee, 1959, pp. 303–4; testimony by J. D. Brown (Dean of the Faculty and Professor of Economics, Princeton University), U.S. Congress, House, Ways and Means Committee, 1959, pp. 372–73.

61. Testimony by Rudolph Friedrich (representative of the American Dental Association), U.S. Congress, House, Ways and Means Committee, 1959, p. 368. Also see testimony by Frank Groner (representative of the AHA), U.S. Congress, House, Ways and Means Committee, 1959, pp. 351–52; testimony by Dr. Frederick Swartz pp. 282–83.

62. Testimony by Frank Groner, U.S. Congress, House, Ways and Means Committee, 1959, pp. 349–51; testimony by Dr. Frederick Swartz, (representative of the AMA), U.S. Congress, House, Ways and Means Committee, 1959, pp. 280–81.

63. Testimony by HEW Secretary Flemming, U.S. Congress, House, Ways and Means Committee, 1959, pp. 21.

widening the discussion to encompass future changes that had been repeatedly rejected in the past as alien to Americans' understanding of the state and health care.

To coincide with American experience, Medicare's opponents argued that the financing of the elderly's health care was "better left within the framework of non-governmental action." Representatives of the AMA and the Eisenhower administration emphasized "the increasing public awareness of the value of voluntary health insurance protection" which had accompanied the rapid growth of such insurance since the war. Instead of designing proposals that would rely on the state, they resuscitated the traditional ideological position that separates Republicans from Democrats: they argued that the appropriate response to the elderly's problem was to "strengthen the voluntary approach."[64]

Nevertheless, Kennedy's insertion of the health issue onto the governmental agenda prompted Medicare opponents to reassess their current political position on health reform. Indeed, some acknowledged privately that some form of national health insurance was inevitable (Harris 1966, 117–18). None were willing to publicly announce their private conclusions, but they did begin to consider openly a possible state role, albeit one highly decentralized and subservient to voluntary approaches. Eisenhower's proposal and HEW's testimony and internal deliberations concentrated on using state involvement to preserve and strengthen nonstate institutions.[65] Even these proposals, though, were unacceptable: to the different factions of Medicare opponents, each proposal—as an HEW administrator concluded—"inevitably involves either an irresponsible use of public funds or an unacceptable degree of Federal regulation of the health insurance business."[66] What Medicare opponents did come to accept was the idea of expanding state involvement in medical relief; they agreed that using the economic status of the individual as the basis of determining need would be consistent with (and reinforce) Americans' enduring unease with state social welfare provisions.[67] It seemed reasonable, then, to rely on negatively perceived poor-law arrange-

64. Testimony by HEW Secretary Flemming, U.S. Congress, House, Ways and Means Committee, 1959, pp. 10–17. Also see testimony by Dr. Larson, U.S. Congress, House, Ways and Means Committee, 1959, pp. 273–80.

65. Testimony by HEW Secretary Flemming, U.S. Congress, House, Ways and Means Committee, 1959, pp. 10–17; JFK Library, DHEW Microfilm, Box 24, Memo from Ida Merriam to David Martin, Allen Pond, R. G. Conley, W. H. Stewart, and Agnes Brewster, 11/2/59, and Memo from W. H. Stewart to Agnes Brewster, R. G. Conley, David Martin, Ida Merriam, and Allen Pond, 11/5/59.

66. JFK Library, DHEW Microfilm, Box 24, Memo from Ida Merriam to David Martin, Allen Pond, R. G. Conley, W. H. Stewart, and Agnes Brewster, 11/2/59.

67. Testimony by George Mustin (representative of the American Nursing Home Association), U.S. Congress, House, Ways and Means Committee, 1959, pp. 67–68.

ments, which would deter the nonpoor (and the nonaged) from coming to expect government financing of health care.[68]

The position of Medicare's opponents converged in the fall of 1960 with that of reformers. Although Kennedy's campaign had increased elite perception of the public's concern over the health issue, Medicare's advocates acknowledged that without a strong, indisputable sign of public opinion, fundamental reform was not yet a viable option (Harris 1966, 117–18). As Democratic congressional leader Mills recalled, "the Kennedy campaign kept telling me about the strong support in the polls for Medicare, but I didn't think that was right at the time."[69] To at least a few reformers like Cohen, an interim solution that capitalized on politicians' recent eagerness to respond to public interest in health reform was the most that could be expected before the election.

In this context, policymakers could agree to address the prominent health care issue by enacting in September 1960 the Kerr-Mills program—an amendment to the Social Security Act that expanded the existing public assistance system to cover the elderly who were unable to afford health care. Originating as a proposal by Mills, the amendment built on the traditional decentralized pattern of public assistance; the central government would funnel matching funds to states, which in turn were to make direct or "vendor" payments to hospitals, nursing, homes and doctors providing care to "charity cases."

In explaining the quick enactment of the Kerr-Mills program, Mills stressed that by the fall of 1960 policymakers had reached a broad consensus in favor of helping the elderly sick poor: state involvement would be expanded but would maintain its weak hierarchical organization. "We could pass Kerr-Mills because there was no objection to it."[70] Thus the AMA, despite its initial reluctance to endorse any expansion of the state into health care, quickly came to herald such expansion as the answer to problems for the sick aged who were truly needy. Moreover, Medicare advocates and in particular Cohen supported and helped design the program because it would help familiarize the public with state involvement in financing medical care. Rather than viewing the Medicare and Kerr-Mills approaches as antagonistic, Cohen persuaded liberals in Congress that both were needed; indeed, he suggested that Kerr-Mills was an important step toward building support for Medicare.[71] In the new political environment of emerging sensitivity to

68. Testimony by HEW Secretary Flemming, U.S. Congress, House, Ways and Means Committee, 1959, pp. 21–30.

69. Mills Interview.

70. Mills Interview; interview with Mills by Charles Morrissey, 4/5/79, Former Members of Congress, Inc.

71. LBJ Library, Interview with Cohen by David McComb, 12/8/68 (tape 1); David 1985, 38–41.

public opinion, policymakers concluded that some response was needed—even if the new policy was geared at this point only to the sick poor.

Major health reform was not a new issue in wartime Britain or postwar America, but ultimately it emerged as a top governmental priority. According to diverse traditions of empirical research, the process by which the health issue was organized into politics should be endogenous to elite thinking; it is expected to reflect elites' free rein—within broad parameters—to define and select policy issues for serious governmental attention. Thus, Weberians expect the capacity of existing institutions to be the primary focus and determinant of elite decisions about setting the governmental agenda and specifying alternatives. Indeed, the initial outcome of American policy discussions is in some respects consistent with Weberian predictions: the existing institutional setting (weak capacity characterized by wide dispersal of authority) coincided with Kerr-Mills's low hierarchical control over the dispersion of government funds.

Extensive primary evidence, however, indicates that the Weberians' causal argument is misspecified. It was public preferences and understandings that propelled major health reform onto the American and British agendas. Policymakers' perception of strong public interest in and support for a change in health care arrangements accounts for the definition and selection of this issue, as well as for the initial formal deliberations over policy alternatives.

In particular, it was after policymakers' perception of public opinion had changed that American and British policy changed. In pursuit of voters and political backing, Kennedy in the United States and the Labour party in Britain attempted to respond to and thereby appeal to public opinion; struggles among exceptionally prominent politicians had a ripple effect, heightening policymakers' sensitivity to public opinion and their attraction to major health reform. After this political shift, politicians and specialists who previously considered major health reform inconceivable now recognized it as practical and worthy of serious governmental discussion. Thus, British policymakers' perception of a change in public opinion led them to dismiss earlier incremental proposals and to begin considering major alterations in administrative arrangements (such as eliminating the panel system).

Why did two broadly similar countries become the sites of dramatically different policy deliberations? The dramatic differences stemmed from important variations in American and British preferences and cultural patterns. Drawing on the public's understandings of state provisions and on its preference that medical services become a state matter, British politicians and policy specialists could consider involving the state in the provision of comprehensive care for the entire country. In the United States, however, policymakers were constrained by their public's comparative unfamiliarity with state social welfare provisions and by Americans' preferences for merely extending the established Social Security system. Reformers such as Wilbur Cohen, who had carefully aligned their proposals with public opinion, sought to maximize the political support for reform by focusing on one service (hospital care) for a restricted population group (the aged), with the state's involvement designed as an extension of a popularly accepted financing system (Social Security). In the United States, it seemed foolish to propose and attempt to focus governmental attention on establishing universal coverage, state provision (rather than financing) of treatment, and extensive GP care; in Britain, centuries of social interaction with institutions had made all of these ideas seem at least conceivable if not yet passable.

PART III

A Search for Consensus

6 | Britain, 1942–1945: Aftermath of the Beveridge Report

Between December 1942, when the Beveridge Report was published, and July 1945, when elections were held to replace the wartime government, British deliberations were framed by two concerns: how to respond to strong public sentiment, symbolized by the outpouring of support for the Beveridge Report, and how to prevent political divisions from rupturing the coalition. The British public strongly favored a new policy direction, one that would reform prewar social welfare policy, particularly health care. In response to strong public attitudes evidenced by the Beveridge Report's reception, the coalition came under heightened political pressure to address the issue of postwar reconstruction. Health reform was the subject of nearly continuous bargaining among leading interest groups, bureaucrats inside and outside the Ministry of Health, and cabinet ministers.[1] British policymakers were prevented, however, from pursuing fundamental reform by political deadlock among competing parties and individuals; they concluded that bold innovation would exacerbate political divisions within the fractious coalition and needlessly diminish their already scarce political capital. Instead, they pursued a low-risk approach, attempting to build a broad consensus behind a compromise plan that would at least partly respond to strong public opinion.

The critical analytic issue is to identify the primary focus of and influence on policymakers as they determined the specific direction of administrative changes and the degree of interest group influence. Weberians claim that

---

1. In the Ministry of Health, the relevant senior administrators included J. Maude, J. C. Wrigley, W. Jameson, and A. N. Rucker. Middle-level officials included J. Hawton, H. A. de Montmorency, A. W. Neville, T. H. Sheepshank, J. Pater, and S. F. Wilkinson.

such decisions to alter institutional arrangements and to respond to interest groups are largely a function of objective administrative capacity. Culturalists, however, emphasize the impact of state actors' perceptions of public preferences and understandings.

THE STRATEGIC UNIVERSE

The publication of the Beveridge Report on December 1, 1942, was a watershed event; it crystallized emerging political and cultural patterns. The report, as Beveridge intended, articulated already established trends in public opinion; the country's unmistakably positive reaction to it altered the calculations of policymakers, intensifying both their sensitivity to public expectations and their commitment to incorporating these expectations into policy deliberations.

Public Opinion

As World War II took a favorable turn with the Allied victory at El Alamein during the fall of 1942, the public—as it had before the Beveridge Report's publication—continued to support major new domestic initiatives. Enduring understandings were echoed in both quantitative opinion surveys and qualitative studies, especially by Mass Observation (MO).[2] These two sources of evidence are complementary: MO's direct recording of ordinary people's thoughts help interpretations of quantitative findings, and polls provide a basis for generalizations from the MO studies.

Public opinion toward social welfare and health policies was characterized by two trends: support for reforming prewar policies and for enlarging the state's role in social welfare and health care. Enthusiasm for reforming prewar arrangements was evident in an April 1943 Gallup poll. The survey reported that 57 percent of respondents would like to see "great changes" in their "way of life after the war"; only a third did not favor this type of substantial reconstruction (Gallup 1976, 75).

Support for major domestic reform built on the favorable understanding of state involvement in domestic life. A June 1944 Gallup poll reported that 68 percent favored the changeover from war to peace occurring mainly

2. MO's studies were based on the responses of a panel to open-ended questions and on random interviews in London and other cities. For a discussion of MO's panel and its interview technique, see Jeffrey 1978 and 1980; Calder and Sheridan, 1984; *Nature*, May 9, 1942: 516–18.

under government control.[3] In a similar vein, a 1943 qualitative study by MO reported that "postwar expectations were increasingly based on . . . the continuation of some measure of state control." Nevertheless, the new understanding of the state was interlaced with a lingering anxiety that "soulless state control" would be introduced; the public favored greater state involvement if it avoided "excessive officialdom, regimentation, and interference with people's lives."[4]

Public interest in, and support for, in the details of major domestic reform had been evident since at least 1940; the Beveridge Report's publication became, in effect, a lightning rod, serving as a focus and indisputable symbol of existing public attitudes. Reflecting these two earlier trends, the report became highly salient across the country, and its proposed change in the direction of policy was strongly supported. A special Gallup poll in December 1942 found that fully 95 percent of the public had heard about the Beveridge Report (British Institute of Public Opinion [BIPO] 1943, 4). Parliament's debate on the report in mid-February 1943 was followed closely by the public, even more so than news about the war; even two years after the report's release, a government survey of chief constables from around the country reported that 76 percent followed the government's handling of Beveridge's recommendations.[5]

The public overwhelmingly supported the Beveridge Report's three major recommendations—a new health service, a children's allowance program, and a full employment plan. Polls confirmed reports that "all shades of public opinion and . . . all sections of the community" welcomed the report's "revolutionary" and "bold" proposals. The special December Gallup survey found "overwhelming agreement that the Beveridge plan *should* be put into effect": 88 percent of respondents favored its implementation (BIPO 1943, 10).[6] The country's support was weakest on the report's specifics, about which the public was reported to be very hazy; the strongest public preferences were directed toward Beveridge's broad objectives. According to parallel inquiries by Gallup and the government's Ministry of Information, the public yearned for the security of a "cradle to grave" comprehensive

3. The question was the following: "During the changeover from war to peace, should the change be done mainly under government control, or should it be left mainly to private business?" Fourteen percent favored using private business, and 18 percent had no opinion; Gallup 1976, 91–92. Also see McLaine, 1979, 180.

4. INF 1/293, "Home Intelligence Special Report: Public Reaction to the White Paper on a National Health Service," by the Ministry of Information, 3/14/44; MO, FR 1921, "Report on Public Attitudes to State Medicine," 10/8/43, pp. 75–76.

5. PIN 8/162, "Public Opinion on the Beveridge Report," 12/42–3/43.

6. See also the Ministry of Intelligence's Home Intelligence Week Report for 12/10/42 in Taylor 1979b, 357; PIN 8/162, "Public Opinion on the Beveridge Report," a series of monthly reports by chief constables from around the country, 12/42–3/43.

program of social services.[7] There was particular support for Beveridge's proposal to make these benefits universally available: 56 percent thought it was "a good idea to include everyone in the scheme," while 30 percent clung to the idea of imposing an income limit (BIPO 1943, 12).

Because the report closely reflected public attitudes, it put into sharp and unmistakable relief the distance between public sentiment and the coalition's reconstruction policy; the public quickly concluded that the government did not share its enthusiasm for Beveridge's recommendations. The British feared, according to MO, that the report "would be sabotaged before it ever got into action" either through compromise or because it would be put into "limbo."[8] Polling data confirmed that the government's treatment of the report in the February 1943 parliamentary debate "brought a profound sense of disillusionment."[9] Almost half the respondents of a March 1943 Gallup poll were "dissatisfied with the government's attitude as explained by the government Ministers in Parliament"; this level of suspicion that "the government was not sincere in its plans for reconstruction" was duplicated in a September 1944 Gallup poll (Gallup 1976, 72, 98). By 1945, this dissatisfaction fueled the public's suspicion that the Government would "shelve" reform proposals to "get back to 'normal' in the 1939 sense."[10]

The public's scrutiny of the Beveridge scheme may help to account for its decidedly mixed evaluation of the wartime government: Britons persistently criticized the coalition for its handling of the domestic policy but expressed strong satisfaction with the government's conduct of the war (as reported in eighteen Gallup polls) (Gallup 1976).

The public's attitudes toward health care mirrored its perception of general social welfare policy. Its strong reaction, in both qualitative and quantitative surveys, to health reform indicates that the issue remained highly salient. Health care's placement on the general, nongovernmental agenda is further indicated by a review of articles published in the *London Times:* the health issue attracted more coverage between 1943 and June 1945 than other domestic policies; in some years the discrepancy was by a factor of five or more.[11]

7. INF 1/293, "Home Intelligence Special Report: Public Feeling about the Beveridge Proposals," by the Ministry of Intelligence, 5/31/44; INF 1/293, "Home Intelligence Special Report: Public Reaction to the White Paper on a National Health Service," by the Ministry of Intelligence, 3/14/44.

8. MO, FR 1634, "MO Bulletin," 3/23/43, p. 6; MO, FR 1617, "Report on Some Opinion Trends among the Forces," 3/4/43, p. 13.

9. MO, FR 1676, "MO Bulletin," 5/10/43, marked "Confidential: circulation very strictly limited," p. 1–2.

10. MO, FR 2234, "MO Bulletin for April–May 1945," pp. 2–3, a bulletin based on the written responses of MO's national panel.

11. Between 1943 and the end of June 1945, health policy was the subject of 274 articles, housing was the subject of 52 articles, and social insurance and unemployment together were

The new understanding of the state, which had gradually evolved from centuries of social interaction with government institutions, was articulated during the early 1940s in the public's strong preference for enlarging state involvement in health care. A respondent in an MO survey observed in 1943: "I've always felt that the state should be responsible for the health of the nation. It's only right that the state should show concern over the people's health, and do their duty."[12] This view was echoed in Gallup polls: a June 1943 survey reported that 70 percent felt that a "state-run medical service would . . . be beneficial for the nation"; in a July 1944 poll, 55 percent favored "a publicly run national health service" while only 32 percent preferred leaving health care arrangements "as they are" (Gallup 1976, 77, 92). In particular, the public seemed to favor central rather than local state involvement: MO found that many of its respondents distrusted local governments; they "would like the [central] State, not the local council, to take over administration, finance and control." Echoing the enduring understandings of local authorities, MO predicted that "opposition to any medical service run or financ[ed] by local councils . . . would be much less strong if a larger, geographically wider body were entrusted."[13]

Nevertheless, the public's favorable understanding of state involvement in health care (as in social welfare generally) was interspersed with concern about red tape. The public did not associate the new meaning of the state with turning doctors into "automatons," who would become "just another civil servant with the civil servant mentality."[14]

The public's general acceptance of stricter state control of the existing medical services was accompanied by strong support for reforming the prewar organization of health care.[15] Beveridge became the focal point of the public's understanding of and preferences for both hospital and general medical care. Gallup's special December survey reported overwhelming endorsement of Beveridge's recommendation of a comprehensive and universally available health service. Eighty-eight percent of the survey respondents favored extending doctors' and hospital services, free of charge, to every person; even among the wealthy, who had the greatest reservations, 81 percent favored this reform (BIPO 1943, 4, 8).

---

the subject of 154 articles. In 1943, the number of articles on health, housing, and social insurance and unemployment were, respectively, 110, 22, and 13. In 1944, the number of articles on health, housing, and social insurance and unemployment were, respectively, 122, 7, and 98. Between January and June 1945, the number of articles on health, housing, and social insurance and unemployment were, respectively, 42, 23, and 45.

12. MO, FR 1921, "Report on Public Attitudes to State Medicine," 10/8/43, p. 29.

13. MO, FR 1921, "Report on Public Attitudes to State Medicine," 10/8/43, pp. 75–76; MO, Topic Collection (TC), Health, Box 1, File F.

14. MO, FR 1921, "Report on Public Attitudes to State Medicine," 10/8/43, pp. 70–71.

15. MO, FR 1921, "Report on Public Attitudes to State Medicine," 10/8/43, pp. 43–56.

The public also had a strong reaction to the coalition's release in February 1944 of a white paper that outlined proposals for establishing a national health service. As in the case of Beveridge's proposals, public support varied according to the level of specificity. Public preferences were hazy on the proposals for specific administrative arrangements. There was strong support, however, for the major principles (free and universally available care) and for the coverage of a comprehensive range of services including hospital and GP care.[16]

The white paper's proposal to extend existing public services to encompass hospital-based specialist services was almost universally approved. Continuing a trend that had emerged before December 1942, a majority felt that hospitals should be taken over completely by the state.[17] In a July 1944 Gallup poll, 42 percent felt that voluntary hospitals should be taken over by a public authority, 21 percent preferred to see them become part voluntary and part public, and another 21 percent favored keeping them entirely voluntary (Gallup 1976, 93). Support for greater state involvement stemmed from hostility to old arrangements for financing voluntary hospitals, such as appeals and flag days: as a respondent in an MO survey observed, "people loathe being pestered to buy flags in support of hospitals."[18]

Moreover, the public favored the white paper's call to reorganize GP care. In particular, a July 1944 Gallup poll found that 69 percent approved of the proposal to reorganize GP care around group practice in health centers.[19] The public apparently believed that health centers would eliminate "the present dual system of private and panel system" in which the patients in the public service "get the second best medical attention."[20]

The public's suspicion of the government's handling of the Beveridge Report was also evident in the area of health care. MO's report that many people expected "merely a glorified extension of the existing panel practice" was confirmed by other studies.[21] A parallel study by the government and

16. INF 1/293, "Home Intelligence Special Report: Public Reaction to the White Paper on a National Health Service," by the Ministry of Information, 3/14/44; MO, FR 1912, "Interim Report on Feelings about a State Medical Service," 9/27/43; MO, FR 1921, "Report on Public Attitudes to State Medicine," 10/8/43, pp. 43–56.

17. INF 1/293, "Home Intelligence Special Report: Public Reaction to the White Paper on a National Health Service," by the Ministry of Information, 3/14/44.

18. MO, TC, Health, Box 1, File M.

19. The question was the following: "Would you approve or disapprove of health centers, where you might get more treatments than you could get at your doctor's surgery, but which might not be so near your home?" Eighteen percent disapproved of health centers; 13 percent reported that they did not know (Gallup 1976, 92).

20. MO, FR 1921, "Report on Public Attitudes to State Medicine," 10/8/43, p. 41; Jeffrey 1980.

21. MO, TC, Health, Box 1, File K, "Investigators' Notes on the Health Survey," 8/5/43.

Gallup reported that the white paper was often seen as an excuse for not accepting the Beveridge proposals.[22]

Political Struggles

The intensification of political struggles over the coalition's domestic policy that followed the Beveridge publication created two irreconcilable political pressures: responding to public support for domestic reform, and minimizing tensions between Labour and Conservatives. The coalition attempted reconciliation by seeking consensus without commitment: it concentrated on areas of popular concern that enjoyed general agreement among ministers while leaving the postwar government with a free hand on reconstruction—"The Government agreed to plan but not legislate."[23] To build consensus and preserve the coalition, the cabinet reinvigorated the previously established process for handling reconstruction. The unintended consequence of this process was to heighten policymakers' sensitivity to public opinion and to create compelling incentives for them to commit the postwar government to major domestic reforms.

Labour and Conservative competing assessments of public opinion were a major source of the cabinet's political divisions over domestic policy. Conservatives, particularly Churchill, were opposed to committing the postwar government to reconstruction because of its undesirable impact on public opinion: promises of reform would create unrealistic expectations. Churchill warned his colleagues that "nothing would be more dangerous than for people to feel cheated because they had been led to expect attractive schemes which turn out to be economically impossible."[24] In addition, Conservatives were convinced that the initial "ballyhoo" over Beveridge was merely the product of "carefully engineered publicity" rather than genuine public sentiment. As Churchill confidently observed, "the Labour Party are seeking to carry, by internal pressure and the use of wartime emergencies, measures that they could never carry at the polls."[25] The Conservatives, then, feared that the "follies of Socialism" would produce an unwanted and "impracticable financial commitment"; they insisted that the coalition "get

22. INF 1/293, "Home Intelligence Special Report: Public Reaction to the White Paper on a National Health Service," 3/14/44.

23. Addison 1977, 224. Also see CAB 65/28, War Cabinet, Minute, WM 150 (42), 11/4/42; CAB 66/30, War Cabinet, Memo, WP (42) 507, "Outline of Statement on Reconstruction Problems," by W. Jowitt, 11/14/42; CAB 66/42, War Cabinet, Memo, WP (43) 465, "Reconstruction Plans," by Lord Cherwell, 10/20/43.

24. CAB 117/75, Personal minute from Churchill to W. Jowitt, K. Wood, H. Dalton, and C. Attlee, 12/17/42. Also see PREM4 89/2, Letter from Lord Cherwell to Churchill, 2/11/43; PREM4 89/2, Memo by K. Wood to Churchill, 11/17/42.

25. PREM4 87/11, Minute to home secretary (H. Morrison), 10/24/43. Also see PREM4 89/2, pt. 2, Letter to Churchill from Lord Cherwell, 11/25/42.

everything ready for [the postwar government] and leave them a free hand to take up or reject a scheme."[26]

In contrast, Labour ministers vigorously argued for a response to public opinion by implementing reconstruction policies during the war. Enunciating his party's interpretation of public sentiment, a senior Labour politician presciently warned Conservative ministers that "the great majority of the public is looking forward expectantly to the adoption of something substantially like the Beveridge Plan"; a "grudging" welcome of Beveridge would be "contrary to the general opinion likely to find strong expression in Parliament and in the country."[27] The benefit of responding to public opinion would be the boost in civilian morale: popular reform represented an "opportunity of genuine re-creation" to reverse the "laziness, the status quo mind, [and the] timidity" that were contributing to the country's "slow national and imperial decline."[28] Questioning the Conservatives' "fatalistically-accepted prospect of [financial] disaster," Labour continually pressured the coalition to enact legislation before the war's conclusion.[29]

Although these diverging positions toward reconstruction and public attitudes were not new, the publication of the Beveridge Report exacerbated tensions to the point of threatening the government's survival. Arguing that "we must not allow our immediate duty [of winning the war] to be obstructed," Churchill stressed the need to "keep the present forces together until...the ship comes into harbor."[30] To prevent the divisive issue of reconstruction from undermining the coalition, the cabinet reinvigorated the process that had earlier been established for policy making: the reconstruction committee's work was elevated to a level of first-rate importance, dominating the attention of senior politicians and bureaucrats.

Following the Beveridge Report's completion, the war cabinet discussed "machinery for organizing...the study of reconstruction problems" and agreed to hold periodic meetings to ensure that planning by specialists was "being undertaken broadly on the right lines"; the result was a new and more high-powered reconstruction committee to provide political supervision of policy specialists.[31] After Parliament's debate on the Beveridge plan in February 1943, the government specified detailed plans for achieving the

---

26. PREM4 89/2, Memo by K. Wood to Churchill, 11/17/42; CAB 66/34, War Cabinet, Memo, WP (43) 65, "Beveridge Report," by Churchill, 2/15/43; PREM4 87/11, Minute to home secretary (H. Morrison), 10/24/43. Also see PREM4 89/2, pt. 2, Letter to Churchill from Lord Cherwell, 11/25/42.

27. CAB 87/13, Memo, PR (43)2, by H. Morrison, 1/20/43; CAB 65/33, War Cabinet Minutes, WM (43) 28th, 2/12/43.

28. PREM4 87/11, Letter from H. Morrison to Churchill, 10/22/43.

29. CAB 87/13, Memo, PR (43)2, by H. Morrison, 1/20/43.

30. PREM4 87/11, Minute to home secretary (H. Morrison), 10/24/43.

31. CAB 65/28, War Cabinet, Minutes, WM 155 (42), 11/19/42.

report's main recommendations. With final decisions made by the cabinet, the revamped reconstruction committee exercised close political supervision over the various departments, including the Ministry of Health and its designs for a new health service. The ministry's specialized deliberations (which included private meetings with major interest groups) produced— after frequent meetings with the reconstruction committee—a white paper that outlined initial decisions about the direction and content of future health policy.

As designed, the cabinet's process for handling reconstruction did identify and build areas of agreement among the coalition's partners. This process for reaching compromises enabled a severely divided coalition to accept the Beveridge Report and four white papers. In terms of the Beveridge Report, the coalition acceded to Labour's insistence that the government respond to public support of reform while honoring Conservatives' refusal to tie the hands of future Parliaments. Similarly, the national health service white paper, according to a former Ministry of Health administrator, was "the product of . . . many compromises in order to get everyone to agree."[32] This consensus-building process, then, produced significant compromises: Conservatives became unwilling partners in a reformist government and Labour ministers sacrificed sacred party principles.

Nevertheless, the process for addressing postwar reform produced precisely what it was intended to avoid—dramatically heightened political tensions. The government's announcement in Parliament of its compromise position on Beveridge left the public and many members of Parliament believing that the government's approach appeared grudging and half-hearted; a significant number of members, including all but two on the Labour backbench, voted against the government at the debate's conclusion. For the coalition's remaining term, politicians and bureaucrats strained to combat the widespread skepticism about the genuineness of the government's professions; to dispel public skepticism, Churchill gave a rare broadcast on plans for "cradle to grave" programs for all classes and all purposes. As a result of this political firestorm, Labour ministers repeatedly warned the cabinet of the growing pressure within their party to withdraw; in May 1945, they did withdraw despite Churchill's interest in prolonging the coalition.[33]

---

32. Pater Interview. Also see MH 80/27, Letter from A. Rucker to Lord Cherwell, 8/1/44; MH 80/25, Memo, "Appendix II: Note on a General Practice Service," handwritten, "J. Maude, 1/28/43"; MH 80/25, Memo, "Notes on a Comprehensive Health Service (to be read with paper submitted to committee on reconstruction priorities)," 2/2/43; MH 80/27, Memo, "The White Paper Scheme," 2/10/44; MH 80/27, handwritten note from F. Clark to J. Hawton, 2/18/44, forwarding memo by H. S. H., "BMA Conference on White Paper."

33. CAB 66/34, War Cabinet, Memo, WP (43) 65, "Beveridge Report," by Churchill, 2/15/43; CAB 65/33, War Cabinet, Minutes, WM (43) 28th, 2/12/43, 29th, 2/15/43, and 31st,

The country's reaction to the coalition's handling of the Beveridge Report and its four white papers presented a general threat to the coalition during the two and a half years following Beveridge's publication. It also had a more concrete impact on state actors: it heightened the urgency that many bureaucrats and politicians attached to major reform as a response to public opinion. Throughout the government, both civil servants and ministers repeatedly stressed the "keen public interest in the Beveridge Report" and the fact that "the public want to be assured that the Government mean business."[34] Public attitudes toward the report were, a former ministry administrator recalled, a constant background concern.[35] This sensitivity to popular interest was evident in the high demand within the government, particularly, the Ministry of Health, for opinion surveys and public relations campaigns.[36]

Cabinet ministers responded to the public's support for the Beveridge Report and its strong suspicion of the government's intentions by insisting that plans for social services be urgently completed to avert a crisis. By October 1943, they reported that proposals were far advanced.[37] Within the Ministry of Health, the recognition of strong public interest in a new health service "galvanized" officials from "merely thinking into... apply[ing] the Ministerial mind seriously."[38] Senior officials' concern with public relations led them to attach great urgency to the new service's formulation and to prepare the white paper's release to appeal to the "man in the street."[39]

2/17/43; CAB 66/36, War Cabinet, WM (43) 140, Minutes, 10/14/43; CAB 66/42, War Cabinet, Memo, WP (43) 465, "Reconstruction Plans," by Lord Cherwell, 10/20/43; CAB 124/233, Memo from Peck to E. Bridges, 12/2/43; Addison 1977, 134; Pater 1981, 46.

34. CAB 87/3, Memo, PR (43) 9, "Draft Interim Report on the Beveridge Report," 2/7/43, and final version of Report, PR (43) 13, 12/13/43; PIN 8/46, Memo, "Introduction of the Social Security Scheme by Stages," by A. Patterson. Also see PIN 8/115, "Official Committee on the Beveridge Report"; Godber Interview.

35. Pater Interview. Also see Godber Interview.

36. MH 80/27, Memo from F. Clark to S. F. Wilkinson, 1/4/44; MH 80/26, Minutes, 12th meeting of the public relations committee, 5/26/43 (present: minister, secretary, parliamentary secretary, and nine other ministry officials); MH 77/28, Memo, "NHS," to S.F. Wilkinson from F. Clark, 1/13/44; CAB 87/7, Memo, "Appendix A. Presentation of the White Paper," annexed to R (44) 24, 1/31/44; MH 77/31, Memo from F. Clark to A. Rucker, 5/12/44; MH 80/27, Letter from A. Rucker to Lord Cherwell, 8/1/44; MH 80/27, Letter from A. Rucker to Lord Cherwell, 8/16/44; MH 80/34, Memo, "Nationwide Campaign for Hospitals," from A. Rucker from J. Hawton, 5/24/44; MH 80/34, Memo, "Nation-Wide Campaign for Hospitals," handwritten, "A. Rucker: for your information, F. Clark, 5/25/44."

37. CAB 123/244, Memo, "Social Security—Future Procedure," by H. Morrison to the committee on reconstruction priorities, 2/22/43; PREM4 89/2, Letter from Lord Cherwell to Churchill, 2/11/43; CAB 66/36, War Cabinet, WM (43) 140, Minutes, 10/14/43; CAB 66/42, War Cabinet, Memo, WP (43) 465, "Reconstruction Plans," by Lord Cherwell, 10/20/43.

38. Pater Interview. See also PREM4 87/9, Table; MH 80/25, Memo, "Notes on a Comprehensive Health Service," probably 2/43; CAB 117/19, Memo, "MH: Degree of Priority Attaching to Reconstruction Problems," approximately 6/43.

39. MH 80/27, Memo from F. Clark to S. F. Wilkinson, 1/4/44. Also see MH 80/26, Minutes, 12th meeting of the public relations committee, 5/26/43.

Many Conservatives (especially members of the party's right wing) were incredulous: the coalition was committing the postwar government to major reforms both by fanning public expectations and by preparing for a heavy legislative program which was believed to be demanded by the general public and Parliament.[40] With Labour ministers beginning to advocate "decisions on reconstruction planning intended for wartime legislative implementation," Conservatives, specifically Churchill, unsuccessfully attempted to slow or even reverse the rising tide of reform proposals.[41] In the coalition's final year, Churchill lashed out at the Exchequer for not resisting the rapid growth of national expenses; he pleaded in cabinet meetings for ministers to resist new financial commitments. Finally, this powerful prime minister was reduced to the awkward position of threatening Labour that a substantial majority of his own party might desert him.[42] To Churchill, the reformist direction was making irresponsibe additions to the annual budget and creating trouble that could break up the coalition.[43]

To challenge the coalition's unmistakable commitment to postwar reform, Churchill stepped in after the national health service white paper had been completed in early 1944 and opposed its publication. But after Conservative ministers emphasized the consequences—Labour's withdrawal and the electoral significance of blatant defiance of public expectations—he acceded to its publication and to the government's deepening involvement in postwar reform.[44] Indeed, during the coalition's last months, the cabinet seriously considered presenting a national health service bill. In response to public expectations and to Labour's lobbying, the Ministry of Health's Conservative minister drafted legislation; by April 1945, he reported that the government was "approaching the stage when [the new service]...may be settled in a Coalition bill."[45]

The new policy-making environment was vividly illustrated by the caretaker cabinet's difficulty in reconciling its policies with public opinion. The Conservative-dominated caretaker government, which governed between the coalition's collapse in May and the July elections, fully recognized—as

40. CAB 75/15, Home Policy Committee Minutes, 11/16/43, 11/23/43, 12/14/43; CAB 75/19, Home Policy Committee, HPC (44) 25, Excerpt from letter from A. Eden to Attlee included in note by Attlee, 3/10/44.

41. CAB 66/38, War Cabinet, WP (43) 255, Memo, "The Need for Decisions," by Attlee, Bevin, and Morrison, 6/29/43.

42. PREM4 89/5, Minute from Churchill to Exchequer, 6/25/44; CAB 65/43, War Cabinet, WM (44) 87, Minutes, 7/4/44; PREM4 88/1, Minute from Churchill to Attlee, 11/20/44; CAB 124/566, "Note for the Record," 1/15/45, marked "Top Secret."

43. Addison 1977, 241–42; PREM4 36/3, Minute, from Churchill to A. Eden, 2/10/44.

44. CAB 124/244, Minute, to Churchill, unauthored but probably A. Eden; CAB 65/41, Minutes, War Cabinet meeting, WM (44) 21st, 2/15/44; MH 80/27, Memo, "The White Paper Scheme," 2/10/44.

45. MH 77/119, Letter from H. Willink to E. Bevin, 4/26/45. Also see MH 80/28, series of memos and letters regarding the drafting of the NHS legislation, 1/45–5/45; CAB 124/275, Memo from J. Maude to Lord Woolton, "Sale and Purchase of Medical Practices," 3/14/45.

one senior Conservative minister explained—that "we must demonstrate to the public the [Conservative's] sincerity" in converting "known preparatory work . . . [into] an actual scheme"; it was particularly important to give "the public . . . evidence of our determination to legislate [a new health insuance plan]."[46] Conservatives, then, were prepared—if Labour campaigned on the health issue—to publicly announce their intention to introduce legislation in the new Parliament. Concerned, however, that modification of the coalition's white paper might not be acceptable to the general public as a whole, Conservative leaders concluded that "politically we should lose a great deal more than we could possibly gain."[47] Churchill decided not to announce their revised scheme. In the new political environment, Conservatives feared that Labour would make damaging criticisms; the grave danger was that Labour would accuse them of "betrayal of all that was promised the nation by the Coalition Government."[48] Even Conservative ministers did not find it politically possible to ignore public expectations. Over all, the fragile consensus of Labour and Conservative ministers produced the greatest reforming administration since the Liberal government of the early 1900s— in spite of the coalition's stated intention of leaving the postwar government with a free hand (Addison 1977, 14).

Policy Discussions

Before the Beveridge Report was even published, the issue of a comprehensive health service was catapulted onto the agendas of the mass public and the government. The political evolution between Parliament's debate over the report in February 1943 and May 1945 added urgency to organized deliberations of Ministry of Health officials, ministers on the reconstruction committee and in the cabinet, and select interest groups. These deliberations raised two critical analytic issues, the variation in state actors' autonomy and the specific changes they proposed in administrative capacity.

46. MH 77/30A, Memo, "NHS: Paper by Minister of Health," draft cabinet paper, 5–6/45; CAB 21/2032, Letter from Lord Woolton to H. Willink, 5/18/45. Also see CAB 65/53, Minutes of Cabinet Meeting, CM (45) 9th, 6/15/45.

47. CAB 21/2032, Memo from Lord Woolton to Churchill, 6/1/45; CAB 21/2032, Letter from Harry to Lord Woolton, 6/7/45. Also see CAB 21/2019, Minutes of meeting of Lord Cherwell, Lord Beaverbrook, H. Willink, Earl of Rosebery, L. H. Belisha, and Lord Woolton, 6/6/45.

48. PREM4 36/4, Note from Churchill to H. Willink, 6/18/45. Also see CAB 21/2019, Minutes of meeting of Lord Cherwell, Lord Beaverbrook, H. Willink, Earl of Rosebery, L. H. Belisha, and Lord Woolton, 6/6/45; CAB 65/53, Cabinet Minutes, CM (45) 9th, 6/15/45; CAB 66/66, Cabinet Memo, CP (45) 32, "NHS," by H. Willink and Earl of Rosebery, 6/11/45.

State Autonomy and Basic Principles

In the course of the Coalition's formulation of a new service, there were significant disagreements between policymakers and interest groups claiming to represent powerful health care producers—national organizations of doctors, voluntary hospitals, and local authorities. Interest group influence on policymakers' resolution of these differences varied: on some basic principles, state actors insisted on exerting independence and disregarded sectional claims, while on others interest groups were quite influential.

State actors and interest groups fundamentally disagreed on two major principles, the universal availability of the service and its free cost. In the face of well-established public attitudes toward free and universal health care, persistent and strong protests by leading interest groups had little influence. The representatives of the BMA persistently argued that access to the new service should be limited to those below a certain income level; they considered covering upper income groups unnecessary because these individuals could provide for themselves.[49] The Ministry of Health, however, was unmoved by the BMA's case; it summarily dismissed such claims as doctors' attempts at "artificially protecting" fees from private patients.[50] Pointing to "public opinion on this decision of the Government," it repeatedly insisted that "most people are glad to see the Government... mak[ing health services] available to all people."[51]

In addition to stressing the popularity of universal coverage, politicians and bureaucrats anticipated that the public would have a strong negative reaction to administrative arrangements that differentiated patients according to financial means. Earmarking certain services for different income brackets "marks the service (like the present panel service) as one for the working classes and not a first-rate affair."[52] Thus, it was argued that "however good [the service] might be, a 90 percent service would be prejudiced from the start, since it would inevitably be regarded as something provided cheaply for the lower classes only, and not good enough for the

49. MH 80/26, Minutes, First meeting with small committee of the medical profession, 5/24/43.
50. MH 80/32, Memo, "The Reasons for a 100 percent Service," probably 1/45; MH 80/28, Memo, "Comprehensiveness in a NHS," handwritten, "To be raised at meeting with Minister 1/23/45. Also see MH 80/26, Memo, "NHS," to secretary of state of Scotland, 6/43, handwritten, "Given to Secretary by G. Henderson, 6/28/43.
51. MH 80/27, Letter from Willink to member of parliament Cobb, regarding his letter to the *Times*, 11/22/44. Also see MH 80/26, Minutes, First meeting with small committee of the medical profession, 5/24/43; MH 80/27, Memo, "Universality," unauthored, undated, probably written winter 1943–44.
52. MH 80/26, Memo, "NHS: Private Treatment by Doctors in the Public Service," from J. Maude to Minister, 9/7/43. Also see MH 80/25, Memo, "Appendix II. Note on a General Practice Service," handwritten, "J. Maude, 1/28/43."

well-to-do."[53] Emphasizing the social meaning of arrangements that differentiate patients, a senior administrator warned the health minister that "many people below the income limit who would be glad enough to avail themselves of a universal service would probably stand aside and continue to pay doctors' bills."[54]

The cabinet and the ministry insisted that the availability of government health care reflect the public's expectations. Even after it made numerous concessions to the BMA following the release of the white paper on health reform, the coalition insisted that the service provide universal availability.[55]

The issue of free health care was also contested. Representatives of the voluntary hospitals opposed the policy of removing all economic barriers to health care, including patient charges. They framed their opposition in terms of popular interest in hospitals: insisting that their objection was not a financial one, they warned that making the service free would remove the mechanism necessary to attract the active interest and support of the public.[56]

The minister of health and the department's civil servants had mixed reactions. They recognized the negative consequences of maintaining patient charges: they would preserve the practice of "relying on the element of fear to stimulate charitable contributions from the public." Some administrators, however, shared the hospitals' concern that a free service would undermine public attitudes toward voluntary hospitals, leading to their collapse. These departmental sympathies were reinforced by the possibility that voluntary hospitals would refuse to join a free service. The ministry recognized that building a new hospital service on the existing municipal hospitals, which were regarded as inferior, would certainly "perpetuate the present dualism."[57] To obtain the voluntary hospitals' participation and to retain their "appeal to the public sentiment," the ministry designed a compromise by which these facilities could charge inpatients a maintenance fee.[58]

53. MH 80/27, Memo, "Universality," unauthored, undated, probably written winter 1943–44.

54. MH 80/26, Memo, "NHS: Private Treatment by Doctors in the Public Service," from J. Maude to Minister, 9/7/43.

55. MH 80/32, Memo, "The Reasons for a 100% Service," probably 1/45; MH 80/28, Memo, "Comprehensiveness in a NHS," handwritten, "To be raised at meeting with Minister 1/23/45."

56. PIN 8/42, "NHS: Payments by Patients in Hospitals," by E. Brown to J. Anderson, 11/8/43; MH 77/30B, Minutes of meeting with voluntary hospital representatives, NHS (44) 16, 10/18/44.

57. PIN 8/42, "NHS: Payments by Patients in Hospitals," by E. Brown to J. Anderson, 11/8/43; CAB 124/422, Letter from Lord Woolton to H. Willink, 1/18/44.

58. MH 77/26, Memo, NHS 10, "Notes on the General Administrative Structure for Discussion with Voluntary Hospital Representatives," 3/43; MH 80/26, Memo, "Charging for Maintenance while in Hospital," probably around 9/43; MH 77/26, "First Rough Outline of a Scheme for a Comprehensive Health Service" (actually, this is probably the fourth draft,

Senior politicians were convinced, however, that the right to free hospital service enjoyed "the great weight of public opinion"; they repeatedly rejected the department's use of maintenance fees to maintain voluntary hospitals' goodwill. Challenging the ministry's tortured distinction between "free total treatment service" and "free maintenance," the reconstruction committee insisted that the entire system of patients' payments be abandoned.[59] The committee recognized that the public's hostility to linking treatment with money would put patient charges "out of harmony with the principle of social security" and lead to public resentment for yet another form of means test.[60] Under the cabinet's directive, the ministry obediently informed the voluntary hospitals that they must simply accept as settled policy that hospital care would be free of any charges at the time of treatment. In the context of evolving public expectations, politicians were convinced that individual payment would become an anachronism.[61]

In short, the influence of interest groups was weak on issues that enjoyed strong public support. On policy questions relating to free and universal access, politicians dismissed interest group pressure and rejected the conciliatory alternatives specified by bureaucrats.

Strong interest group influence. The remuneration arrangements for doctors and the role of private practice in the new service were two contentious issues on which interest groups exerted significant influence. On these issues, policymakers made substantial concessions to interest groups because they perceived the mass public as apathetic, uninformed, or even potentially supportive of interest group warnings of excessive state expansion.

Bureaucrats and politicians disagreed with interest groups over whether

---

which was completed 2/17/43); MH 77/26, Memo, NHS 27, "National Health Service," notes of a meeting of J. Maude, H. George, J. Hawton, J. Pater, B. D., and J. Wrigley, 7/2/43; MH 80/34, Memo, "NHS: Payments by Patients in Hospitals," by J. Maude, 12/11/43; CAB 87/ 12, Minutes of the Reconstruction Committee, PR (43) 24th, 10/15/43, and 29th, 11/1/43; CAB 87/5, Minutes of Reconstruction Committee, R (44) 2nd, 1/10/44.

59. MH 77/26, Notes of third meeting with medical profession, 5/17/43. The committee rejected the maintenance fee proposal during the fall of 1943 and January 1944. CAB 87/12, Minutes of the Reconstruction Committee, PR (43) 24th, 10/15/43, and 29th, 11/1/43; CAB 87/5, Minutes of Reconstruction Committee, R (44) 2nd, 1/10/44.

60. CAB 87/13, Memo to the Reconstruction Committee, PR (43) 76, "NHS," by T. Johnston (secretary of state for Scotland), 10/12/43. Also see CAB 87/13, Memo to the Reconstruction Committee, PR (43), 88, "NHS—Maintenance of Patients in Hospital," by T. Johnston (secretary of state for Scotland), 10/29/43.

61. CAB 87/5, Minutes of Reconstruction Committee, R (44) 3rd, 1/10/44; MH 80/34, Letter from Ministry of Health to J. Wetenhall, probably January or early February 1944; MH 77/30B, Minutes of meeting with voluntary hospital representatives, NHS (44) 16, 10/18/44; CAB 124/442, Minutes, Meeting between ministers and representatives of the voluntary hospitals, 1/18/44; CAB 124/422, Letter from Lord Woolton to H. Willink, 1/18/44; CAB 87/7, Memo to the Reconstruction Committee, Appendix B to R (44)24, "Main Changes in the White Paper Resulting from the Committee's Meetings of January 10th and 11th," 1/31/44; MH 80/34, Memo, "Voluntary Hospital Finance," probably spring 1944.

doctors should be remunerated by salary or on a capitation basis (i.e., the current NHI system of relating the reimbursement of doctors to their number of patients). Attempting to draw on potential public anxiety over excessive state development, the BMA fiercely opposed even partial payment by salary because it would reduce doctors to regimented civil servants. Instead of providing "an incentive to good work," the BMA charged that "making the doctor a salaried servant" would "tend to encourage stereotyped mediocrity in the medical profession."[62] The only alternative was to continue capitation payment.

There were pockets of strong opposition within the Ministry of Health to maintaining capitation fees precisely because they would reinforce competition among doctors. In spite of these objections, though, senior officials were sympathetic to the BMA's argument given the general public's low interest in the issue. As a senior official stressed, not "many patients are likely to be so well informed as to know how the doctors are being remunerated in the new service."[63] In the absence, then, of strong public interest in the details of the doctors' remuneration, bureaucrats and politicians tried to work out an alternative to a salaried service, something that combined basic salary and capitation fees. Although Conservatives pushed for enlarging the role of capitation and Labour ministers advocated a greater salary component (which their party had consistently supported), the coalition backed the compromise arrangement.[64]

The role of private practice by doctors in the new service was second major issue on which interest groups won significant government concessions. Attempting to stir public anxiety over the state's growing role, the BMA insisted that doctors working in the new state service have the right to decide whether they would practice privately.[65] Ministry officials recognized that the medical profession's position was motivated not just by financial concerns but by "finding themselves under much closer control" and by a "vague sense of the 'civil service' bogey." The BMA attempted to fuel the public's anxiety by warning that "all the individuality of the doctor's professional work will be throttled with regulations and controls."[66]

Again, ministry officials were not of one mind on this issue. A theme in

62. MH 80/26, Letter to secretary from Dr. Anderson (secretary, BMA), 5/12/43.
63. MH 80/25, Memo on attitudes of doctors, handwritten, "J. Hawton, 3/5/43."
64. CAB 87/5, Minutes of Reconstruction Committee, R (44) 3rd, 1/10/44; MH 80/26, Memo, "NHS. Summary of Main Happenings of the Year," handwritten, "J. Hawton, 11/43."
65. MH 80/26, Memo, "NHS," to secretary of state of Scotland, 6/43, handwritten, "Given to Secretary by G. Henderson, 6/28/43"; MH 80/26, Memo, "NHS: Summary of Main Happenings of the Year," handwritten, "J. Hawton, 11/43."
66. MH 80/25, Memo, "Appendix II: Note on a General Practice Service," handwritten, "J. Maude, 1/28/43"; MH 77/26, Memo, "National Medical Service: Whole-time v. Part-Time Service," 3/43, handwritten, "Internal Distribution Only."

departmental debates was the fear that allowing doctors to work simultaneously in the new service and in private practice would have an undesirable impact on the public. The aim of the new service, administrators argued, was that "it becomes, and is seen by all to be, a full health provision of the first class lines ... [and] it has no sort of taint of poor relief or social distinction."[67] Permitting doctors who joined the new service to conduct private practice at the same time would be "tantamount to admitting that the public service is a second best affair."[68] Instead of encouraging public recognition that the new system was quite unlike the panel system, the decision to allow doctors to run both private and public practices would "fix the notion of two kinds of medical consultation, two classes of patients." "We are led," one senior administrator predicted, "straight to the old conception of a second-rate [government] service for the working classes and a first-rate [private service] for those who can afford to pay for it."[69] Allowing public and private practice to coexist, then, would "ruin any chance we have of gradually getting the bulk of the population to look on the NHS as the first-line medical service for all, ... and not as something to be faintly ashamed of using, socially."[70]

In spite of these reservations, politicians and senior administrators remained preoccupied with the BMA's fierce opposition because they feared it would dampen public support for the new service and prompt the best doctors to refuse to join the new program. As a senior ministry official explained "it would be both right and politic to go to the utmost limit of concession" by mixing public with private practice.[71] The government presented its first major compromise in the white paper. Young doctors would have to enter the government health service full-time or not at all; but as a "concession to ease established doctors ... from the old ideas to the new," they could work simultaneously in the new service and in their private practice.[72] By April 1945, though, the minister fully capitulated to the BMA's

67. MH 77/26, Memo, "National Medical Service: Whole-time v. Part-Time Service," 3/43, handwritten, "Internal Distribution Only."

68. CAB 87/13, Memo to Reconstruction Committee, PR (43) 3, "A Comprehensive Medical Service," by E. Brown and T. Johnston (secretary of state for Scotland), 2/2/43.

69. MH 80/25, Letter from J. Maude to G. Henderson, 4/12/43. Also see MH 80/25, Memo on attitudes of doctors, handwritten, "J. Hawton, 3/5/43."

70. MH 77/26, Memo, "National Medical Service: Whole-time v. Part-Time Service," 3/43, handwritten, "Internal Distribution Only." Also see MH 80/31, Memo, "GP Service. Some Argumentative Points," by McNicol, 2/26/43; MH 80/26, Memo, "NHS: Private Treatment by Doctors in the Public Service," from J. Maude to Minister, 9/7/43.

71. MH 80/25, Memo, "Appendix II: Note on a General Practice Service," handwritten, "J. Maude, 1/28/43."

72. MH 77/26, Memo, "National Medical Service: Whole-time v. Part-Time Service," 3/43, handwritten, "Internal Distribution Only." Also see MH 80/26, Memo, "NHS: Summary of Main Happenings of the Year," handwritten "J. Hawton, 11/43"; MH 80/26, Memo, "NHS," to secretary of state of Scotland, 6/43, handwritten, "Given to Secretary by G. Hen-

unrelenting opposition; he agreed to allow even young doctors entering the state service to practice privately.[73]

The influence of medical producers on the formulation of basic principles contradicts Weberians' treatment of state autonomy; moderately strong capacity was associated with low state autonomy. Marmor's hypothesis that physicians' preferences determine governmental methods of payment (1983, 121) is confirmed by British policymakers' capitulation on the issues of remuneration and private practice. The formulation of basic principles is not, however, simply the story of interest group domination; instances of significant sectional influence were intermingled with state actors' adoption of policies (such as free and universal access) that defied fervent opposition from medical interest groups. When state actors concluded that "obstruction [by]... sectional interest [would] not be tolerated by public opinion," they readily took positions independent of medical producers despite the actual or implied threat by doctors and hospitals to withhold their services.[74]

The alternating weakness and strength of medical interest groups is not explained by the state's administrative capacity, which remained uniform within this single policy area; it is more adequately accounted for by state actors' balancing of public sentiment and interest group claims. The extent to which the state's continuous interaction with health care producers translated into actual influence varied according to policymakers' perception of public preferences and understandings. When the public was uninformed or "hazy," policymakers compromised; but they defied medical producers on issues that were "generally approved... by Parliament and public opinion."[75]

State Capacity and Administrative Arrangements

In addition to addressing the major principles of the new service, policymakers also specified and decided among detailed alternatives for its administrative structure. Ongoing discussions among interest groups, Ministry of Health officials, and cabinet ministers concentrated on altering the state's capacity—its specialization in, and hierarchical control over, health care.

---

derson, 6/28/43"; MH 80/26, Memo, "NHS: Private Treatment by Doctors in the Public Service," from J. Maude to Minister, 9/7/43; CAB 87/13, Memo to the Reconstruction Committee, PR (43) 55, "NHS," by E. Brown, 9/10/43; CAB 87/5, Minutes of Reconstruction Committee meeting, R (44) 13th, 2/5/44; CAB 65/41, Minutes of the War Cabinet, WM (44) 17th, 2/9/44; MH 80/27, Memo, "The White Paper Scheme," 2/10/44.

73. MH 77/119, Letter from H. Willink to E. Bevin, 4/26/45.

74. MH 77/31, Memo, "Notes for the Minister's Speech at Croydon," 5/12/44. Also see MH 80/27, Memo, "NHS," probably by F. Clark, 6–8/44.

75. MH 77/31, Memo, "Notes for the Minister's Speech at Croydon," 5/12/44. Also see MH 80/27, Memo, "NHS," probably by F. Clark, 6–8/44.

After Parliament's debate on the Beveridge Report in February 1943, politicians and policy specialists intensely debated the overall administrative framework, which would become the basis for subsequent policy discussions. The minister of health and his civil servants strongly advocated abandoning the inefficient prewar administrative structure, which had dispersed authority to decentralized government and private bodies; instead, they favored "going over to a rational system whereby one organization took care of health as a whole."[76] To strengthen the state's hierarchical control over health care, the ministry proposed that authority over the administration and planning of all health services be unified in a new "Health Authority." Under this proposal, all health services within specified regions would be placed under a single governmental body, which would be created by combining existing local authorities.

However attractive from a technical viewpoint, this proposal for a more firmly ordered system of authority ignored the political need to build consensus. In addition to intense interest group opposition,[77] cabinet ministers on the reconstruction committee were alarmed at the ministry's apparent disregard for public attitudes. Disregarding the minister of health's pleas about the merits of his capacity-enhancing proposals and the travesty of weakening them, the committee demanded a new set of proposals in July 1943.[78] By November 1943, a new minister more willing to pursue a consensus approach that weighed interest group concerns and public opinion had been appointed, the Conservative Henry Willink.

In spite of the ministry's confidence in and aggressive campaign for unified administration, politicians backed an organizationally weaker compromise. Separate administrative arrangements were designed for the service's three branches: hospital, GP, and clinic care. Public preferences and enduring understandings dominated the decision to adopt this tripartite organization and thereby disperse government authority. In particular, policymakers wrestled with two opposing sets of public attitudes toward state institutions, especially on the local level: widespread hostility toward local authorities because of their long-standing association with poor-law provisions, and

76. MH 80/26, Comments on the home secretary's note, probably in response to note in preparation for reconstruction committee's 7/30/43 meeting.
77. CAB 87/13, Memo to Reconstruction Committee, PR (43) 46, "NHS," by E. Brown, 7/28/43. The rejection of the ministry's proposals by the three interest groups is contained in MH 77/26, MH 80/25, and MH 80/26.
78. CAB 87/12, Minutes of Reconstruction Committee meeting, PR (43) 18th, 9/8/43; MH 80/26, Memo, "The Effect of the Decision of the Cabinet Committee," handwritten, "J. Hawton, 8/20/43"; MH 80/26, Memo, "NHS," by Department of Health for Scotland, 6/8/43; MH 80/26, Memo, "National Health Service," from J. Maude to minister, 9/4/43; MH 80/26, Comments on the home secretary's note, probably in response to note in preparation for reconstruction committee's 7/30/43 meeting; CAB 87/12, Minutes of the Reconstruction Committee, PR (43) 24th, 10/15/43.

widespread familiarity with these authorities, who were defended as embodying the democratic principles of popular participation.[79]

The proposed tripartite structure was intended to maintain local involvement in services of long-standing interest (hospital and clinic care) while not directly associating voluntary hospitals and GPs with management by these traditional poor-law authorities. Within this structure, GP services would be largely administered through a central body and clinic services left under their traditional local management; the new regional health authorities would manage the hospital branch, thereby allowing continued local government involvement without putting voluntary hospitals "under" direct local control.

After the summer of 1943, specialists generated and politicians chose among detailed proposals for a tripartite structure; perhaps the most important and controversial deliberations involved the service's two largest branches, hospital and GP care.[80]

Administrative arrangements for hospital service. Bureaucrats, politicians, and interest groups debated whether and to what degree the new service ought to establish a firmly ordered system of central authority over the country's two main systems of hospital care, its government facilities and its voluntary hospitals. These discussions were framed by new social understandings of the state (especially at the national level) and by public preferences for a state-run medical service that would take over voluntary hospitals, which were viewed as a nuisance that pestered the country for contributions.

Policymakers failed to take into account public support for the state's takeover of voluntary hospitals; they assumed that it was vital to preserve the independence and autonomy of voluntary hospitals. To preserve the two existing systems, they proposed bringing voluntary hospitals and the local authority hospital into a single system that would be operated by new regional health authorities.[81] These new amalgamations of existing local authorities would be given financial responsibility for both private and public hospitals. To policymakers who were simultaneously weighing public familiarity with local government services and popular unease with local

79. CAB 87/12, Minutes of Reconstruction Committee meeting, PR (43) 16th, 7/30/43; MH 80/26, Memo, "NHS: Summary of Main Happenings of the Year," handwritten, "J. Hawton, 11/43"; MH 80/26, Memo, "The Effect of the Decision of the Cabinet Committee," handwritten, "J. Hawton, 8/20/43"; CAB 87/13, Memo to Reconstruction Committee, PR (43) 49, "Administration of the New NHS," by H. Morrison, 8/17/43; CAB 87/12, Minutes of Reconstruction Committee meeting, PR (43) 17th, 8/18/43; BIPO 1943, 8–9; Eckstein 1958, 158–59.

80. See Webster (1988) for an exhaustive discussion of the full range of services that were designed.

81. MH 80/27, Memo, "The White Paper Scheme," 2/10/44; Pater Interview.

authorities, the new regional health authorities were attractive as "administrative devices of a new kind"—they "would not be a local government service as presently understood."[82] Under this compromise arrangement, the government's hierarchical control over hospitals would be marginally improved because all hospitals would be under government (albeit local) authority.

Representatives of the voluntary hospitals strongly opposed these regional health authorities because control over reimbursement was too decentralized. They feared that making hospitals rate-aided (dependent on local government financing) would cause the public to consider private facilities a poor-law service. Pinpointing the core of the difficulty, voluntary hospitals complained of the "psychological effect on the subscribing public" of "any direct payments by a particular local authority to a particular voluntary hospital"; it would create the "impression with the public that the hospitals were to be 'carried' by public funds according to need." Emphasizing the importance of avoiding "direct payment from *a* local authority to *a* voluntary hospital," they explained that "there was all the difference in the world between the private person's knowledge that a hospital was 'State-aided' and his knowledge that it was 'rate-aided'."[83]

As an alternative, the voluntary hospitals insisted on centralizing control over reimbursement to their facilities: they proposed that public funds given them come from the central exchequer and not from local authorities.[84] Drawing on new social understandings of the state, the voluntary hospitals' proposal was intended to maintain their respectability by distancing themselves from the stigma of local authority provisions.

Politicians' and bureaucrats' perception of public sentiment, however, led them to reject the voluntary hospitals' argument for greater hierarchical control over their reimbursements. In particular, Ministry of Health officials resisted the voluntary hospitals' demands to be singled out for central government reimbursement because such an arrangement would perpetuate the public's perception of a two-class hospital system. There was wide agreement within the ministry that such an arrangement would continue the old administrative system—local authorities funding only municipal hospitals—and would reinforce prevailing cultural patterns by

82. MH 77/26, Memo, "NHS 3," 3/2/43; MH 77/26, Minutes, "NHS 22," notes of second meeting with representatives of the medical profession, 4/15/43. Also see MH 80/26, Memo, "GP Service," by A. E. Hickinbotham, 8/23/43; CAB 87/12, Minutes of Reconstruction Committee meeting, PR (43) 16th, 7/30/43.
83. MH 80/26, John Hawton, "NHS: Summary of Main Happenings of the Year." 11/43; MH 80/32, Letter from J. P. Wetenhall to Minister, 11/8/44.
84. MH 80/26, Memo, "NHS: Summary of Main Happenings of the Year," handwritten, "J. Hawton, 11/43"; MH 80/32, Letter from J. Wetenhall, 11/8/44; MH 77/30B, Minutes of meeting with voluntary hospital representatives, NHS (44) 13, 10/5/44.

which municipal hospitals were perceived as poor-law institutions. As a senior official explained to hospital representatives,

> if all payments to voluntary hospitals from public funds came from central sources, there would grow up a dichotomy in the hospital services—the voluntary hospitals becoming regarded as "State-aided," the local authority hospitals as "rate-aided." The result would be a distinction in people's minds between two separate hospital systems, a tendency directly contrary to the general aim of achieving a single planned hospital system.[85]

Initially, at least, ministry officials marginally improved the state's hierarchical control. They specified arrangements to establish government authority over the administration and financing of both voluntary and local government hospitals, refusing to "establish one as a centrally arranged and centrally paid service, the other as a local one."[86]

Minister Willink, however, became consumed after the white paper's publication with "secur[ing] the whole-hearted co-operation" of health care providers; his strategy for pursuing reform amidst political deadlock was predicated on not "upsetting the existing state of affairs and existing interests."[87] His search for interest group goodwill not only reinforced policymakers' continuing misperception of public opinion (especially regarding voluntary hospitals) but also resulted in even weaker administrative arrangements. Despite his staff's continuing confidence in their department's organizational capacity, Willink further sought to calm voluntary hospitals' anxiety over public perceptions. He forced the ministry to gut the administrative authority of the new regional bodies; the new bodies' responsibility would be limited to planning, with administrative control left with the existing operators. To further appease voluntary hospitals, the ministry proposed reimbursing hospitals through a regional clearing house rather than through local authorities.[88]

The outcome, then, of policymakers' efforts was a weak administrative structure: they specified new hospital arrangements that failed either to

85. MH 77/30B, Minutes of meeting with voluntary hospital representatives, NHS (44) 13, 10/5/44.

86. MH 80/34, Letter from Minister of Health to J. Wetenhall, probably January or early February 1944. Also see MH 77/30B, Minutes of meeting with voluntary hospital representatives, NHS (44) 15, 10/17/44.

87. CAB 87/9, Memo to the Reconstruction Committee, R (44) 167, "NHS: Some Points Emerging from Recent Discussions with Local Authorities and Other Interests," by H. Willink, 9/27/44; MH 77/30B, Memo for meeting with voluntary hospital representatives, NHS (44) 8, "The Joint Authority and Hospital Services," probably spring 1944.

88. MH 80/34, Memo in connection with meeting with voluntary hospital representatives, NHS (45) 16, 2/28/45.

concentrate authority in the national government or even to establish local governmental authority over all hospitals.

Administrative arrangements for GP service. There is a significant parallel between discussions of the new hospital branch and deliberations over the GP service: in seeking to preserve existing arrangements for GP care, policymakers compromised the state's specialization and hierarchical control. The policy network's deliberations were framed by public support for extensive state involvement in GP care, as evident in the public's backing of health centers, and its fear that reform would produce only a glorified extension of the disliked panel system.

Under political pressure to build consensus, senior politicians and ministry administrators attempted simultaneously to preserve existing arrangements and to respond to strong public hostility to the panel system: the new alternative had to "secure the maximum amount of goodwill while at the same time enabling us to say that the new service is a distinct improvement over the old."[89] To reassure the public, policymakers insisted on salient changes that would "mark" the service's GP branch as drastically modified. Thus, ministers embraced the highly popular proposal to create health centers as "the declared policy of the Government."[90] But to garner the respect of the medical profession, the ministry and its political superiors decided that the new service could be based on the "simple extension of NHI technique"; reform would simply mean improving the efficiency of the existing system.[91] In particular, the "main responsibility for GP service would rest with the central Department" and, specifically, with the Minister-directed Central Medical Board (CMB). The CMB was to develop the institutional specialization to serve as the contracting and employing body for doctors; one of its functions was to control the distribution of doctors and to prevent "further doctoring in over-doctored areas."[92]

But Willink and other politicians reacted to criticism of the white paper by gutting plans for strengthening the state's hierarchy and specialization. Cabinet ministers joined the BMA in drawing on public unease over "soulless state control" to successfully attack the ministry's proposals because it would "establish ... a large bureaucratic machine." In his quix-

89. MH 80/26, Memo, "NHS," by Department of Health for Scotland, 6/8/43.
90. CAB 87/5, Minutes of Reconstruction Committee meeting, R (44) 4th, 1/11/44.
91. MH 80/26, Memo, "NHS: Summary of Main Happenings of the Year," handwritten, "J. Hawton, 11/43."
92. MH 80/26, Memo, "NHS: Summary of Main Happenings of the Year," handwritten, "J. Hawton, 11/43"; CAB 87/12, Minutes of the Reconstruction Committee, PR (43) 24th, 10/15/43. The board's policies would ultimately be directed by the minister, but doctors would be well represented; CAB 87/7, Memo to the Reconstruction Committee, Appendix B to R (44)24, "Main Changes in the White Paper Resulting from the Committee's Meetings of January 10th and 11th," 1/31/44; CAB 87/5, Minutes, R (44) 5th, 1/11/44.

otic pursuit of consensus amidst deadlock, Willink disregarded his administrators' arguments that charges of civil direction were a bogey and a "gross travesty of what is in . . . the White Paper."[93] Instead, he directed the ministry to address the medical profession's "instinctive dislike of a 'state' service."[94] In particular, the department curtailed the authority and specialized tasks of the Central Medical Board: it dropped some of the board's most important administrative powers and compromised its capacity to make expert decisions by granting the medical profession (through independent advising bodies) an important voice in the framing of policy. Only Labour's intervention prevented Willink from granting these advisory bodies the right to appoint their own members and publish their views, a prerogative that the ministry's own public relations official warned would "result [in] . . . political and every other kind of chaos."[95] Nevertheless, once in the caretaker government and unfettered by Labour, Willink eliminated the board altogether.

Between the Beveridge Report's publication and the coalition government's breakup in the spring of 1945, bureaucrats specified new principles and administrative arrangements and politicians made initial authoritative choices. These decisions, contrary to Weberian expectation, were not primarily determined by objective organizational capacity. Rather, public understandings and preferences were the primary focus of policy discussions. The cabinet's process for safely managing the reconstruction issue altered the calculations of politicians and specialists, convincing them that their interests were tied to policy formulation that responded in some measure to public opinion. Moreover, the coalition's behavior contradicts the Weberian claim that state autonomy from interest groups is a function of existing capacity. Moderately strong administrative capacity was associated with low state autonomy rather than the independence anticipated by Weberians; the government abdicated in the face of doctors' demands to mix public with private practice and to be paid on a capitation basis. With administrative resources remaining constant, the influence of medical interest groups varied according to policymakers' perception of public opin-

93. CAB 65/41, Minutes of the War Cabinet, WM (44) 17th, 2/9/44; MH 80/27, Memo, "White Paper on a NHS: Notes on Some of the Main Criticisms Expressed by Doctors in the Press and Elsewhere," probably early 1944.

94. MH 80/25, Memo on attitudes of doctors, handwritten, "J. Hawton, 3/5/43."

95. MH 80/27, Memo from F. Clark to S. F. Wilkinson, 1/4/44. Also see MH 77/119, Letter from Willink to E. Bevin, 4/26/45; CAB 87/5, Minutes of Reconstruction Committee, R (44) 2nd, 1/10/44; MH 80/26, Memo from A. Rucker to minister and secretary, 12/23/43; MH 80/27, Memo, "General," probably spring 1944; CAB 87/6, Minutes, Meeting of the Reconstruction Committee, R (44) 65th, 10/2/44; CAB 87/6, Minutes, Meeting of the Reconstruction Committee, R (44) 65th, 10/2/44; CAB 87/5, Minutes of Reconstruction Committee, R (44) 3rd, 1/10/44.

ion. In particular, state actors' sensitivity to strong and weak public sentiment was inversely related to sectional influence.

Finally, Weberian analysis indicates that the British state's moderately strong capacity should lead to stronger administrative arrangements. Indeed, bureaucrats were quite confident in their institution's capacity: anticipating contemporary complaints about today's fragmented and inefficient administrative arrangements, they proposed that the state enhance its specialization in and hierarchical control over health care. Nonetheless, the coalition sacrificed administrative strength and responded to perceived public opinion. It adopted a tripartite rather than unified framework and limited the state's organizational resources in the new hospital and GP branches; ultimately, the new hospital authority was reduced to a planning body and the Central Medical Board was elminated from the GP service. The result, in the words of several former senior civil servants, was a "dog's breakfast": with "one thing after another... conceded that shouldn't have been," implementing the service "would have been an administrative nightmare," requiring "a Ministry staff of arch-angels to work."[96]

Contrary to culturalist expectations, though, the coalition was in important respects unresponsive to public opinion; political deadlock and the pressure to pursue consensus contributed to elites' adoption of policies that contradicted public attitudes. Either misperceiving or deliberately defying public sentiment, policymakers insisted on preserving voluntary hospitals. Following Parliament's Beveridge debate, the public was suspicious of the coalition's intentions; this cynicism was well founded. Politicians and bureaucrats designed the new GP to be "founded on the familiar 'panel' system," with the popular health centers only "tried out gently."[97] Public preferences and understandings, then, could not simply be transmitted into government decisions.

Ultimately, the odds were stacked against the consensus approach attracting the necessary support to overcome persistent political division and pass major social welfare legislation. Endless compromises to split the difference between contending political and professional positions created the perception that the new service's costs and benefits would be unfairly distributed. From the public's perspective, the costs would be borne by all, but Britons also suspected that benefits—because of government timidity and sectional influence—would disproportionately favor the powerful. Interest groups disliked the new program because it promised to benefit others while shunting the burden of lost revenue and increased government infringement

96. Pater Interview; Godber Interview.
97. MH 80/26, Memo, "National Health Service," from J. Maude to Minister, 9/4/43; MH 80/26, Memo, "NHS: Summary of Main Happenings of the Year," handwritten, "J. Hawton, 11/43."

onto them. To formulate a reform package that demonstrably promised benefits to a large number of people required a different political context—one not divided between Conservatives, who were intent on leaving the postwar government with a free hand, and Labour, which advocated a redistributive program that responded to public demands. It would take a major shift in Britain's political climate before policymakers became willing and able to respond more fully to the mass public's support for major health reform.

7 | United States, 1960–1964: Kennedy's Inauguration and Johnson's Succession

Between November 1960, when John Kennedy was elected president, and the November 1964 presidential election, Americans' preferences and understandings of health care remained consistent: they strongly favored significant reform in the direction of Medicare's social insurance approach. The response of the national government was, however, neither immediate nor direct; rather, it was refracted through the prism of institutional and political conflict. Deliberations over Medicare were simultaneously promoted by presidential attempts (especially by Kennedy) to marshal existing public opinion and ensnared in political deadlock. Presidential appeals could not eliminate congressional opposition to bold Medicare reform, but the tandem of promotional politics and ongoing negotiations encouraged members of Congress to become more sensitive to public concerns. As a result of this heightened sensitivity to public opinion, members of Congress (including a majority of senators) joined administration efforts to build consensus behind a compromise health reform bill.

THE STRATEGIC UNIVERSE

Kennedy's prominent public appeals for Medicare's enactment were a critical catalyst in linking strong, sustained public opinion toward health reform with the legislative and executive decisions on interest group demands and future health policy.

Public Opinion

Following their established pattern of beliefs, Americans in the early 1960s identified health care for the elderly as a major problem and favored Medicare's proposed change in policy. These two trends in public preferences surfaced both in published polls and in the White House's private state-level surveys by Louis Harris and later Oliver Quayle III.[1]

Harris's private polls for Kennedy indicate that old-age problems and particularly medical care continued, as it had during the late 1950s, to be a highly salient issue. In his June 1962 study of New York state, for instance, Harris reported that interest in the elderly's health care was rising steadily.[2] Moreover, although newer issues relating to the economy, race, and peace gained increasing prominence as the 1964 election approached, the question of the elderly's medical care remained among the most frequently identified concerns in Quayle's surveys of six states.[3]

A tabulation of the issues covered in the *New York Times* provides a broad, indirect, indicator of the health issue's placement on the public's policy agenda; the *Times* gave it more extensive coverage between 1961 and 1964 than it gave other competing policy issues.[4] "With the possible exception of civil rights," the *Times* observed, "no domestic issue in recent years has produced a response from a greater cross-section of American opinion than Medicare" (quoted in David 1985, 108).

The public not only consistently identified the elderly's health care as a major concern but also continued to favor a particular policy direction, a reform of existing health care arrangements which enlarged the state's role via the Social Security system. In his state-level surveys leading up to the 1962 elections, Harris reported that the Medicare issue was "working for Democrats from one end of the country to the other."[5] In the important 1962 California gubernatorial race, for instance, Harris observed a dramatic rise of older people's problems as an issue: 31 percent favored Pat Brown's position, while only 11 percent backed Nixon's; by a more than 10 percent margin, respondents preferred the Democratic candidate's specific position

1. Harris studied fifteen states in the country's four major regions, with many being surveyed several times. See Jacobs 1990 for more detail. JFK Library, POF, Boxes 104, 105, and 106; R. F. Kennedy Papers, Attorney General's Correspondence, Box 15.
2. JFK Library, POF, Box 106, "A Study of Races for Governor and Senator from New York State," by Louis Harris, 6/62.
3. LBJ Library, CF PR16, Box 80, "Surveys of Public Opinion in New York, California, Oklahoma, Ohio, Indiana, Maryland," by Quayle, 4/64.
4. During the years 1961–1964, medical assistance and health insurance were mentioned 822 times in the articles and editorials of the *Times:* 191 times in 1961, 336 in 1962, 82 in 1963, and 213 in 1964. During this period, education and federal education policies were mentioned 262 times: 71 times in 1961, 61 in 1962, 60 in 1963, and 70 in 1964. The salient issue of federal aid for education was mentioned on 596 occasions: 313 times in 1961, 133 in 1962, 85 in 1963, and 65 in 1964.
5. JFK Library, POF, Box 104, "A Study of the First and Fourth Congressional Districts in West Virginia," by Louis Harris, 1/62. The White House and its pollsters regularly interpreted respondents' support for "helping the aged" and providing "medical care for the aged" as backing for the Medicare approach of building on the Social Security system.

on medical care for the aged. In Florida, Harris found that public support for medical care for the aged was still tremendously strong and a valuable issue for the incumbent senator to capitalize on.[6] His June 1962 analysis of New York concluded that a majority of respondents supported medical care reform and that such reform was one of the country's most popular issues: "The most promising two specific issues for the Democrats on national grounds are medical care for the aged and civil rights."[7]

Confirming these private reports, a published Gallup poll reported that 67 percent supported Medicare in May 1961.[8] Even more convincing evidence of public preferences before the elections was provided by a series of four Gallup polls in the spring and summer of 1962: when considering alternative approaches to financing the elderly's medical care, the public preferred the Medicare approach over that of private voluntary programs.[9]

Reforming the elderly's medical care continued to be a popular idea after the mid-term elections. In a rating of the administration's performance on several national issues, a majority of voters in five of the six states Quayle polled favored Kennedy and Johnson's efforts on behalf of Medicare.[10] The findings of the White House's private state-level surveys were confirmed by published data. Gallup polls reported that in October 1964 58 percent supported Medicare. A November 1964 survey by Michigan's Survey Research Center found that 75 percent would favor a federal law to provide medical care for the elderly.[11] In general, public support for health reform was stronger than it had been a decade earlier: based on his extensive review of opinion surveys, Schiltz concluded that Medicare clearly enjoyed greater popular support in the early 1960s than did national health insurance proposals in the 1950s (1970, 139).

The major alternative for addressing elderly health care, traditional public assistance to the poor, was quite unpopular. By the early 1960s, polls had tracked public attitudes about government financing of the poor's medical

6. JFK Library, POF, Box 105, "A Study of the Gubernatorial and Senate Elections in California, Wave II," by Louis Harris, 12/61, and "A Second Survey of the Political Climate in Florida," by Louis Harris, 12/61.

7. JFK Library, POF, Box 106, "A Study of Races for Governor and Senator from New York State," by Louis Harris, 6/62.

8. As Schiltz notes, the general form of the question was the following: "Would you favor or oppose having the Social Security tax increased in order to pay for old age medical insurance?" (1970, 140).

9. In March 1962, 55 percent preferred the Medicare approach while 34 percent favored private schemes; in May, 48 percent supported Medicare and 41 percent the private approach; in July 1962, the difference was 44 percent to 40 percent; finally, in August, the spread was 45 percent to 37 percent (Schiltz 1970, 170; Erskine 1975, 134).

10. LBJ Library, CF PR16, Box 80, "Surveys of Public Opinion in New York, California, Oklahoma, Ohio, Indiana, Maryland," by Quayle, 4/64.

11. The discrepancy in the findings of the October and November 1964 polls probably reflects the differences in question wording (Erskine 1975, 132).

expenses for nearly thirty years; the first poll conducted after the passage in the fall of 1960 of the Kerr-Mills bill recorded the lowest percentage of approval for public medical relief *and* the highest rate of disapproval for government financing of the poor's health care (Schiltz 1970, 128).

Public support for major health reform was anchored in Americans' emerging understanding and acceptance of the state's involvement in social welfare. This receptiveness was expressed in terms of Social Security, the most familiar and popular form of state social welfare provision. A June 1961 Gallup poll found that 67 percent favored increasing the Social Security tax to pay for health insurance for the aged. Providing even more convincing support, an April 1962 Gallup poll reported that a majority favored handling the medical care of the aged through Social Security rather than through private arrangements. Reiterating these findings, Harris reported after the Kennedy administration's first year in office that "putting [the elderly's health care costs] under Social Security is indeed a popular issue ... in every State we have surveyed in 1961."[12] He recommended that the Medicare issue be posed as a "moderate government program in the tradition of Social Security."[13]

Like the British, the American public was uninformed or hazy on Medicare's specific features. As Schiltz suggests, polling data indicated a very low level of public understanding of the details involved (1970, 142–43). It seems likely, then, that public support for Medicare was directed at the general principle of financing the elderly's health care through the familiar and popular Social Security system.

In the context of Americans' enduring understandings, however, the expectation of an expanded state role coexisted—far more intensely than in Britain—with an uneasiness over the prospect of excessive interference with accepted practices. Pinpointing Americans' ambivalence, a private poll in Kennedy's files reported that, "on balance, most people ... want something done—they have doubts only about the method."[14]

Political Struggles

Between the 1960 and 1964 presidential elections, national political struggles simultaneously encouraged prominent presidential appeals for public support of Medicare and negotiations between the administration and members of Congress to avoid deadlock. Kennedy was inaugurated into an

12. JFK Library, R. F. Kennedy Papers, Attorney General's Correspondence, Box 15, "A Study of the Primary Outlook in South Carolina," by Louis Harris, 12/61.
13. JFK Library, POF, Box 105, "Race for U.S. Senate in Indiana," by Louis Harris, 1962.
14. JFK Library, POF, Box 104, "A Study of Attitudes in North Dakota," by John Kraft, 4/63.

unenviable political position; he was saddled with a weak electoral mandate and a bipartisan conservative coalition in Congress. For a weak president, marshaling existing public opinion became an attractive strategy for enhancing his otherwise marginal influence on the governing process. Although members of Congress were unwilling to approve bold Medicare legislation, the White House found significant receptiveness to building consensus on a compromise bill: moderate Republicans were motivated by liberal sympathies and Democratic congressional leaders were eager to construct a record of their party's leadership. Under the accumulated impact of the White House's public appeals and its commitment to negotiation, policymakers became committed by 1964 to responding to public opinion with compromise legislation.

In spite of the vigor suggested by the "thousand day" blitz of "New Frontier" proposals that began his term, Kennedy's influence on domestic policy was unusually constrained. The narrow margin of his election victory gave him only a fragile mandate to govern; as Harris warned soon after the inauguration, the Republicans had seized the initiative on reading the mandate of the election.[15] The president was being challenged by Democratic members of Congress as well as Republicans. He found himself isolated and at odds with his own political party's majorities in the House and, after 1962, the Senate. Bipartisan conservative majorities, a member of Congress predicted to Kennedy shortly after the 1960 election, would defeat the administration's legislative program.[16] With the White House's domestic leadership stymied by congressional opposition, government policy was left—as Harvard political scientist Samuel Beer soberly explained—to be made by "a crazy quilt of feudal baronies where men with the mind of the American Dark Ages hold sway."[17]

Embattled but intent on influencing policy, administration officials engaged in a heated and protracted debate over two strategies for leading congressional deliberations on Medicare—prominent public appeals or relatively quiet negotiations among insiders. The insider strategy and its major proponent, Wilbur Cohen, accepted the political position of the president and Congress as a given until the next election; this approach concentrated on negotiation among politicians and specialists to build a broad congressional coalition. Another group contended that the president's political position was not an unyielding structural fact; they argued that by rousing existing public opinion the president could shake up the existing stalemate

15. JFK Library, POF, Box 30, Memo to president from L. Harris, 3/21/61.
16. JFK Library, POF, Box 49, Memo, "Enactment of the Kennedy 1961 Program in the Senate," attached to letter for president from Joe Clark, 12/15/60.
17. JFK Library, POF, Box 65, Letter to A. Schlesinger from Samuel Beer, 2/5/63 (forwarded to Kennedy); Interview with C. Daly by C. Morrissey, 4/5/66; Sorensen 1965.

and convert congressional opponents of his legislative proposals into supporters.[18] Partly because of political and personality conflicts, many Administration officials and members of Congress viewed the two strategies as mutually exclusive. But in fact they complemented each other; each drew attention to Medicare's prominence—one to its salience outside Washington, the other to its distinction within. Presidential appeals heightened policymakers' sensitivity to existing public opinion and negotiation highlighted the growing congressional interest in reform. By 1964, influential members of Congress made tactical adjustments to the point of nearly accepting compromise legislation.

A group of White House officials persistently counseled Kennedy that congressional opposition should be met with an orchestrated campaign. "The major need ahead for the Administration," a White House aide explained to the president, "is a deliberate program to marshal public support for our legislative proposals."[19] Instead of abiding by the outdated notion of the president as a "mysterious figure operating behind closed doors," White House press secretary Pierre Salinger emphasized the political benefit of "mak[ing] some direct appeals to the people"; these appeals would mobilize Americans to fight for their interests.[20] Arthur Schlesinger, Jr., similarly urged Kennedy to abandon the old habit of "tell[ing] the public as little as decently possible" in favor of extensive "public information"; the new style of "open government" would "rouse mass support" for "lively, innovating governments."[21] And pollster Harris joined the chorus: once the president's "fundamental constituency" (namely, the general public) had become "aroused and mobilized, Congress, business and all groups [would] respond as a man to the reverberating chorus."[22]

The White House fully realized that careless public appeals could fritter away scarce political capital and antagonize Congress on issues (such as economic policy) on which it would need legislative cooperation. Choosing from a large pool of conceivable issues, Kennedy took the calculated risk of renewing his previous identification with Medicare; he was lured back to Medicare because private polls and leading politicians' observations suggested that it was what people across the country wanted. With the White

---

18. The strongest advocates of rousing the public within the administration were the undersecretary of HEW, Ivan Nestingen, and White House official Dick Donahue, a close aide of Lawrence O'Brien. In addition to Arthur Schlesinger, Frederick Dutton and Pierre Salinger were White House aides who expressed general support for the president exercising popular leadership.

19. JFK Library, POF, Box 63, Memos from Dutton to president, 2/28/61 and 3/5/61; Ex FG1, Box 108, Memo from Dutton to president, 3/23/61.

20. JFK Library, Salinger Papers, Box 11, Memo from Salinger to Sorensen, 4/17/61.

21. JFK Library, POF, Box 65, Memo to president from A. Schlesinger, 3/16/61.

22. JFK Library, POF, Box 30, Memo to president from L. Harris, 7/26/62.

House regularly analyzing Harris polls, Kennedy and his aides accepted the pollster's report that medical care for the aged continued to be one of the dominant issues and "a veritable skyrocket... with the electorate."[23] Kennedy explained to one senator that, while other "issues had become so complicated the public had great trouble understanding them," Medicare was one of the few simple issues that he could talk to the people about.[24]

Administration supporters along with HEW and White House officials convincingly argued that presidential leadership which demonstrably crystallized existing public support could enhance Congress's receptiveness to Kennedy's health care proposal.[25] Although Congress typically concentrated on narrow, particularistic interests, an indisputable symbol of public support would (much as the Beveridge Report had) focus the attention of policymakers on a coherent and popular new direction for health policy; reaching outside Washington would unify forces within. As Harris and others explained, "if handled quietly, [Medicare] will die aborning in the legislative chambers" because special interests were "neither silent nor inactive"; but if "the President takes [this issue] directly to the people," members of Congress will focus on the general public's attitudes and special interests "will in short order [be] overpower[ed]."[26] Attracted by the public's continuing support of Medicare, Kennedy decided to once again get "personally involved and identified with the [Medicare] issue" by waging a "great fight across the land" for Medicare's enactment.[27]

The centerpiece of the administration's strategy was a week of over thirty rallies held across the country in May 1962.[28] These rallies culminated in a major speech by Kennedy to a sellout crowd in New York City's Madison Square Garden and to millions who watched it on one of the three national television networks. Kennedy was persuaded that the rallies represented a useful instrument for generating "eloquent demonstrations of the mass de-

23. JFK Library, POF, Box 105, Memo to president from L. Harris, 10/4/62. Also see POF, Box 50, "Notes for Congressional Sessions," 1/17/62, typed in upper corner, "TCS"; R. F. Kennedy Papers, Attorney General's Correspondence, Box 15, Table, "Trends of Public Opinion on Kennedy Administration," 2–12/61; POF, Box 105, "Public Reaction to the President during the First 60 Days," by Louis Harris, 3/22/61; POF, Box 30, Memo to president from L. Harris, 7/26/62.

24. JFK Library, Interview with Senator Gaylord Nelson by E. Bayley, 7/1/64.

25. Nestingen Interview.

26. JFK Library, POF, Box 105, "Public Reaction to the President during the First 60 Days," by Louis Harris, 3/22/61; Salinger Papers, Box 11, Memo from Salinger to Sorensen, 4/17/61.

27. JFK Library, M. Feldman File, Box 27, Letter to P. McNamara from the president, 8/30/61. Nestingen Interview.

28. Related attempts by the administration to draw on public support for Medicare include the following: the construction of vocal grass roots organizations; prominent presidential actions such as speeches, special messages to Congress, and press releases; and Democratic party distribution of information. David 1985, 55–58, 67–69; JFK Library, Ex LE/IS1, Box 483, Letter to R. Donahue from B. Carstenson, 2/28/63.

mand for this program."[29] An unquestionable sign of existing public opinion, it was hoped, would convince members of Congress to accept the administration's (accurate) interpretation—presented in both public and private forums—that no other domestic program had as much support as Medicare.[30]

The strategy of rousing the public failed, as even its advocates conceded, to create a conclusive sign that Americans overwhelmingly favored Medicare.[31] Pointing to the mere "ripple of interest" that met Kennedy's May 1962 speech, Samuel Beer suggested to Schlesinger that it was naive and futile to attempt to manufacture "great waves of public opinion" or even to assume that galvanizing the public would switch congressional votes and remove Congressional obstruction.[32] In fact, Mills concluded during the early 1960s: "I don't think that there was any . . . majority feeling for it." When pressed to approve Medicare, he questioned whether there was enough interest to justify increasing taxes to finance the program.[33] The administration's failure seemed to vindicate the charges of Medicare's opponents: there was no public clamor for the reform; it was "not in step with [the views] of the rest of the American people."[34] But, however disappointing these presidential appeals were, Kennedy did keep the spotlight of national media on Medicare; the glare was too much for many politicians to ignore altogether.

To proponents of the insider approach like Wilbur Cohen, the advocates of promotional politics were interlopers who disrupted negotiations and created a great deal of difficulty.[35] Whereas the strategy of prominent pres-

29. Nestingen Interview; JFK Library, POF, Box 38, Speech Files, "New York Rally, 5/20/62."

30. Testimony by A. Ribicoff (Secretary, HEW), U.S. Congress, House, Ways and Means Committee, 1961, p. 187; JFK Library, Interview with C. Daly by C. Morrissey, 4/5/66; POF, Box 50, "Notes for Congressional Sessions," 1/17/62, typed in upper corner, "TCS"; POF, Boxes 104, 105, and 106; R. F. Kennedy Papers, Attorney General's Correspondence, Box 15; POF, "A Study of the New 14th Congressional District in New York," Report no. 1171, by Louis Harris, 6/62; POF, Box 104, "A Study of the First and Fourth Congressional Districts in West Virginia," by Louis Harris, 1/62.

31. Nestingen Interview.

32. JFK Library, POF, Box 65, Letter to A. Schlesinger from Samuel Beer, 2/5/63 (forwarded to Kennedy).

33. Mills Interview. Also see JFK Library, Feldman Papers, Letter to president from Anderson, 8/8/62, regarding letter from Seymour Harris that president forwarded to Anderson; testimony by W. Reuther (President, United Auto Workers), U.S. Congress, House, Ways and Means Committee, 1961, p. 1652; testimony by G. Meany (President, AFL-CIO), U.S. Congress, House, Ways and Means Committee, 1964, pp. 1210–12; exchange between Mills and W. Wirtz (Secretary, Department of Labor), U.S. Congress, House, Ways and Means Committee, 1963, pp. 213–15.

34. Statement by committee member B. Alger, U.S. Congress, House, Ways and Means Committee, 1964, p. 1881. Also see JFK Library, Name File (Wilbur Mills), Box 1896, Letter to Mills from Congressman C. MacGregor, 7/20/62.

35. LBJ Library, Interview with Cohen by D. McComb, 12/8/68 (Tape 2).

idential appeal was to channel policymakers' attention outside Washington, the tactic of negotiation was directed at the politicians and specialists in Washington—at building common ground for reform. In particular, advocates of the insider approach sought to capitalize on a potential convergence of interest in reform: they labored to design compromises that would attract moderate Republicans and congressional leaders who were committed to constructing a record of Democratic leadership.

Efforts to build consensus through negotiation were an ongoing component of the administration's activities, evident in three critical arenas: within the administration, in the House Ways and Means Committee, and in discussions stemming from two votes on the Senate floor. Because Kennedy entered the White House committed to the enactment of Medicare, HEW began to formulate specific proposals shortly after the November election; these detailed arrangements were transmitted to the White House in the form of a draft bill subsequently presented to Congress in February 1961.

After this initial but critical set of deliberations, policy discussions shifted to Congress, where potential areas of compromise were explored. The Ways and Means Committee's two sets of hearings (summer 1961 and November 1963) became the focal point of negotiations among politicians, interest groups, and policy experts (the November hearings were resumed in January 1964 after Kennedy's assassination). Committee members, especially Republicans and conservative southern Democrats, were exceptionally deferential to their chairman Mills's political judgment and expertise. Cohen in particular worked with Mills to neutralize the opposition on both the committee and the House floor in order to get a compromise bill reported out.[36] In spite of optimistic forecasts by Cohen and other administration officials, Ways and Means never approved a bill and, as a result, the House never voted on Medicare before the 1964 election. Mills claimed that the coalition favoring Medicare was not large enough to justify the risk of bringing a bill to the House floor.

Although Ways and Means' control over tax policy ensured that it would be a focus of all policy deliberations, the administration twice attempted to force its hand by going to the Senate floor with Medicare amendments to House-passed bills, in July 1962 and September 1964.[37] Touting the outcome

36. Interview with Cohen by D. McComb, 12/8/68 (Tape 2); Cohen Interview; Nestingen Interview.
37. JFK Library, Interview with Mrs. Richard Bolling by R. Grele, 3/1/66; Ex LE, Box 467, "Possible Items for Discussion with the Legislative Leaders," 1/16/62; Nestingen Interview. Mills himself was reported to have privately recommended pressing for a Senate vote as a way to prompt favorable action in the House: JFK Library, Feldman Papers, Box 11, Memo to M. Feldman from W. Cohen, 1/4/62; O'Brien Papers, Box 10, Memo to president from M. Feldman, 1/6/62.

of inside negotiation, Cohen recommended to Sorensen in July 1962 that the White House seriously consider a compromise bill he had fashioned with moderate Republican senator Jacob Javits.[38] Although the White House was initially hesitant, it did decide to take the calculated risk of committing the president to the Senate amendment. This 1962 attempt at consensus building fell short, however, as the bipartisan opposition to Medicare—especially twenty-one southern Democrats—was enough to defeat the amendment.

Despite some White House criticism for unnecessarily tending to compromise, Cohen continued to pursue negotiations after the July 1962 Senate vote. Mills's seemingly critical decision in November 1963 to back Cohen's strategy of working out a compromise was derailed by Kennedy's assassination.[39] President Johnson was initially reluctant to endorse a compromise bill. Echoing the concerns of Conservatives in the British caretaker government, Johnson feared that endorsing a compromise would invite damaging political criticism for departing from his predecessor's commitments. Reversing his earlier ambivalence, Johnson made Kennedy's original bill a top priority in order to demonstrate that he was carrying on Kennedy's programs and was worthy of inheriting his predecessor's political base.[40] Cohen's drive for a compromise was put on hold; even reports of Mills's "great interest in fashioning a [revised] bill that will pass" did not alter Johnson's insistence on doing "what Kennedy wanted to do."[41]

By the fall of 1964, however, attention had shifted from the previous fall's tragic events to the approaching election. With Ways and Means abruptly concluding its deliberations in June without reporting out a bill, the administration and its supporters resumed negotiations with senators and designed another compromise package to be introduced as a floor amendment to a House-passed bill.[42] Unlike the 1962 vote, the Senate's September 1964 vote approved the Medicare amendment, marking the first time that one of the legislative chambers had passed a health insurance bill. The political stakes rose as the Medicare legislation was sent to a conference

38. JFK Library, Sorensen Papers, Box 36, Memo to Sorensen from Cohen, 7/6/62.
39. Nestingen Interview. JFK Library, POF, Box 39, Speech Files, Press release, "Remarks of the President," 7/17/62; Sorensen Papers, Box 35, "HEW Legislative Highlights (as of 11/22/63)," by Secretary Celebrezze; Cohen Interview; Mills Interview.
40. LBJ Library, Interview with Elizabeth Goldschmidt by M. Gillette, 11/6/74 (Tape 2); JFK Library, Interview with C. P. Anderson by John Stewart, 4/14/67; LBJ Library, Ex LE, Box 1, Memo to T. Sorensen from P. Hughes (Assistant Director, BOB), 12/24/63; Ex FG1, Box 9, Report, "The 1964 Johnson Legislative Program"; Panzer Papers, Memo to president from P. Southwick, 1/13/64; Ex LE/IS1, Box 75, "Suggested Draft of a Two-Minute Script for President Johnson to Be Included in a Film on Medicare"; Ex LE/IS1, Box 75, Remarks president delivered to group of Medicare supporters, 1/15/64; CF FG1, Box 16, Memo to president from Donald Cook, 11/27/63.
41. LBJ Library, Ex LE/IS1, Box 75, Memo to president from L. O'Brien, 1/27/64; Cohen Interview.
42. LBJ Library, Wilson File, Box 3, Memo to L. O'Brien from H. Wilson, 7/21/64.

committee to reconcile the House and Senate bills. Johnson and senior administration officials feared that failure to approve a Medicare scheme would be "seized upon by the press as a *major* and the *only* defeat for the President's legislative program."[43] As election day loomed closer, Cohen stepped up private negotiations in order to hammer out a compromise and Johnson was urged to pull out all the stops in pressuring the conferees to accept the compromise bill.[44] Nevertheless, the Medicare amendment died in the conference committee; Mills refused to agree to any compromise package.

Thus, in both the United States and Britain the consensus approach failed to build sufficient political support for health reform. Although it did not produce new legislation, deliberation over compromise arrangements did have an important impact on the policy-making atmosphere: it focused policymakers' attention on reform and on public opinion toward the issue. In the United States, the accumulated impact of Kennedy's promotional leadership and Cohen's negotiation with members of Congress produced growing pressure within Congress to respond to the public's embracing of Medicare. Policymakers' concern with attitudes outside Washington was heightened by Johnson's decision during the fall of 1964 to select Medicare as the centerpiece of his presidential election campaign. By the fall of 1964, influential members of Congress, including a southern senator, were convinced that Medicare was the hottest and most emotional domestic issue.

By 1964, even the risk-averse chairman of the Ways and Means Committee perceived growing public and congressional interest in the issue and freely acknowledged to the White House that a compromise approved by the House Conferees could be enacted.[45] Mills's rationale, then, for deadlocking the conference committee was not to permanently kill health reform. On the contrary, he no longer questioned either the existence of public support or the need for holding hearings; in the new policy-making atmosphere, he sought to design a "total package" that would respond to popular expectations and be "accepted as a solution of the problem." Mills's fear now was that the administration's narrow focus on hospital and catastrophic care would begin an uncontrollable process of piecemeal additions; he warned in 1964 that, after "people wake up to the fact that

43. LBJ Library, Ex LE/IS1, Box 75, Memo to L. O'Brien from Cohen, 9/24/64, forward to Johnson, 9/24/64.
44. LBJ Library, Wilson File, Box 3, Memo, "A Possible Compromise Social Security Bill," 9/9/64, attached to memo to M. Mantos and H. Wilson from Cohen; Memo to president from B. Moyers, 9/8/64.
45. LBJ Library, Mantos Papers, Memo to L. O'Brien from M. Mantos, 9/16/64; Ex LE, Box 2, Memo to L. O'Brien from H. Wilson, 9/11/64, forwarded to president, 9/11/64; Wilson File, Box 3, Memo to president from L. O'Brien, 9/13/64; Cohen Interview.

we're taking care of 25% of [the elderly's] medical costs," there would be great public disappointment and demand for further reforms. Mills adjourned the conference committee not with a defiant rejection of Medicare but with the promise that he would bring the proposal before the Ways and Means Committee as the first order of business in 1965.[46] In short, Mills and other politicians who had previously been ambivalent toward Medicare made tactical adjustments to reflect the new policy-making atmosphere.

POLICY DISCUSSIONS

By the time Kennedy edged out Nixon as Eisenhower's successor, major health care reform was a prominent item on the agendas of the mass public and of such government institutions as Congress and HEW. The political climate's evolution after the 1960 election encouraged politicians and specialists to specify and choose among alternatives for financing the elderly's health care. Policy discussions within the administration only days after Kennedy's election initiated formal debate on Medicare, and the critical deliberations of administration officials, members of Congress, and representatives of leading interest groups occurred in the hearings of the Ways and Means Committee.

State Autonomy and Basic Principles

State actors and major producer groups such as the AMA profoundly disagreed on two basic principles, Social Security financing and the elderly's access to health care. Polling data and historical evidence suggest that the country enthusiastically supported enlarging the state (via the Social Security system) in order to finance the elderly's health care. Americans were highly supportive of the Medicare approach and disliked the alternative, which restricted access by using a means test and financed benefits through the government's general revenues. In this context of established public sentiment, interest group attacks on the principles of access and Social Security financing had little influence.

In the debate over state involvement in financing the elderly's health care, a senior presidential adviser explained that the basic issue between the AMA and the administration was whether a means-tested public

46. Mills Interview; JFK Library, Interview with Mills by J. O'Connor, 4/14/67; LBJ Library, Moyers papers, Box 78, Memo to Secretary from Cohen, 7/2/64; Interview with Wilbur Mills by J. Frantz, 11/2/71; Ex LE/IS1, Box 75, Memo to L. O'Brien from Cohen, 9/24/64, forward to Johnson, 9/24/64; Marmor 1973, 56–57.

assistance program should be the basic program of protection for the aged.[47] The AMA and other groups erroneously claimed that the public supported their position of restricting state involvement to the poor-law arrangements created by the 1960 Kerr-Mills law.[48] In addition to claiming that the public preferred Kerr-Mills, conservatives on Ways and Means portrayed Medicare's assumption that "everyone is entitled to good health by an agency of the Federal Government" as alien to enduring public understandings. Medicare was not only out of step with public opinion, it threatened to undermine American values: interfering with "many million[s] [of older people] who do not need help" would "destroy the [country's] . . . moral fiber" and undermine the traditional "concept of individual and family responsibility."[49] In place of the unwanted and dangerous Medicare approach, the AMA and its allies insisted that Kerr-Mills deserved a chance to prove itself.[50]

By November 1964, the administration and influential members of Congress had arrived at a different interpretation of public sentiment, one that led them to dismiss interest group arguments. Consistent with polling data and the uniformly negative meaning attached to poor-law arrangements, politicians and administrators argued that "giv[ing] benefits only to *some* of [the elderly] who meet an income test would . . . change the character of the program from social insurance to 'welfare' " and would be perceived by Americans as "humiliating" and "undignified."[51] It was feared that reliance on the Kerr-Mills poor-law arrangements would not only prompt many of the aged to forego greatly needed medical care but would also alienate public support; it would invite a backlash among the general public reminiscent of recent popular demonstrations against recipients of means-tested benefits.[52] Convinced that Americans had "outgrown the philosophy of the Elizabethan poor laws" and would resent returning to them, Kennedy

---

47. JFK Library, Sorensen Papers, Box 36, Memo to president from M. Feldman, 6/7/62.

48. For example, see the testimony by Dr. E. Annis (President, AMA), U.S. Congress, House, Ways and Means Committee, 1963, p. 783.

49. Statement by committee member T. Curtis, U.S. Congress, House, Ways and Means Committee, 1961, pp. 406; statement by committee member B. Alger, U.S. Congress, House, Ways and Means Committee, 1961, pp. 1449.

50. JFK Library, Interview with Mrs. Richard Bolling by R. Grele, 3/1/66.

51. JFK Library, POF, Box 79A, Memo to president from Cohen, 5/10/63; JFK Library, Feldman Papers, Box 27, Letter to president of the Senate from the president, 2/13/61. Also see statement by committee member A. Ullman, U.S. Congress, House, Ways and Means Committee, 1961, pp. 314–15; testimony by A. Celebrezze (Secretary, HEW), U.S. Congress, House, Ways and Means Committee, 1963, pp. 30–31; JFK Library, POF, Box 42, Speech Files, Annual message to Congress on state of the union, 1/14/63.

52. Testimony by A. Hayes (President, International Association of Machinists), U.S. Congress, House, Ways and Means Committee, 1961, p. 1092; JFK Library, Sorensen Papers, Box 36, "Comments on AMA . . . Telecast Opposing Kennedy-Anderson Bill—for President's Press Conference," 5/28/62.

and other senior officials were adamant—even as they pursued consensus—that the introduction of a means or income test was not in the area of acceptable compromise.[53]

As an alternative to the Kerr-Mills approach, the president relied on the "sound and proven Social Security principles" because they were "one of the most popular approaches in America."[54] In place of demeaning means tests, Medicare would provide financing "on terms that older people find acceptable."[55] Medicare advocates argued that, in addition to appealing to the elderly, the program was "tailor made for Mr. Average American": by simply "exten[ding]" the "*tried and tested* insurance method," the program would be "familiar" and "desirable" to Americans in general.[56] The administration and influential members of Congress, including Mills, defied interest group opposition; they remained convinced that Social Security's principle of "eligibility and entitlement for all, regardless of income" would have wide popular appeal.[57]

Discussion of Medicare's coverage—what group of aged should have access—was another contested principle; it raised two specific questions: What test of retirement should trigger eligibility? Should the aged who were not insured under Social Security be covered or "blanketed-in"? Beneficiaries' eligibility would be triggered by reaching retirement age. Noting that sixty-eight was the average age of retirement, an HEW administrator reasoned in early 1961 that it might therefore be a more logical starting point than sixty-five. Concerned not to violate Americans' expectations that working people could meet their health costs through nongovernmental means, he suggested that "includ[ing] 1 to 2 million persons who are regularly employed merely because they have passed their 65th birthdays seems . . . to belie [Medicare's] premise."[58]

53. JFK Library, Sorensen Papers, Box 36, "Suggested Opening Statement by the President for Next Press Conference," 6/12/62; POF, Box 79A, Memo to president from Cohen, 5/10/63.

54. JFK Library, Feldman Papers, Box 27, Letter to president of the Senate from the president, 2/13/61. Also see DHEW Microfilm, Roll 25, Letter to F. Hayes (Housing and Home Finance Agency) from R. G. Conley (HEW civil servant), 12/62; Ex IS1, Box 381, Letter to *Medical Tribune* from president, 5/21/62.

55. Testimony by A. Ribicoff (Secretary, HEW), U.S. Congress, House, Ways and Means Committee, 1961, pp. 28–29.

56. Statement by committee member A. Ullman, U.S. Congress, House, Ways and Means Committee, 1964, pp. 1878–79; JFK Library, Salinger Papers, Box 12, "Health and Social Security for the American People," 1/10/61. Also see testimony by A. Ribicoff (Secretary, HEW), U.S. Congress, House, Ways and Means Committee, 1961, pp. 184–85; testimony by A. Celebrezze (Secretary, HEW), U.S. Congress, House, Ways and Means Committee, 1963, pp. 32–33.

57. JFK Library, Feldman Papers, Box 27, Letter to president of the Senate from the president, 2/13/61; DHEW Microfilm, Roll 25, Letter to F.Hayes (Housing and Home Finance Agency) from R. G. Conley (HEW civil servant), 12/62.

58. JFK Library, DHEW Microfilm, Roll 24, handwritten, "Health Insurance Bill, A. W. Willcox, 1/15–16/61."

Senior officials in HEW and the White House, however, offered a different interpretation of public understandings; they emphasized the public perception of Social Security, which set eligibility at sixty-five. Although lowering the retirement age from sixty-eight to sixty-five would cost a third more, the administration's primary concern was to build on existing public expectations; policymakers decided to "avoid public misunderstanding" by establishing the same age base for eligibility for medical benefits as for monthly insurance benefits.[59]

The issue of whether the elderly who were not insured under Social Security should be "blanketed-in" was also raised; because the uninsured had not contributed to the program, general revenues would be used to finance their protection. The opposition to blanketing-in the uninsured included not only the AMA but also some Medicare advocates. Doctors warned that encompassing all Americans over sixty-five was the first step to universal coverage. Reformers took a different angle, cautioning that blanketing-in would undermine public attitudes, which undergird the Social Security system. "Treating contributors and non-contributors alike," Cohen advised, "might raise questions about the whole contributory basis of the system" and weaken "public acceptance . . . that the right to benefits is acquired through . . . contributions"; Cohen asked, "Why pay if you can get the same protection anyway?"[60]

Authoritative policymakers ultimately were not swayed by these reservations; instead, they focused on the public's exceptional interest in the elderly's hardships and its expectation that Social Security cover all Americans over sixty-five. By 1964, the White House and Mills modified their earlier positions and agreed to establish equal access regardless of whether beneficiaries are presently insured.[61] In the face of strong public support, then, state actors adopted basic principles that were opposed by leading interest groups.

---

59. DHEW Microfilm, Roll 24, "Reasons Pro and Con for Social Security Administration's Recommended Changes in the Anderson-Kennedy Bill," 1/3/61, "for meeting with Secretary-designate," 1/5/61. Also see JFK Library, DHEW Microfilm, Roll 24, "Proposed Specifications for Medical Insurance Benefits," 12/16/60; Feldman Papers, Box 27, Attachment to letter for president from HEW secretary (A. Ribicoff), 2/10/61; DHEW Microfilm, Roll 24, Memo from W. Stewart (Public Health Service) to Ellen Woolplert (Surgeon General's Office), 12/7/60.

60. JFK Library, DHEW Microfilm, Roll 24, Letter to Senator C. P. Anderson from Cohen, 9/11/61.

61. JFK Library, DHEW Microfilm, Roll 24, and Feldman Papers, Box 27, Memo to director of the BOB from Labor and Welfare Division, 1/22/61; DHEW Microfilm, Roll 15, "Significant Improvements in Anderson Bill (S. 909) made by Anderson Amendment to the Welfare Bill (HR 10606)," probably originally completed in the early summer of 1962, handwritten, "Revised later in Senator Anderson's Office, 9/27/62"; DHEW Microfilm, Roll 25, Memo to Cohen from R. Ball, 1/9/63; DHEW Microfilm, Roll 25, Letter to David Bell (Director, BOB) from A. Celebrezze (Secretary, HEW), 11/9/62; Feldman Papers, Box 11, Memo to T. Sorensen from Cohen, 12/19/62; LBJ Library, Ex LE/IS1, Box 75, Memo to president from L. O'Brien, 5/11/64.

Strong interest group influence. On two other contentious issues, however, policymakers perceived the public as apathetic or potentially supportive of sectional claims: limiting coverage of services to hospital care and charging patients a deductible. On these issues, policymakers reached compromises that substantially replied to interest group concerns.

Members of the health policy network disagreed over whether services covered under Medicare should be limited to hospitalization or extended to provide comprehensive protection, including the services of doctors. Both the BOB and the Public Health Service division within HEW pushed for coverage of comprehensive medical care. To these administrators, it seemed irrational to create a new program that "le[ft] many oldsters subject to economic deprivation"; failure to cover care outside hospitals could also increase Medicare's cost by creating a "necessity or temptation to institutionalize" beneficiaries and provide expensive hospital treatment.[62] Administration officials were joined by Mills, who recommended to Kennedy and later Johnson that "the way to start" the program was to "take care of the costs of the doctor bill and other related services."[63]

Nonetheless, reformers successfully resisted efforts to liberalize Medicare by including comprehensive care. In Britain, the long-standing social interactions with hospitals as well as Friendly Societies and NHI panels created public expectations of a comprehensive health service, which policymakers could not ignore. But American politicians and specialists formulated policy in a profoundly different cultural context. Given Americans' ambivalence toward the state and comparatively limited understanding of health care, policymakers naturally did not detect strong public demand; in this comparative silence, interest group attacks on Medicare seemed deafening.

The AMA in particular fiercely criticized Medicare for threatening to impose control on hospitals, doctors, and patients; the result would be "production lines of disinterested physicians."[64] The catchphrase "socialized medicine" was viewed by the AMA as a "big help in prejudicing the public" and in reminding policymakers of Americans' uneasiness with the state.[65]

American policymakers addressed interest group charges, but they did

62. JFK Library, DHEW Microfilm, Roll 24, and Feldman Papers, Box 27, Memo to director of the BOB from Labor and Welfare Division, 1/22/61; DHEW Microfilm, Roll 24, "Public Health Service: Recommendations for Legislation for Health Benefits for Aged Persons," handwritten, "Sent to Governor A. Ribicoff... on 12/28/60."

63. Mills Interview; LBJ Library, Interview with Wilbur Mills by J. Frantz, 11/2/71.

64. Testimony by Dr. E. Annis (President AMA), U.S. Congress, House, Ways and Means Committee, 1963, pp. 652–53; testimony by Representative F. Bow, U.S. Congress, House, Ways and Means Committee, 1964, p. 1095; testimony by Dr. F. Groner (President, AHA), U.S. Congress, House, Ways and Means Committee, 1961, p. 250.

65. Harris 1966, 128. Also see statement by committee member T. Curtis, U.S. Congress, House, Ways and Means Committee, 1961, pp. 404–6; testimony by Dr. E. Howard (AMA), U.S. Congress, House, Ways and Means Committee, 1961, pp. 1436–37.

not expect (as their British counterparts did) to win interest group goodwill; they fully anticipated that the great majority of physicians, would oppose any Medicare bill, no matter how carefully designed. Accordingly, they narrowed Medicare's scope in order to blunt the AMA's potential appeal to the public; as a high ranking HEW administrator explained, "avoid[ing] payments to physicians...makes the AMA opposition less relevant."[66]

To make interest group criticism "less relevant," Medicare's coverage was limited to focus on hospital costs and exclude doctor services. Preoccupied with "what we thought the country was ready at the time to accept," policymakers consciously patterned Medicare—as a liberal senator explained to Kennedy—"after that type of health insurance which has experienced by far the greatest acceptance on the part of the American people— insurance against hospital costs."[67] Medicare advocates within the Administration and Congress aligned their reform proposals with Americans' acceptance of the elderly's hospital costs as the most important problem.[68]

Reformers' insisted that Medicare not cover the cost of services performed within the hospital by private doctors, namely, radiologists, anesthetists, pathologists, and physiatrists. The administration's initial decision to include these specialists drew support from one of Medicare's nominal opponents, the AHA, which testified that excluding them from legislation would "reduce the hospital element to a nursing home with an operating room."[69] Covering a patient's stay in the hospital without including specialized treatment seemed ludicrous.

Concerned, though, that the public might be potentially alarmed by AMA objections about socialized medicine, administration and congressional officials came to agree with an HEW administrator that it was "better to omit all physicians' services than to open the bill to attack on that ground."[70] At an exceptional meeting of reformers following the Senate's defeat of Medicare in 1962, no one suggested expansion of the program to cover doctor service.[71] Policymakers insisted on distancing Medicare from the

66. JFK Library, DHEW Microfilm, Roll 24, "Health Insurance Benefits," attached to covering slip from R. Ball to S. Saperstein, 1/16/61; DHEW Microfilm, Roll 24, "Social Security Administration Comments on Public Health Service Recommendations," 1/4/61; Feldman Papers, Letter to president from Anderson, 8/8/62, regarding letter from Seymour Harris that president forwarded to Anderson.
67. JFK Library, Feldman Papers, Letter to president from Anderson, 8/8/62, regarding letter from Seymour Harris that president forwarded to Anderson.
68. Testimony by A. Ribicoff (Secretary, HEW), U.S. Congress, House, Ways and Means Committee, 1961, pp. 186–87.
69. Testimony by Dr. F. Groner (President, AHA), U.S. Congress, House, Ways and Means Committee, 1961, pp. 256–57.
70. JFK Library, DHEW Microfilm, Roll 24, "Issues in the Health Insurance Bill," approximately 1/24/61. Also see DHEW Microfilm, Roll 24, Memo to Cohen from S. Saperstein, 1/24/61.
71. The meeting, which consisted of HEW officials and Medicare advocates from outside

appearance of state domination and being able to credibly declare that no services performed by physicians would be affected; to do so, they were willing to capitulate to AMA criticism and exclude all doctor services including those performed by the specialists.[72]

On the issue of including a deductible provision in Medicare, interest groups also significantly influenced policy. A group of politicians and specialists asserted that Medicare should cover the "first dollar" of the elderly's financial cost rather than require beneficiaries to pay part of the initial cost through a deductible. White House and HEW officials argued that instead of encouraging treatment, a deductible in effect imposed a means test. Beneficiaries would have to pay a charge to receive treatment; in consequence, many sick individuals would be deterred from obtaining timely medical care.[73] In addition to introducing the despised means test, patient charges would defeat "one of the basic purposes of the health insurance proposal": deductibles would drive the retired back to public assistance (to meet the cost of the deductible, many beneficiaries would have to retreat to poor-law programs).[74] If deductibles were enacted, "the public [would] ... feel it has been deluded." Although policymakers promised that Medicare would "assure care to the aged as a matter of right, regardless of financial need," patient charges would either have the deterrent effect of a means test or actually force the elderly to rely on public assistance.[75]

In the absence of an outpouring of public support for free care (as in Britain), administration officials and their supporters concluded that it was politic to include deductibles as a concession to medical interest groups and their sympathizers in Congress. Disregarding the reservations about deductibles, the White House joined the secretary of HEW and Cohen in bowing to "strong feeling in Congress [that] ... the aged should have some financial responsibility for meeting the costs of their health care."[76] In Brit-

government, concentrated on reassessing the bill's prospects after the Senate defeat in July; JFK Library, DHEW Microfilm, Roll 25, Letter to Hirst Sutton from Cohen, 11/7/62, forwarding minutes of meeting of consultative group on the administration's proposed health insurance program for the aged on 10/29/62.

72. Testimony by A. Celebrezze (Secretary, HEW), U.S. Congress, House, Ways and Means Committee, 1963, pp. 34–35; JFK Library, DHEW Microfilm, Roll 25, "Brief Summary of the President's Proposal for Hospital Insurance for the Aged," prepared by Social Security Administration, probably 1963.

73. JFK Library, Feldman Papers, "Improvements Needed in Anderson-King Bill (HR 4222)," F. Dutton forwarded to M. Feldman, 4/3/61.

74. JFK Library, DHEW Microfilm, Roll 25, Memo to Cohen from R. Ball, 1/9/63.

75. Testimony by Dr. F. Groner (President, AHA), U.S. Congress, House, Ways and Means Committee, 1961, pp. 250–52.

76. JFK Library, DHEW Microfilm, Roll 25, Letter to Hirst Sutton from Cohen, 11/7/62, forwarding minutes of meeting of consultative group on the administration's proposed health insurance program for the aged on 10/29/62. Also see DHEW Microfilm, Roll 24, "Major Modifications of Bill to Amend Title II of the Social Security Act to Provide Health Insurance Benefits," attached to memo for T. Sorensen from secretary, probably sent early 1/61.

ain, policymakers' sensitivity to their country's expectations led them to reject such arguments as heard in the United States—that patient charges would instill a "desirable deterrent to excessive care and . . . [an] element of individual responsibility." In the United States, the absence of widespread public support for free care convinced policymakers that satisfying interest group demands and appeasing congressional concerns would be more politic.[77]

American policymakers, then, strictly adhered to principles that enjoyed strong popular backing, while conceding to interest group claims when the public seemed hazy or potentially supportive of those claims. Episodes of seemingly inexplicable government concessions (like excluding coverage of specialists from coverage of specialist-oriented hospital care) coexisted with policymakers' stubborn defiance of interest groups when they clearly contradicted the "people's will." Contrary to Weberian expectations, the moderately weak American state exercised significant autonomy from major producers on important principles. Politicians' and bureaucrats' independence from interest groups, then, was a function not of "objective" organizational capacity but of policymakers' perception of public preferences and understandings.

State Capacity and Administrative Arrangements

Debate on the use of the Social Security approach, an HEW official complained shortly after Kennedy's election, "grossly overshadowed other important policy questions relating . . . to the administration of the program."[78] After Kennedy's inauguration, administration officials, members of Congress, and interest groups began to address this imbalance by specifying and deciding among detailed alternatives for changing the state's health care administrative structure. In particular, there were significant disagreements within the policy network over two issues related to changing administrative arrangements—the expansion of the central state into new areas and the significance of such expansion for the program's future.

Policymakers intensely disagreed about whether and to what degree the state ought to establish hierarchical control over and specialization in the new financing program for the elderly. These deliberations simultaneously drew on and were constrained by Americans' ambivalence between contin-

77. JFK Library, DHEW Microfilm, Roll 24, "Reasons Pro and Con for Social Security Administration's Recommended Changes in the Anderson-Kennedy Bill," 1/3/61, "For meeting with Secretary-designate, 1/5/61; DHEW Microfilm, Roll 24, "Major Modifications of Bill to Amend Title II of the Social Security Act to Provide Health Insurance Benefits," attached to memo for T. Sorensen from secretary, probably sent early 1/61.

78. JFK Library, DHEW Microfilm, Roll 24, "Issues to Be Resolved," "Draft, 12/22/60, M. Pond."

uing suspicion of state provisions and growing acceptance of the Social Security system. The administration and its congressional supporters were committed to responding to strong public preferences for Medicare by using Social Security to expand the state's role. Medicare advocates persistently strove to design new administrative arrangements for the program that would not arouse the public's uneasiness over state interference. Their solution was to forge a new state role but on an administratively weak foundation.

In January 1961, the recently elected Kennedy administration pulled together the Medicare proposal it would send to Congress. During this critical period, officials within HEW and especially the BOB outlined the consequences of establishing a new government program and strenuously argued for direct and strong central state control over the disbursement and use of that program's funds.

HEW was confident about its capacity to perform the necessary specialized tasks. To control the quality of care, HEW was certain that it could and should prescribe standards for participating providers of service; such standards would assure Medicare beneficiaries a minimum level of care. Moreover, HEW found it entirely feasible to negotiate contracts with producers that would minimize unnecessary services and unreasonable costs. As an HEW official matter-of-factly explained: "Negotiation of . . . rates of payment to hospitals is a relatively simple fiscal and cost accounting procedure"; "[it] can be accomplished expeditiously and at [relatively low cost] . . . by the use of electronic processing equipment of the [Social Security Administration]."[79] The BOB shared HEW's confidence in the central state's administrative capacity and in the prospect that the health department could readily carry out the function of reimbursing hospitals directly. HEW, BOB, and others were confident, then, in the state's organizational capacity to provide "direct Federal administration"; it seemed feasible and "necessary for the government to develop an entirely new machinery."[80]

Senior BOB administrators emphasized to the White House and Kennedy himself that failure to develop and utilize a strong federal administrative organization would have dire future consequences; without one, the new program would contribute to further inflation of medical costs. Compared

79. JFK Library, DHEW Microfilm, Roll 24, "Reasons Pro and Con of the Use of Private Health Insurance Agencies in the Administration of a Health Insurance Program," 1/4/61, handwritten, "For meeting with Secretary-designate, 1/5/61." Also see DHEW Microfilm, Roll 24, "Proposed Specifications for Medical Insurance Benefits," 12/16/60; DHEW Microfilm, Roll 24, "Summary of Health Insurance Proposals," attached to letter for Senator Anderson's assistant from Cohen, 2/8/61; Feldman Papers, Box 27, Memo to director of the BOB from Labor and Welfare Division, 1/22/61.

80. JFK Library, DHEW Microfilm, Roll 24, "Issues to Be Resolved," "Draft, 12/22/60, M. Pond."

to the government's substantial organizational capacity, institutions outside Washington, civil servants warned, "may not be strong from an administrative standpoint and may not be as responsive or desirable for a program where . . . the costs are to be paid by the Federal Government."[81]

These technical arguments for strong, direct administration were, however, disregarded by politicians and specialists. Instead, policymakers agreed that gaining public acceptance for a government health insurance plan made it necessary to deflect rather than fuel attacks on Medicare for expanding the state.

In particular, the AMA and others directly appealed to the public's anxieties by charging that Medicare would trample on the "traditional American system" and introduce "a Government-controlled and compulsory system."[82] Soon after Medicare's passage, hospitals and doctors would be entombed in "the definitions, the requirements, the restrictions" concomitant with state domination.[83] The AMA reasoned that, because "control follows money when the Government steps in," "numerous rules and regulations must be promulgated" to "assur[e] the Government that the services have been rendered satisfactory."[84] These new state controls would strike at the heart of the "constitutional American way": they put "patient freedom . . . at stake"; "the patient's choice to freely select his doctor and his hospital" would be limited by Medicare's requirement that he choose a facility under contract to the government.[85]

Administration officials and congressional officials fully realized that the AMA's warnings about socialized medicine were merely "a bogeyman . . .

---

81. JFK Library, DHEW Microfilm, Roll 24, and Feldman Papers, Box 27, Memo to director of the BOB from Labor and Welfare Division, 1/22/61. Also see Feldman Papers, Box 27, Note to T. Sorensen and M. Feldman from David Bell, 1/24/61; DHEW Microfilm, Roll 24, "Reasons Pro and Con of the Use of Private Health Insurance Agencies in the Administration of a Health Insurance Program"; testimony by A. Celebrezze (Secretary, HEW), U.S. Congress, House, Ways and Means Committee, 1963, p. 162.

82. Testimonies by Dr. L. Larson (President, AMA), and Dr. E. Annis (representative of the AMA), U.S. Congress, House, Ways and Means Committee, 1961, pp. 1302–3, 1308–9, 1439; statements by committee members J. Byrnes and B. Alger, U.S. Congress, House, Ways and Means Committee, 1961, pp. 1818, 1824.

83. Testimony by L. Stetler (AMA staff member), U.S. Congress, House, Ways and Means Committee, 1961, pp. 1430–31. Also see testimony by Representative F. Bow, U.S. Congress, House, Ways and Means Committee, 1964, p. 1095

84. Testimony by Dr. E. Annis (President, AMA), U.S. Congress, House, Ways and Means Committee, 1963, pp. 652–53; testimony by Representative F. Bow, U.S. Congress, House, Ways and Means Committee, 1964, p. 1095. Also see testimony by Dr. E. Howard (AMA), U.S. Congress, House, Ways and Means Committee, 1961, pp. 1436–37; testimony by Dr. F. Groner (President, AHA), U.S. Congress, House, Ways and Means Committee, 1961, p. 250; statement by committee member T. Curtis, U.S. Congress, House, Ways and Means Committee, 1961, pp. 404–6.

85. Testimony by Dr. E. Howard (AMA), U.S. Congress, House, Ways and Means Committee, 1961, pp. 1436–37; testimony by Dr. L. Larson (President, AMA), U.S. Congress, House, Ways and Means Committee, 1961, pp. 1444–45; Harris 1966, 123.

to scare the American people," but they concluded that such warnings might indeed be successful in arousing public unease and dampening support.[86] To defuse potential public unease, they ignored the recommendations for enhancing state capacity and instead pursued three strategies for dispersing authority and ceding specialized functions to private organizations.

Sensitive to Americans' ambivalence toward state provisions, bureaucrats repeatedly refrained from performing one of their central functions: clearly specifying the details of proposals. Civil servants in HEW successfully argued that it was preferable to sacrifice the clarity of the language and risk administrative problems than to include services and provisions that could be perceived as socialized medicine.[87] They repeatedly recommended that Medicare exclude government services such as veteran administration hospitals and "omi[t] . . . some or all of the detail" including "statutory references to the Secretary and his regulatory authority."[88]

In a second strategy to defuse potential public anxiety over state control, policymakers decided to create an "intermediary" between hospitals and the federal government by decentralizing reimbursement and relying on familiar private agencies such as Blue Cross to negotiate rates and pay hospital bills. The use of Blue Cross to establish a "buffer" between hospitals and government was expected to enjoy "virtually universal acceptance" by hospital administrators. More important, this buffer was expected to be favorably perceived by the general public; it ensured that the "individual recipient would . . . appear as an independent, voluntary subscriber and not as a ward of the Government."[89] The White House as well as influential members of Congress, then, supported the use of private agencies because they would defuse the "widespread and vocal concern" about government control or interference.[90]

Politicians and specialists received ample high-level warnings that dis-

---

86. Testimony by A. Ribicoff (Secretary, HEW), U.S. Congress, House, Ways and Means Committee, 1961, pp. 181–82. Also JFK Library, Sorensen Papers, Box 36, "Suggested Opening Statement by the President for Next Press Conference," 6/12/62; testimony by A. Celebrezze (Secretary, HEW), U.S. Congress, House, Ways and Means Committee, 1963, pp.34, 134.

87. JFK Library, DHEW Microfilm, Roll 24, handwritten, "Health Insurance Bill, A. W. Willcox, 1/15–16/61."

88. JFK Library, DHEW Microfilm, Roll 25, Memo to A. David from S. Saperstein, 2/13/63. This concern was echoed in JFK Library, DHEW Microfilm, Roll 24, "Issues in the Health Insurance Bill," approximately 1/24/61, and Memo to Cohen from S. Saperstein, 1/24/61.

89. Testimony by Dr. D. Wilson (representative of the AHA), U.S. Congress, House, Ways and Means Committee, 1963, pp. 352–54; JFK Library, DHEW Microfilm, Roll 24, "Health Insurance Benefits," attached to covering slip from R. Ball to S. Saperstein, 1/16/61.

90. LBJ Library, DHEW Microfilm, Roll 24, Letter to Hirst Sutton from Cohen, 11/7/62, forwarding minutes of the 10/29/62 meeting of consultative group on the administration's Medicare proposal. Also see Mantos File, Box 9, Memo to L. O'Brien from M. Mantos, 9/15/64; JFK Library, POF (Box 79A) and Sorensen Papers, Box 36, Memo to president from A. Ribicoff, 6/2/62.

persing HEW's administrative responsibilities by using Blue Cross agencies would begin an irreversible process of rapid cost escalation, with the anticipated result "a more costly and less satisfactory service." Nevertheless, policymakers were simply more concerned with addressing the public's perception of the state than with the consequences of weak administrative arrangements; they sensed little support and potentially broad opposition to direct administration by the federal government itself and concluded that the "public relations advantages" of establishing a buffer would "outweigh some of the basic advantages of greater speed, flexibility and control which come from a direct-line operation."[91]

A third strategy for blunting the AMA's appeal to public unease was to give Medicare beneficiaries the option of choosing whether their contribution would entitle them to receive insurance coverage from a government plan or from a private scheme. Cohen and other HEW officials counseled against the option provision: instead of serving beneficiaries, it would force millions of people to make difficult decisions. Outlining a public relations and administrative nightmare, these policy specialists warned that the option provision would invite "general confusion . . . [and] exploitation" and result in "large-scale dissatisfaction from people who had made 'wrong choices'."[92] In effect, Cohen and HEW officials were alarmed that the option provision would nullify a large part of the state's role: the government could be reduced to merely a collection agency for private insurance companies, with its authority dispersed to nonstate bodies throughout the country.

Nonetheless, politicians decided that giving the individual a clear choice and some "freedom" provided another, if admittedly "unworkable," mechanism to mitigate potential public anxiety. After 1963, Kennedy and the Senate and conference committee agreed that the option provision demonstrated Medicare's reliance on freedom of choice and voluntary rather than compulsory provisions. Reflecting policymakers' preoccupation with the constraints of American culture, Cohen compromised his administrative judgment and counseled the White House and members of Congress to "forget about whether it will work for the time being."[93]

In short, presidents Kennedy and Johnson, as well as members of Congress, insisted on fundamentally compromising Medicare's administrative organization in order to bolster its argument that government meddling in

91. JFK Library, DHEW Microfilm, Roll 24, "Health Insurance Benefits," attached to covering slip from R. Ball to S. Saperstein, 1/16/61; DHEW Microfilm, Roll 24, and Feldman Papers, Box 27, Memo to director of the BOB from Labor and Welfare Division, 1/22/61.
92. JFK Library, DHEW Microfilm, Roll 15, "An Option to the Three Choices for Basic Benefits under Private Insurance," unauthored and probably 6/62; Cohen Interview.
93. Cohen Interview. Also see testimony by A. Celebrezze (Secretary, HEW), U.S. Congress, House, Ways and Means Committee, 1963, p. 59; David 1985, 90–91.

health care would not be possible.[94] Policymakers fled from unambiguous statements of new government authority and embraced Blue Cross and the option provision; all these decisions were aimed at undermining the state's hierarchical control and specialization: its authority was radically dispersed and private organizations were entrusted to provide the necessary expertise. To demonstrate that Medicare would pose no "threat to the freedoms we cherish," politicians and specialists willingly ceded control over enormous sums of government-collected funds to nonstate organizations which would "serv[e] less as the Government's agent than as the representative of the hospitals."[95]

Administrative arrangements and potential for future development. A second major issue in policy deliberations involved the future significance of new admnistrative arrangements; at the core of this debate was Medicare advocates' peculiar approach to reform—an approach that dramatically departed from that pursued in Britain. In a British coalition racked by divisions between Labour and Conservative ministers, politicians and bureaucrats ultimately agreed on the objective of future health policy: the entire population would be entitled to a comprehensive range of health services. Labour and other supporters of reform hoped to use the country's overwhelming acceptance of this objective, enshrined in the Beveridge Report, to gradually build support for the necessary means—a significant state role in financing and providing health care. In the United States, Medicare's advocates took a nearly opposite approach: reformers used the public's acceptance of the means (the Social Security system) to gradually build support for their unspoken but firmly held objective of creating a universal and comprehensive health insurance.

American reformers concluded after the successive defeats of health insurance plans that the objective of comprehensive, universal coverage was inconsistent with American attitudes and should not be openly discussed. To align health reform with existing public opinion, they pursued an incremental strategy of building on the public's enthusiasm for the Social Security system and hospital care; once the Social Security approach to financing the elderly's hospital costs was established, reformers would make

94. Testimony by A. Celebrezze (Secretary, HEW), U.S. Congress, House, Ways and Means Committee, 1963, pp. 34, 134; JFK Library, POF, Box 79A, Memo to L. O'Brien from A. Ribicoff, just prior to 6/2/62; DHEW Microfilm, Roll 25, "Brief Summary of the President's Proposal for Hospital Insurance for the Aged," prepared by Social Security Administration, probably 1963.

95. JFK Library, Sorensen Papers, Box 36, "Suggested Opening Statement by the President for Next Press Conference," 6/12/62. JFK Library, DHEW Microfilm, Roll 24, Letter to Hirst Sutton from Cohen, 11/7/62, forwarding minutes of the 10/29/62 meeting of consultative group on the administration's Medicare proposal. Also see testimony by A. Ribicoff (Secretary, HEW), U.S. Congress, House, Ways and Means Committee, 1961, pp. 181–82.

small improvements until the entire population and range of services were covered. Medicare's advocates, then, conceived of the program not as an end in itself but rather as a means or, to borrow the phrase of its opponents, as a "first step" toward the unannounced objective of comprehensive, universal health insurance. This incremental strategy had an unintended consequence: the means came to define the ends. After Kennedy's election, political expediency repeatedly persuaded reformers to foreswear the real objective and to insist that the "provision of complete medical care ... was never the philosophy of our bill."[96] In pursuit of what was supposed to be the means (Medicare), reformers effectively sacrificed their long-term objective by deliberately, even eagerly, designing Medicare to prevent the program's future development.

In an odd switch of roles, Medicare's opponents were left to identify the objective of health reform—in order of course to assail it. The AMA and others charged that, as the first step in imposing socialized medicine, Medicare would lay the basic groundwork for later expansions. Once Medicare was implemented, public expectations would rise and reformers would agitate for extending coverage both to doctor and other health costs and to other groups and perhaps ultimately the whole population.[97]

To dampen public anxiety and assure skeptical congressional leaders that "hospital insurance for the aged ... is where it will stop," Medicare's advocates designed and supported administrative arrangements that would establish a "safeguard" or "built-in governor on the political escalation of the whole program."[98] In particular, policymakers sought to limit Medicare's development by designing two safeguards that would be securely anchored in public attitudes.

The first safeguard was to make Medicare fully financed by contributions.[99] Cohen explained that relying on self-financing methods would put a "brake on increasing costs ... because you have to raise the employee

96. JFK Library, Feldman Papers, Letter to president from Anderson, 8/8/62, regarding letter from Seymour Harris that president forwarded to Anderson. Also see DHEW Microfilm, Roll 24, "Observations on the Medical Assistance for the Aged Program," 1/4/61, handwritten, "For meeting with Secretary-designate, 1/5/61; Sorensen Papers, Box 36, "Possible Question by John Herling," "TCS—Press Conference, 6/7/62"; testimony by A. Ribicoff (Secretary, HEW), U.S. Congress, House, Ways and Means Committee, 1961, pp. 219–20; LBJ Library, Ex LE/IS1, Box 75, Memo to president from L. O'Brien, 1/27/64.

97. Statement by committee member T. Curtis, U.S. Congress, House, Ways and Means Committee, 1961, pp. 200–201; testimony by Dr. F. Groner (President, AHA), U.S. Congress, House, Ways and Means Committee, 1961, p. 250.

98. Testimony by A. Celebrezze (Secretary, HEW), U.S. Congress, House, Ways and Means Committee, 1963, pp.36–37,163–64; testimony by Senator J. Javits, U.S. Congress, House, Ways and Means Committee, 1964, pp. 1270–71.

99. JFK Library, Salinger Papers, Box 12, "Health and Social Security for the American People," 1/10/61.

contribution to pay Social Security."[100] To ensure that Medicare would in fact and appearance be a self-financing program, the administration and members of Congress decided to create a separate trust fund for the collection and disbursement of Medicare's contributions.[101] Reformers made incremental expansion less likely by demonstrably linking concentrated benefits with distributed costs: future change would require large numbers of wage earners to bear increased taxes for benefits targeted to isolated groups.

The second safeguard involved the Kerr-Mills program. Rather than seeking the elimination of the decentralized poor-law system, senior administration officials emphasized to apprehensive members of Congress that Kerr-Mills would play an important supplemental role in the country's overall health care.[102] Demand for additional health care benefits, would be controlled by the public's negative perception of poor-law programs: those needing services not covered by Medicare would have to turn to Kerr-Mills and its means-tested programs. Thus, while British policymakers eliminated the poor-law system, their American counterparts emphasized its constructive role in deterring future requests for more benefits.

According to Weberians, the influence of producer groups and the direction of future institutional changes are primarily a function of policymakers' assessment of the state's objective administrative capacity. Indeed, the outcome of this stage of Medicare's formulation (low hierarchy and specialization) is in part consistent with Weberian expectations concerning the direction of institutional change in a weak state; in the British state, which enjoyed comparatively more extensive administrative capacity, policymakers specified and seriously considered stronger organizational arrangements.

Although the outcome may be somewhat unsurprising, the story of health policy formulation under the British coalition government and the Democratic White House is unexpected. It was state actors' perception of public

100. JFK Library, Ex LE/IS1, Box 75, "Social Security: The Conservative Approach," talk Cohen gave to a medical profession audience, 10/64. Also see testimony by Cohen (Assistant Secretary, HEW), U.S. Congress, House, Ways and Means Committee, 1963, pp. 88–89. Cohen's argument was reiterated by the secretary: testimony by A. Ribicoff (Secretary, HEW), U.S. Congress, House, Ways and Means Committee, 1961, pp. 181–82.

101. LBJ Library, Wilson File, Box 3, "Possible Modifications in King-Anderson Bill," attached to 1/24/64 minutes of meeting with Mills; Cohen Interview; David 1985, 90–91.

102. JFK Library, Feldman Papers, Letter to president from Anderson, 8/8/62, regarding letter from Seymour Harris that president forwarded to Anderson; DHEW Microfilm, Roll 24, "Observations on the Medical Assistance for the Aged Program," 1/4/61, handwritten, "For meeting with Secretary-designate," 1/5/61; Sorensen Papers, Box 36, "Possible Question by John Herling," "TCS—Press Conference, 6/7/62"; testimony by A. Ribicoff (Secretary, HEW), U.S. Congress, House, Ways and Means Committee, 1961, pp. 219–20; LBJ Library, Ex LE/IS1, Box 75, Memo to president from L. O'Brien, 1/27/64; testimony by A. Celebrezze (Secretary, HEW), U.S. Congress, House, Ways and Means Committee, 1963, pp. 30–31.

preferences and understandings that was the primary focus of—and influence on—policymakers' decisions regarding interest group influence and new institutional changes.

Although political struggles in the United States and Britain occurred in fundamentally different contexts, they had a similar impact on policymakers' strategic calculations; political struggles heightened state actors' sensitivity to public opinion and their willingness to make authoritative choices among alternative principles and administrative arrangements. In particular, politicians' and bureaucrats' perception of public opinion produced complex negotiating patterns with interest groups. This bargaining defies simple categorization in terms of the organizational capacity of either the entire state or the departments responsible for health care: the variable outcome was related not to administrative resources, which remained constant, but to alternating levels of strong and weak public opinion.

Moreover, American and British policymakers specified and accepted dramatically different institutional changes; these changes in state capacity were primarily produced by variations in public preferences and understandings. American policymakers drew on public enthusiasm for Social Security to forge a major new role for the national government, but they remained reticent state builders, acutely sensitive of the public's enduring ambivalence toward the state. To counter the AMA's warnings of socialized medicine, presidents Kennedy and Johnson as well as members of Congress attempted to downplay the appearance of government control and to emphasize that in both the short and long term there would be no interference with the established practices for providing health care. Thus, while the British policymakers were discussing a massive state role and comparatively strong administrative arrangements, their American counterparts profoundly compromised Medicare's authority over and specialization in the distribution of government funds.

Deliberations over Medicare and NHS also present evidence that contradicts Weberian expectations. Politicians and bureaucrats in the moderately weak American state should—according to Weberians—exert minimal independence, settling into a relationship with producer groups that is dominated by cooperation and concessions. In the case of Medicare, however, American policymakers persistently exercised high independence from interest groups on specific issues. Moreover, contrary to Weberian expectations, administrators in HEW and the BOB did have high confidence in their institution's capacity, and they aggressively lobbied President Kennedy for direct federal administration. But the White House and members of Congress did not seriously consider these capacity-enhancing arguments because they were preoccupied with enduring public attitudes. The Medicare case, then, is characterized by the coexistence of strong confidence in state capacity and proposed institutional changes that would establish weak administrative arrangements.

Although policy decisions in the United States and Britain diverged substantially, both countries pursued a consensus approach that ultimately proved ineffective in enacting legislation. Consensus builders vainly struggled to fashion compromises that would win broad support for wide distribution of new health benefits. But building consensus through compromise antagonized more than it pleased; by 1945 in Britain and 1964 in the United States, there only seemed to be losers.

PART IV

*Bold Innovation
in Ongoing
Policy Discussions*

8 | Britain, 1945–1946: The Labour Government and the National Health Service Act

After landslide results in Britain's July 1945 elections and America's November 1964 races, politicians and bureaucrats decided the final shape of health legislation. The elections provided indisputable evidence of public support for innovative legislation; this perception created nearly irresistible incentives for policymakers to pursue reform. With public opinion becoming their central concern, they continued to weigh the long-standing claims of medical producers but significantly altered their previous bargaining relations with these groups.

Historic episodes of legislative innovation in the United States and Britain have typically been interpreted as representing either radical change or continuity: they have been presented alternately as radical transformation or implementation of an already formed consensus.[1] This bifurcation of historical interpretation has obscured the most significant aspect of watershed legislation, the intermingling of strong elements of both change and continuity. Landslide victories create strong pressures on policymakers to respond to public opinion by pursuing bold and lasting innovations, but even during these extraordinary periods politicians and bureaucrats build on and therefore preserve long-standing public understandings and practices. In terms of Medicare and NHS, the final alternatives specialists generated and politicians chose represented breakthrough innovations in ongoing discussions and established arrangements. The most important characteristic, then,

---

1. For the general debate on continuity and change in Britain's postwar government, see Addison 1977 and Morgan 1984. For discussion of these themes in terms of the NHS, see Fox 1986; Webster 1988; Klein 1983; and Pater 1981. There is no comparable debate for Medicare; the themes of continuity and change are expressed in a somewhat different form in Beard 1913 and Hofstadter 1955 and 1948; see also Morone 1990.

of major reform is the admixture of strong commitments to both bold change and continuity.

Labour's showing in the British elections in July 1945 was among the rarest of political events, a landslide upset. After the election, the previous pattern of public opinion remained stable; Britons continued to support reform of prewar social welfare arrangements, specifically health policy. Labour's landslide, though, did significantly affect the political context. By dramatically propelling Labour out from under Conservative party domination and into a position of dominance in national politics, the elections motivated policymakers to respond to the seemingly indisputable shift in public attitudes.

The Labour government found an exceptionally receptive political environment for making two bold departures from previous discussions and arrangements: it formulated major new reforms (like nationalization of hospitals) and introduced proposals to Parliament which the coalition government had discussed but been unable to draft into bill form. The pursuit of innovation, though, coexisted with a commitment, by even the government's most ardent reformers, to continuity and to avoiding an abrupt break. Labour's health legislation emerged from organized, ongoing bargaining among cabinet ministers and Ministry of Health officials;[2] although continuing to weigh medical producers' long-held claims, policymakers restructured the policy network to significantly curtail direct interest group participation.

The Strategic Universe

By the collapse of the coalition government in the spring of 1945, clear patterns of public opinion toward health reform had developed, but the health policy network was unwilling or unable to respond effectively. As an unmistakable expression of public opinion, Labour's landslide profoundly altered policymakers' calculations, intensifying their sensitivity to public concerns and their commitment to bold changes. The formulation of the NHS was most directly affected by developments between July 1945 and March 1946, when the government submitted its bill to Parliament.

2. Senior Ministry of Health officials during this period included W. S. Douglas, followed by W. Jameson, J. C. Wrigley, A. N. Rucker, and J. Hawton. Middle-level officials included J. Pater, S. F. Wilkinson, and A. E. Hickinbotham.

Public Opinion

The Conservative and Labour parties entered the 1945 election favoring pragmatic reform of health care and avoiding divergent positions: the Conservatives feared criticism for abandoning the Beveridge Report; Labour expected its opponents to portray the party as radical and irresponsible (Addison 1977, 261–64). In spite of what was said, or left unstated, each party's electoral message was dominated by the public's wartime perception of the two parties; voters seemed to face a distinct choice between returning to prewar arrangements or introducing bold reforms.

Because of the Conservatives' wartime opposition to domestic reconstruction, the public—as evident in polls and MO reports—feared that the party was eager to "get back to normal in the 1939 sense." The the Conservatives seemed to be the party that had been lukewarm on the Beveridge Report (Marwick 1970, 365–66). In stark contrast, Labour alone seemed to project the new mood, to express the "new foundations of public opinion." During the war, the Labour party had been perceived as a committed advocate of reform, as evident by the overwhelming rank-and-file opposition to the coalition's tepid handling of the Beveridge Report. Analysis of polls and election results by British historians suggests that Labour was uniquely identified with social welfare reform and greater state involvement (Addison 1977, 261–64; Morgan 1984, 44–45).

Although preelection polls repeatedly reported strong preferences for a Labour government (Gallup 1976), "practically no one," according to a qualitative study by MO, had "any suspicion of what the results would be."[3] "Everyone saw Churchill," a senior Ministry of Health official recalled, "as 'the War Hero' and everyone thought that people were going to vote for 'the War Hero'."[4] But for British voters, there were apparently two distinct governments—one associated with foreign policy and the other with domestic affairs. Support for "the man who won the war" was separate from and subsumed by deep-seated public fear of a return to prewar conditions. The consequence of this split in voters' evaluations "completely astonished" the country;[5] in a staggering upset, Labour won a 146-seat majority, its first (and to this date largest) independent majority in the House of Commons.

Labour's victory represented a popular mandate to provide innovative

3. MO, File Report 2270 A, "A Report on the General Election, June–July 1945," 10/45, pp. 124.
4. Pater Interview.
5. MO, File Report 2270 A, "A Report on the General Election, June–July 1945," 10/45, pp. 125.

leadership. The Conservative's lopsided loss reflected, according to MO's prewar analysis, a "movement of allegiance *away* from the Old Order" and "*away* from the established institutions ... implicated in the bitter, anxious past."[6] Polls confirmed MO's report that Labour's victory expressed a "real hope for the future [and for] ... something new that was to be seriously and earnestly tried out."[7] A Gallup poll shortly after the election found that 56 percent felt the "election results mean that the British people want the Labour party ... to introduce sweeping changes such as nationalization"; only 30 percent viewed them as indicating that the party should "govern along existing lines only more efficiently."[8]

Labour received a mandate to lead in a particular policy direction. Echoing the consistent findings of sixteen Gallup polls between December 1943 and May 1949, MO reported that the "top civilian grumbles after six years of war centered on food, shopping, clothing difficulties and housing troubles."[9] Labour received strong public support for its decision to immediately generate legislation to address pressing domestic problems. During the active period after the election, polling respondents consistently gave high marks to Labour's prime minister, Clement Attlee, and the cabinet itself, which in November 1945 was approved by 57 percent and disapproved by only 16 percent (Gallup 1976, 121).

There was, then, strong public concern regarding the essentials for survival—food, clothing, and shelter. Although Britons did not identify health care on their short list of essentials, they nonetheless did express strong interest in and support for Labour's handling of medical reform. Reflecting the high salience of the health reform issue, an April 1946 Gallup poll reported that 65 percent were following Parliament's discussion of the NHS (Gallup 1976, 130–31). Health care's exceptionally high placement on the country's agenda was indirectly reflected in the *London Times* coverage of policy issues. The health issue received far more newspaper coverage between July 1945 and the end of 1946 than other major domestic policies: it attracted twice the coverage of social insurance and unemployment combined.[10]

In addition to remaining salient, health legislation that promised to en-

6. MO, File Report 1676, "M-O's Bulletin," 5/10/43; File Report 2234, "M-O Bulletin for April–May 1945." Harrisson 1944.

7. MO, Flle Report 2270A, "A Report on the General Election, June–July 1945," 10/45, 129.

8. The question was the following: "Do you think that the election results mean that the British people want the Labour party to govern along existing lines only more efficiently, or to introduce sweeping changes such as nationalization?" (Gallup 1976, 112).

9. MO, File Report 2376, "M-O Bulletin New Series no. 1," 3–4/46.

10. Between July 1945 and December 1946, health policy was the subject of 316 articles; social insurance and unemployment attracted 153 pieces.

large the state's role and introduce free, comprehensive care continued to enjoy strong popular backing. In an extensive Gallup poll in April 1946, respondents agreed by a 3-to-1 margin that the government's health care proposal would result in better health services for the country as a whole.[11] Health reform was supported by a majority of respondents across all age and economic groups, as well as by all political groupings except Conservative party supporters. The popularity of the proposal rested in large part on its commitment to the principle of universality: respondents felt that the reform would result in better health services mainly because it would create the "same chance of good treatment for all, rich and poor" (Gallup 1976, 130–31).

Political Struggles

In reaction to voters' startling swing away from the "old order," politicians and bureaucrats were determined to respond to public opinion and its endorsement of bold reform. But the Labour government had little leeway to fulfill its popular mandate for innovative leadership: it was handcuffed by extraordinary emergencies in the country's finances and in such basic services as housing. The Cabinet identified national health care legislation as one of its few opportunities to respond to strong public opinion.

Paralleling the general public's reaction, politicians viewed the election results as both surprising and indicative of popular opposition to the "old order." For most politicians, Labour's landslide victory was an "unbelievable" or "profound shock": "most of the political world," one historian observed, was "convinced that Churchill's charisma would carry the day" (Addison 1977, 14–15). This "rare seismic landslide" shattered the received wisdom about public opinion; policymakers became convinced that voters both preferred bold changes and expected Labour to satisfy this popular mandate (Morgan 1984, 40–41).

The Labour government's attempt to fulfill its popular mandate was, however, neither automatic nor consensual. Rather, cabinet ministers had significant misgivings and disagreements over how to weigh the benefits of bold reform against the risks of significant controversy.

Not long after the Labour cabinet was formed, health reform became a central focus of intense divisions. Leading government officials fully expected the NHS bill to be highly controversial among both Labour sup-

11. The 65 percent of respondents who reported keeping track of Parliament's discussion of NHS were asked the following question: "Do you think that the government's plans will or will not result in better health services for the country as a whole?" Forty-one percent felt that the reform would result in better health services, 14 percent responded that it would not and 10 percent had no opinion. (Gallup 1976, 130–31).

porters and leading interest groups; it seemed certain to be opposed through all its stages.[12] The chief ministerial critic of NHS proposals, the quite influential Herbert Morrison, repeatedly predicted in cabinet meetings that passage of a bill would be blocked or, at the very least, delayed by fierce opposition. Even the left-wing minister of health, Aneurin Bevan, who naturally downplayed the threat of opposition, conceded that NHS legislation would "undoubtedly meet with considerable opposition" and "several very big points of controversy."[13] Emphasizing the political danger of putting the government's prestige directly behind a controversial proposal, a civil servant counseled ministers to consider the political consequences "if public opposition leads to a significant modification of the plan."[14] In addition to embarrassing Labour, bold reform could also strain Labour's relations with such key supporters as local governments, particularly the London County Council.

After a series of divisive meetings, the cabinet finally decided to back a bold NHS bill; ministers calculated that the benefit of responding to the popular mandate far outweighed the risks of controversy; to do otherwise courted certain disappointment. Faced with a series of intractable domestic problems that defied short-term solutions (such as reconstruction of the country's housing and industry), the government identified major health reform as one of its few opportunities to "deliver" a sweeping change. The fiery minister of health refused merely to adopt wartime proposals because they "contain[ed] too many compromises with the existing situation"; he persuaded the cabinet of the political attractiveness of "call[ing] for something bolder than a mere extension and adaptation of existing services."[15] As the government's top civil servant explained to Prime Minister Attlee, Bevan's plan could "constitute a bold, clear-cut scheme which will catch the imagination of the public and of Parliament."[16]

The prime minister and the balance of the cabinet decided, then, that the immediate introduction of a bold NHS bill was of the "utmost importance" to fulfill the "political program of the Government."[17] They rejected at-

---

12. MH 80/29, "The Time-Table for the Hospital Bill," 8/45.

13. CAB 128/2, CM (45) 65th, Minutes of Cabinet Meeting, 12/20/45; CAB 129/6, CP (46) 3, Memo, "NHS," by Bevan, 1/3/46. Also see CAB 129/3, CP (45) 205, Memo, "NHS: The Future of the Hospital Services," by Bevan, 109/5/45.

14. CAB 21/2019, Memo from B.W.G., 1/5/46, regarding Bevan's January 3d cabinet paper.

15. MH 80/30, NHS (46) 2, "NHS," minutes of meeting with representatives of the Trade Union Congress, 1/8/46; CAB 129/5, CP (45) 339, memo, "Proposals for a NHS," by Bevan, 12/13/45.

16. PREM 8/288, Memo to Prime Minister from N. Brook, 12/19/45.

17. CAB 134/697, SS (45) 15th, Minutes of Social Services Committee, 12/17/45; CAB 75/22, HPC (45) 80, by Greenwood, 8/24/45; PREM 8/288, Memo from N. Brook to Attlee, 3/7/46. Also see CAB 75/21 HPC (45) 29th, Minutes of Home Policy Committee meeting, 11/6/45.

tempts by ambivalent or politically conservative ministers to carry the NHS bill over into the next session. Warnings by Morrison and others that introducing bold health legislation would crowd out some of the other bills fell on deaf ears; the prime minister and cabinet refused to accept that other legislation was more urgent and insisted that the health care legislation proceed in the current session. "There seems to be little doubt," the government's top civil servant advised Attlee, "that the [health] Bills must go on."[18]

The government's determination to respond to public opinion with bold reform was reflected in two major changes in the policy-making process. To enable cabinet ministers to exercise significant control over the formulation of bold reforms, Attlee fundamentally reorganized the cabinet to funnel decision making from the departments through a set of cabinet committees up to the government's apex—the "inner inner" cabinet consisting of the prime minister, Herbert Morrison, and Ernest Bevin. Through the cabinet's interlocking committees, groups of ministers actively supervised individual departments' formulation of major legislation. An unusually receptive extracabinet environment meant that this internal policy-making process enjoyed an exceptional degree of independence and control in shaping legislation: in addition to facing no serious obstruction from opposition forces, the government enjoyed near unified support from the normally fractious Labour movement and its representatives in the House of Commons (Morgan 1984, 61–63,92–93,500–4). Because the cabinet wielded an unusual degree of control over policy formulation, the crucial policy decisions on NHS were made before legislative consideration—between the election and March 1946, when a bill was submitted to Parliament.

Nevertheless, the cabinet's deliberations involved bruising political conflict that pitted clusters of politicians and bureaucrats against each other. With consideration of health reform beginning in the Ministry of Health, divisions quickly emerged among administrators. By early fall, the minister of health ironed out the divisions within his department and presented the pivotal components of his NHS scheme to the cabinet's Social Services Committee. The Social Services Committee served as the primary intermediary between the cabinet and the Ministry; after its review and supervision of the department's proposals, the cabinet began considering Bevan's plan in October 1945.

18. PREM 8/288, Memo from N. Brook to Attlee, 3/7/46. Also see CAB 75/21, HPC (45) 29th, Minutes of Home Policy Committee meeting, 11/6/45; CAB 134/697, SS (45) 15th, Minutes of Social Services Committee, 12/17/45; CAB 66/67, CP (45) 94, Memo, "King's Speech on the Opening of Parliament," 8/4/45; CAB 75/22, HPC (45) 80, Memo for the Home Policy Committee, "Legislative Programme," by Greenwood, 8/24/45; CAB 128/2, CM (45) 65th, Minutes of cabinet meeting, 12/20/45, comments by A. Greenwood; CAB 129/7, CP (46) 94, Memo, "NHS," by Morrison and Greenwood, 3/6/46.

A series of divisive cabinet meetings were necessary to resolve intense disagreements over the designing of specific features of NHS legislation, especially the issue of nationalizing hospitals. To minimize the threat to the government's cohesion, Attlee carefully orchestrated the cabinet's consideration of health reform, gradually easing it into a commitment on a bill. After the NHS proposal was shuttled back and forth between the Ministry of Health and the Social Services Committee, a divided cabinet approved its central principles during meetings in October and November. But in its December meeting the cabinet refused to authorize the drafting of a bill: to the Ministry's chagrin, it required Bevan to submit more detailed information to enable ministers to closely monitor the legislative content of his proposals. By early January, the cabinet accepted, though not without significant opposition among senior ministers, the main features of the proposal and authorized the drafting of a bill. Finally, in early March, a less fractious cabinet easily approved a bill for presentation to Parliament.[19]

With the important battles fought within the government's revamped policy making structure, the cabinet's bill was overwhelmingly carried in Parliament with no significant alterations; it was signed into law in November 1946. As a former Ministry of Health administrator recalled, "the real crunch was in the fall of 1945 and after that it was smooth sailing."[20]

The Labour government, then, carefully structured its internal policy-making process to control the formulation of bold reform; a second major indication of the government's commitment to fulfilling its popular mandate was its decision to restructure the health policy network to restrict interest group participation. Morrison and others who objected to Bevan's proposals urged that health policy be generated, as it had been under the coalition, through organized ongoing bargaining between government officials and major interest groups; groups representing narrow, particularistic interests should remain influential participants. The Ministry of Health, Morrison contended, should enter into "protracted" negotiations with the interests concerned before beginning actual preparation of a bill.[21]

Bevan successfully countered that, although leading interest groups should have the opportunity to express their views, their input should be limited to "work[ing] out details." In a democratic system, he maintained, it is the elected government's responsibility to decide "all the main features of the

19. CAB 128/2, CM (45) 65th, Minutes of cabinet meeting, 12/20/45; CAB 129/5, CP (45) 339, "Proposals for a NHS," by Bevan, 12/13/45; CAB 128/5, CM (46) 3rd, Minutes of cabinet meeting, 1/8/46; CAB 128/5, CM (46) 22nd, Minutes of cabinet meeting, 3/8/46.
20. Pater Interview. See Pater 1981 for a detailed discussion of the bill's relatively easy passage through Parliament.
21. CAB 128/2, CM (45) 65th, Minutes of cabinet meeting, 12/20/45, comments by H. Morrison; CAB 128/1, CM (45) 40th, Minutes of cabinet meeting, 10/11/45, comments by A. Greenwood.

proposals" and to insist that "no concessions could be made on the main principles."[22] The voters' representatives, he was suggesting, should be responsible to broad publics rather than to narrow special interests.

The cabinet endorsed Bevan's position that "prolonged negotiations were out of place"; he approached major interest groups on the basis that negotiation would center on "administrative detail" rather than "the main structure [and] the main concepts."[23] In stark contrast to the wartime governments' quixotic pursuit of interest group goodwill, ministry officials were determined to fight for their proposal: it now seemed inconceivable to politicians and bureaucrats that they would be "cowered by the threat of the medical profession to oppose [the government's proposal]."[24] Still, however determined Labour was to restrict direct interest group participation and lobbying, the government nonetheless felt constrained to weigh in its private deliberations long-standing sectional claims; after all, the new program would depend on medical producers to actually provide the new services.

To respond, then, to the public's demand for change, Labour endorsed bold NHS legislation and streamlined its policy-making process. But this reformist orientation coexisted with an attentiveness to previous arrangements and policy discussions. On the most practical level, Ministry of Health officials suggested that passing a bill in the current Parliament meant that wartime proposals must "still [be] substantially usable"; meeting a tight timetable was impossible if the entire structure of the scheme had to be changed.[25] In addition, Bevan and other senior government officials insisted on anchoring NHS in arrangements that would be familiar to the public; they avoided reforms that would be *"too abrupt a break from established practices"* (my emphasis).[26] "Administrators," a former ministry official recalled, "were thinking that the public acceptance of radical change would

22. CAB 129/3 CP (45) 205, Memo, "NHS: The Future of Hospitals" by Bevan, 10/5/45; CAB 128/5, CM (46) 3rd, Minutes of cabinet meeting, 1/8/46; CAB 128/2, CM (45) 65th, Minutes of cabinet meeting, 12/20/45. Also see MH 77/100, Letter to B. Docker (representative of the BHA) from Bevan, 11/9/45; MH 77/119, Letter from Bevan to C. Hill, 11/13/45; MH 80/29, NHS (45) 47, "NHS," minutes of meeting between the Ministry of Health and representatives of the medical profession's negotiating committee, 12/4/45; CAB 129/3, CP (45) 231, "NHS: The Hospital Services," by minister of health, 10/16/45; MH 77/119, NHS (46) 3, "NHS," minutes of meeting between the Ministry of Health and the medical profession's negotiating committee, 1/10/46; CAB 129/5, CP (45) 339, Memo, "Proposals for a NHS," by Bevan, 12/13/45.
23. Pater Interview and MH 80/32, NHS (46) 30, Minutes of meeting with medical profession's negotiating committee, 5/13/46. Also see PREM 8/288, Memo to prime minister from N. Brook, 1/7/46; MH 80/30, Memo, "NHS: Discussion of the Government's Proposals," handwritten, "3/46."
24. Pater Interview.
25. MH 80/29, "The Time-Table for the Hospital Bill," 10/45.
26. MH 80/30, NHS (46) 2, "NHS," minutes of meeting with representatives of the Trade Union Congress, 1/8/46.

only go so far."[27] Even as they considered bold innovations, then, politicians and bureaucrats remained committed to incorporating established arrangements and avoiding a truly radical departure: the new was to be firmly anchored in the old. As a result of the Labour government's calculated strategy for pursuing bold reform, it became the "most effective of any British government since the passage of the 1832 Reform Act" (Morgan 1984, 503–4).

POLICY DISCUSSIONS

Health reform was on the public's policy making agenda even before the Beveridge Report was published in December 1942, but final authoritative decisions on NHS legislation were not made until after July 1945. These critical decisions emerged from the organized deliberations of ministers and bureaucrats; policymakers curtailed medical producers' direct participation but in their private deliberations still considered their well-known support for established practices.

State Autonomy and Basic Principles

The Labour government inherited contentious matters of basic principle; on some issues politicians and bureaucrats pursued reforms that were independent of and in opposition to the interests of major societal groups, which favored maintaining established practices. In particular, state actors continued to disagree with medical producers' well-established positions concerning the universal availability of health services and their free cost. Universal and free coverage were the most popular aspects of the Beveridge Report and the coalition's 1944 white paper; polling data as well as Labour's landslide victory appeared to confirm the public's strong support for these highly salient principles. In this context, continued interest group opposition seemed almost indecent to policymakers *and* interest groups. Indeed, the BMA's president pragmatically recommended that "denigrat[ing]" and presenting "direct opposition to the Bill ... [was] unsound"; doctors should "confine [them]selves to obtaining modifications of certain parts of the Bill."[28] Faced with the country's new mood, doctors steered away from objecting to universal coverage; in the new environment, the BMA no longer vocally advocated an income limit that would restrict care to those in "need."

27. Godber Interview.
28. MH 77/119, Statement by Henry Souttar to BMA council, discussed in letter from ministry official A. Rucker to Souttar, 6/6/46.

Although aspects of the NHS were fiercely contested within the cabinet, ministers readily agreed to adopt the principle of universal coverage. Pointing to the public support for making everyone eligible, Bevan reminded the cabinet of the "mandate the Government had received to establish a comprehensive health service... available for all."[29] Indeed, Ministry of Health administrators advised Bevan to draw on public enthusiasm for universal coverage in presenting the government's bill to Parliament and the prees: while prewar arrangements meant that "only the breadwinner had been entitled to a family doctor service," Labour's scheme made available a "full and first-class health service for every man, woman and child in this country."[30]

A second major principle, the free cost of the service at the point of treatment, also enjoyed strong public support and had a similar reception. In this context, interest groups effectively abandoned their wartime position of favoring patient charges and the cabinet fully embraced Bevan's proposal to adopt the 1944 white paper's objective of a free service.[31] Bureaucrats and ministers accepted Labour's landslide as a "mandate" to provide health care without charge and anticipated a palpable "relief at no longer being under threat for meeting the cost of health care."[32] To stir public enthusiasm for the cabinet-approved bill, Bevan was advised to emphasize to the country that health care would for the first time be divorced from the ability to pay: it would be "freely available to all who need it."[33]

Labour's adoption of a free and universal health program was not viewed by Bevan and other ministers as an isolated decision but rather as related to the establishment of a popular "new pattern of social services." Focusing on the unpopularity of the poor laws, officials emphasized that "many people in genuine need of assistance have been deterred from seeking it... and many who have been obliged to seek assistance have done so under a degradation." By introducing free and universal coverage, the new health service would challenge the "persist[ence]...[of] deeply grounded...prejudices"; the outcome would be the "final break-up" of the "outmoded and dying poor law." Ministers concluded that introducing a new pattern of social welfare provision was politically essential: Labour's most enduring

29. MH 80/30, NHS (46) 2, "NHS," minutes of meeting with representatives of the Trade Union Congress, 1/8/46. Also see CAB 129/5, CP (45) 339, Memo, "Proposals for a NHS," by Bevan, 12/13/45. Godber Interview.

30. MH 80/30, Memo, "NHS Bill: Lobby Conference.... Notes for Minister," handwritten, 3/21/46.

31. CAB 129/5, CP (45) 339, Memo, "Proposals for a NHS," by Bevan, 12/13/45.

32. MH 80/30, NHS (46) 2, "NHS," minutes of meeting with representatives of the Trade Union Congress, 1/8/46; Godber Interview.

33. MH 80/30, Memo, "NHS Bill: Lobby Conference.... Notes for Minister," handwritten, 3/21/46. Also see Klein 1983, 24–25; CAB 129/6, CP (46) 3, "Appendix: Needs of a Bill," by Bevan, 1/3/46.

legacy would be the bold transition toward dealing with "the problem of need...afresh," that is, in a way that the public perceived positively.[34]

Strong interest group influence. On two contentious issues, remuneration arrangements for doctors and the role of private practice in the new service, policymakers did not perceive strong public support and instead focused on interest group claims. But in the new political environment created by Labour's landslide, they made concessions but were unwilling to abdicate—as wartime governments did—to interest group demands for continuing established practices.

Policymakers and interest groups took opposing positions on whether doctors should be remunerated by salary or on a capitation basis (the NHI system of relating reimbursement of doctors to their number of patients). Within the Labour party, especially in its left wing, there existed long-standing support for introducing full salaried reimbursement (Webster 1987). Senior administrators in the Ministry of Health echoed these concerns of the organized labor movement, arguing that salary reimbursement would reduce financial competition between doctors.[35] While the Labour party and its supporters pressed for change, the BMA revived its previous push to continue capitation payment; framing its claims in terms of public preferences and understandings, the BMA noted that "the amount of money offered by the Government in compensation is irrelevant." Attempting to draw on lingering public wariness over excessive state development, the BMA warned that salary reimbursement went against the "public interest"; it would "affect the freedom of the medical profession" and reduce doctors to "servants of the [central] state or local authorities."[36] Fierce interest group opposition led Bevan to predict to the cabinet that the reimbursement arrangement would be one of the main issues in the parliamentary debates.[37]

Despite reservations within the government and the organized labor movement, senior policymakers acknowledged the BMA's warnings against creating "full-time salaried servants." Bevan argued persuasively that full salary

34. CAB 134/698, Social Services Committee (SS) (46) 13, Cover memo on "Report of the Inter-Departmental Committee on the Break-Up of the Poor Laws," by Bevan, J. Wilson (President of the Board of Trade), and J. Griffiths (Minister of National Insurance). Also see CAB 124/561, Office of Lord President: Legislative Programme, Memo by Bevan and J. Griffiths, 3/46; MH 80/47, Minutes of meeting, 3/27/46 (chaired by Greenwood and attended by Bevan, J. Wilson, J. Griffiths and several civil servants—A. Rucker, G. Henderson, and W. S. Murrie); CAB 134/298, FL (46) 1st and 3rd, Minutes of the Future Legislation Committee, 2/5/46 and 3/19/46.
35. MH 80/30, NHS (46) 2, Minutes of meeting with the Trade Union Congress, 1/8/46.
36. MH 77/119, Letter from Charles Hill to Bevan, 3/8/46; MH 80/32, Memo, "The Minister's Proposals for a NHS: The [BMA] Negotiating Committee's Observations," probably mid-January 1946.
37. CAB 129/7, CP (46) 86, Memo, "NHS Bill," by Bevan, 3/1/46.

remuneration would be seen as too abrupt a break from firmly established customs. In addition to potentially fueling BMA campaigns to spark public unease, full-salaried reimbursement ignored—Bevan and other officials acknowledged—socially shared meanings that linked work with "financial incentives" and the "principle of payment by results." Although Labour's left-wing health minister intended ultimately to create a full-time salaried service, he conceded that it would be "impracticable to make such a major change in established practice at once." Doctors were too thoroughly imbued with society's market-oriented values to be "ripe" for it.[38]

Searching for an alternative to a full-salaried service, the Labour government revived the coalition's concession to doctors; it decided to combine salary and capitation methods, with the salary component limited to new entrants during their first three years. Bevan concluded that this admixture of new and old would proceed "as far as it was desirable to go at present" toward "eliminat[ing] the worst features of the capitation rate system."[39] While the wartime government's quixotic pursuit of professional goodwill had often led to a series of concessions, Labour refused to abdicate its initial compromise in the face of vociferous attacks by the House of Lords and the BMA.[40]

The role of doctors' private practice in the new service was another issue on which medical producers won significant government concessions. In particular, the dispute centered on permitting GPs to practice privately and, especially, on requiring publicly owned hospitals to set aside "pay beds" for specialists. The BMA argued for continuity and against "destroying private specialist practice." In a bid to spark public anxiety over the state's expansion, it warned that doctors working in the new service needed the "right" to practice privately and consequently needed government-owned hospitals to set aside pay-beds for them to use.[41]

38. CAB 128/5, CM (46) 3rd, Minutes of cabinet meeting, 1/8/46; CAB 134/697, SS (45) 15th, Minutes of Social Services Committee, 12/17/45; MH 80/32, Memo, "How to Pay Doctors in the GP Service," probably between 7/45 and 2/46. Also see CAB 128/2, CM (45) 65th, Minutes of cabinet meeting, 12/20/45; MH 80/30, NHS (46) 2, Minutes of meeting with the TUC, 1/8/46; MH 77/177, Memo, "Remuneration of General Practitioners," probably around January 1946, located in files of the Spens committee on the remuneration of GPs.

39. CAB 128/2, CM (45) 65th, Minutes of cabinet meeting, 12/20/45. Also see MH 80/32, Memo, "How to Pay Doctors in the GP Service," probably between 7/45 and 2/46; CAB 134/697, SS (45) 15th, Minutes of Social Services Committee, 12/17/45.

40. CAB 128/6, CM (46) 93rd, Minutes of cabinet meeting, 10/31/46; MH 80/30, "BMA: Notes on Main Points in BMA Council's Report on Bill," handwritten, "February," probably 1946; MH 80/32, NHS (46) 30, Minutes of meeting with representatives of the BMA, 5/13/46.

41. MH 80/32, NHS (46) 30, Minutes of meeting with representatives of the BMA, 5/13/46. Also see MH 80/32, NHS (46) 31, Minutes of meeting with representatives of the medical profession, 5/20/46; MH 80/32, Memo, "The Minister's Proposals for a NHS: The [BMA] Negotiating Committee's Observations," probably mid-January 1946. For the BMA's public appeals, see Eckstein 1958.

Elements within the government and the labor movement opposed compromise with doctors; the continuation of private practice would have an undesirable impact on public opinion: it would preserve public attitudes associated with the poor laws and maintain "undesirable class distinctions" between paying and nonpaying patients.[42] Voicing concerns within the labor movement, Ministry of Health administrators and cabinet ministers warned that allowing private practices outside the government's facilities would lead "the public to presume that they gave a better service." Giving the "impression that better treatment might be obtained privately" would defeat the purpose of the bill. The result would be to "prejudice the success of the national scheme": "segregat[ing] . . . State patients from [paying] patients" would threaten the cabinet's desire to "emphasize . . . universality."[43]

In spite of these reservations, however, the cabinet and senior administrators revived the coalition's concession to medical producers and permitted the mixing of public and private practice. In the absence of unmistakably explicit public interest in the issue, policymakers emphasized that eliminating private practice would have a powerful indirect effect on public opinion: this radical departure would drive many doctors elsewhere (especially the most talented), which in turn would isolate government care as a separate, inferior system. The result would be to preserve the class distinction between paying and nonpaying patients. The cabinet agreed with Bevan, then, that compromising by allowing GPs to practice privately and specialists to use hospital pay-beds was "essential if we are to attract some of the best specialists into the service from the outset."[44]

Bolstered by its resounding electoral mandate and by evolving public understandings of the state, Labour refused to capitulate (as had the coalition) in the face of medical producers' unrelenting demands that private practice be fully preserved.[45] Instead, Labour insisted on reversing the country's traditional priorities; the government unambiguously declared that the "medical needs [of the public service] must first be served." For instance, it restricted the number of pay-beds and decided that even those allowances

42. CAB 134/698, SS (46) 4th, Minutes of the Social Services Committee, 3/4/46.
43. CAB 128/5, CM (46) 3rd, Minutes of cabinet meeting, 1/8/46; MH 80/29, Memo, "NHS—Hospital Scheme," handwritten, "August 1945. Copy of Secretary's Minute."
44. CAB 129/7, CP (46) 86, Memo, "NHS Bill," by Bevan, 3/1/46. Also see CAB 134/698, SS (46) 4th, Minutes of the Social Services Committee, 3/4/46; PREM 8/288, Memo from A. Greenwood to Attlee, 3/6/46, regarding "NHS Bill"; MH 80/32, NHS (46) 30, Minutes of meeting with representatives of the BMA, 5/13/46; MH 80/30, NHS (46) 17, Minutes of meeting with medical profession, 2/4/46.
45. MH 80/32, NHS (46) 31, Minutes of meeting with representatives of the medical profession, 5/20/46.

for private practice could be "overridden if it is needed urgently for a non-paying patient under the public service."[46]

State Capacity and Administrative Arrangements

The coalition government's political deadlock made consensus building seem necessary; in the "entirely new situation" created by Labour's sweep, policymakers were convinced that wartime compromises had produced excessive administrative complications.[47] Ministry of Health bureaucrats, politicians including the chancellor of the exchequer, and major interest groups all reiterated the argument for creating a unified structure and opposing the coalition's tripartite scheme of establishing separate administrative arrangements for the service's three branches. In particular, these diverse groups and individuals favored strengthening the state's specialization and, especially, hierarchical control in order to increase efficient administration. The BMA charged that dividing administration into several compartments would perpetuate or create barriers to proper coordination of the country's medical services.[48] Government officials similarly argued that the central state's new responsibilities required "very close financial control by the Health Departments and the Treasury"; the cabinet was amply warned of alarming fiscal consequences if "effective control of expenditure" was compromised by dispersing the central state's authority into separate branches.[49]

The administrative argument for establishing a firmly ordered system of authority was neither a primary focus of nor influence on the cabinet and other officials. Policymakers adopted the tripartite administrative structure because it offered a pragmatic response to two opposing patterns of public preferences and understandings toward state institutions; the undesirable consequences of weak organizational arrangements were accepted as "unavoidable."[50]

On the one hand, ministers and bureaucrats attempted to incorporate the public's familiarity with local government and voluntary participation in the provision of social welfare. Bevan and others acknowledged that the

46. CAB 129/7, CP (46) 86, Memo, "NHS Bill," by Bevan, 3/1/46; MH 80/30, NHS (46) 23, "NHS: Meeting with the Representatives of the Voluntary Hospitals," 2/11/46.

47. MH 80/30, NHS (46) 2, "NHS," minutes of meeting with representatives of the Trade Union Congress, 1/8/46; CAB 129/5, CP (45) 339, Memo, "Proposals for a NHS," by Bevan, 12/13/45.

48. MH 80/32, Memo, "The Minister's Proposals for a NHS: The [BMA] Negotiating Committee's Observations," probably mid-January 1946.

49. CAB 134/697, SS (45) 15th, Minutes of Social Services Committee, 12/17/45; CAB 128/2, CM (45) 5th, Minutes of cabinet meeting, 12/20/45, comments by the chancellor of the exchequer; MH 80/29, Memo, "NHS—Hospital Scheme," handwritten, "August 1945. Copy of Secretary's Minute."

50. Godber Interview; Pater Interview.

"whole scheme would break down" if administrative arrangements failed to "carry over from the old system to the new the spirit of voluntary service" and to "keep up a healthy local interest in administration."[51] Government officials agreed with interest groups that divorcing the central state from day-to-day administration was essential to "attract personal interest" in the new administrative units.[52] "Considerable delegation" by the central government would preserve "scope ... [for] people with local experience and knowledge" and preclude the minister's emergence as the "sole administrator" who suffocated local involvement through "direction" and "detailed central scrutiny."[53]

On the other hand, policymakers recognized that local authorities' provisions retained the shadow of the poor laws; with the national government free of this stigma, Bevan explained to the cabinet that "all the population" would expect the central state to take charge of the new service.[54] To vividly demonstrate that neither the hospital nor the GP branches were under the traditional poor-law authorities, the government decided that the central state would at least formally dictate the "general policy for all services" and "ensure coordination" between the three branches.[55]

Labour chose the tripartite structure, then, to institutionalize these opposing patterns of public attitudes: carving out a "place both for local and for central government" would "reconcile [central] state organization of the

51. CAB 129/5, CP (45) 339, Memo, "Proposals for a NHS," by Bevan, 12/13/45; MH 80/30, NHS (46) 23, "NHS. Meeting with the Representatives of the Voluntary Hospitals," 2/11/46. Also see MH 80/30, NHS (46) 19, Minutes of meeting with the King Edward's Hospital Fund for London, 2/5/46; MH 80/30, Memo, "NHS Bill: Lobby Conference.... Notes for Minister," handwritten, 3/21/46; PREM 8/288, Memo from N. Brook to Attlee, 12/19/45, regarding CP (45) 339 and 345.

52. MH 80/32, NHS (46) 30, Minutes of meeting with representatives of the BMA, 5/13/46; MH 80/30, Memo, "NHS Bill: Lobby Conference.... Notes for Minister," handwritten, 3/21/46; CAB 129/5, CP (45) 339, Memo, "Proposals for a NHS," by Bevan, 12/13/45; CAB 128/1, CM (45) 40th, Minutes to cabinet meeting, 10/11/45; CAB 129/3, CP (45) 205, Memo, "NHS: The Future of the Hospital Services," by Bevan, 10/5/45; MH 80/36, Memo, "BHA's 'Six-Point Plan' for a Hospital Service," by the Ministry of Health, probably spring 1946.

53. MH 80/30, NHS (46) 7, probably spring 1946; MH 77/119, NHS (46) 3, Minutes of meeting with medical profession, 1/10/46. Also see MH 80/29, Memo, "NHS Bill Notes on Hospital Proposal," handwritten 7/45; MH 80/30, NHS (46) 17, Minutes of meeting with medical profession, 2/4/46; MH 80/32, NHS (46) 30, Minutes of meeting with representatives of the BMA, 5/13/46; CAB 129/6, CP (46) 3, "Appendix: Needs of a Bill," by Bevan, 1/3/46; CAB 129/5, CP (45) 339, "Appendix: Summary of Proposals for a NHS," by Bevan, 12/13/45.

54. CAB 129/3, CP (45) 205, Memo, "NHS. The Future of the Hospital Services," by Bevan, 10/5/45.

55. MH 80/30, NHS (46) 7, "NHS: Questions Put to Minister by Negotiating Committee of Medical Profession and the Minister's Replies," probably spring 1946; MH 80/32, NHS (46) 32, 5/27/46. Also see MH 80/29, Memo, "NHS Bill. Notes on Hospital Proposal," handwritten 7/45; MH 77/119, NHS (46) 3, Minutes of meeting with medical profession, 1/10/46; MH 80/30, NHS (46) 17, Minutes of meeting with medical profession, 2/4/46; MH 80/32, NHS (46) 30, Minutes of meeting with representatives of the BMA, 5/13/46.

Service with personal interest and the participation of individuals locally."[56] To underscore its dual commitment to maintaining local authorities' involvement and doctors' and hospitals' respectability, Labour modified the coalition's proposal in order to administratively strengthen each of the three branches. In particular, it strengthened the state's hierarchical control and specialization *within* each branch: executive councils were to manage general medical services, regional hospital boards and hospital management committees were to control hospitals,[57] and local health authorities were to administer clinic treatment. Under Labour's scheme, each of the three branches would take control of its own planning and execution. But the government effectively abandoned policy experts' long-standing commitment to coordinating care *across* the separate branches. The detailed proposals for the two largest branches, the hospital and GP services, sparked the greatest controversy.

Administrative arrangements for hospital service. Bureaucrats, politicians, and major interest groups continued to disagree over whether and to what degree the new service ought to establish central state authority over the country's two main systems of hospital care—its local government facilities and its private voluntary hospitals. These discussions were framed by public opinion that favored a state-run medical service and, as Gallup reported, "sweeping changes such as nationalization" (1976, 112).

The government and, specifically, Bevan began their deliberations with the "one big question": whether to nationalize or to preserve (as the coalition proposed) the two established hospital systems. No idea received criticism from as wide a range of sources as nationalization. Cabinet ministers led by Morrison, bureaucrats, and leading interest groups—especially representatives of the voluntary hospitals and the local authorities—maligned the plan for radically breaking from established public understandings and practices. Within the Ministry of Health, several bureaucrats warned that it "will look like wholesale confiscation" by a "completely centralized system."[58] Representatives and supporters of voluntary hospitals similarly argued that the "liquidation" of existing hospitals bore "no relation to our accumulated experience or to the historical evidence"; nationalization would mean "obliterating" "local personal interest."[59] Local authorities

56. CAB 129/5, CP (45) 339, Memo, "Proposals for a NHS," by Bevan, 12/13/45; MH 80/30, NHS (46) 23, "NHS: Meeting with the Representatives of the Voluntary Hospitals," 2/11/46. Also see MH 80/30, NHS (46) 19, Minutes of meeting with the King Edward's Hospital Fund for London, 2/5/46.

57. Authoritative control over the hospital service was compromised by the government's agreement to cede control over teaching hospitals to special boards of governors.

58. CAB 21/2019, Memo from B.W.G., 1/5/46, regarding CP (46) 3; MH 80/29, Memo, "NHS—Hospital Scheme," handwritten, "August 1945. Copy of Secretary's Minute."

59. MH 77/100, Letter from J. Wetenhall, 2/14/46; MH 80/32, Memo, "The Minister's

and Morrison shared this emotional indignation about nationalization's "drastic" change. Morrison doggedly claimed that strong public attachment to local government should *"outweigh the arguments based on grounds of administrative convenience and technical efficiency"* (my emphasis).[60] In particular, Morrison and others contended that "bringing the hospitals under bureaucratic Whitehall control" ignored the "social advantages of the local government system": it would "impair" or "los[e] the spirit of voluntary public service" and terminate local governments "as a school of political and democratic education."[61]

In its boldest departure from prewar arrangements, the cabinet decided to "decisively and openly" "take over—into one national service" both local authority and voluntary hospitals.[62] Contrary to Morrison's claims, this bold decision was not based on administrative convenience and technical efficiency. Just the opposite; precisely because of public understandings and preferences policymakers "adopt[ed] a solution which would admittedly not be perfect." Accurately gauging public opinion, ministers and bureaucrats were attracted to the popularity of nationalization; it was a "bold scheme . . . [that] would have the backing of Government supporters throughout the country."[63] Ministry officials observed that they would be "very much mistaken" to assume that "people of this country are satisfied with . . . hospital care"; Bevan persuaded his colleagues that "imaginative" responses to this kind of dissatisfaction were "exactly what we were returned to [do]."[64]

Labour decided that nationalization would be popular because it accurately reflected the public's resentment of both voluntary hospitals and local government provisions. Breaking with wartime perceptions, politicians and bureaucrats now recognized that voluntary hospitals' continual campaigns

Proposals for a NHS: The [BMA] Negotiating Committee's Observations," probably mid-January 1946. Also see MH 80/34, "File: S. A. Anderson's Memo. J. Hawton to See," undated, but probably late summer 1945; MH 80/30, NHS (46) 23, "NHS. Meeting with the Representatives of the Voluntary Hospitals," 2/11/46.

60. CAB 128/1, CM (45) 43rd, Minutes of cabinet meeting, 10/18/45. Also see CAB 129/3, CP (45) 227, Memo, "NHS: The Future of the Hospital Service," by Morrison, 10/12/45.

61. MH 80/29, Memo, "NHS—Hospital Scheme," handwritten, "August 1945. Copy of Secretary's Minute"; PREM 8/603, Memo from Morrison to Attlee, 3/5/46; CAB 128/5, CM (46) 44th, Minutes of cabinet meeting, 5/9/46; CAB 129/3, CP (45) 227, Memo, "NHS: The Future of the Hospital Service," by Morrison, 10/12/45; CAB 21/2032, Memo from John Maude to lord president, 10/8/45, regarding cabinet meeting the following day on the future of the hospital service.

62. CAB 129/3, CP (45) 205, Memo, "NHS: The Future of the Hospital Services," by Bevan, 10/5/45.

63. MH 80/34, Memo, "Reform of the Voluntary Hospital System," probably late summer 1945; MH 80/29, Memo, "NHS—Hospital Scheme," handwritten, "August 1945. Copy of Secretary's Minute"; CAB 128/1, CM (45) 43rd, Minutes of cabinet meeting, 10/18/45.

64. CAB 129/3, CP (45) 231, Memo, "NHS: The Hospital Services," by Bevan, 10/16/45; MH 80/30, Memo, "NHS Bill. Lobby Conference. . . . Notes for Minister," handwritten, 3/21/46.

for financial support were widely resented as a form of "begging"; it was necessary to "do away with the current methods of seeking contributions."[65] Focusing on the negative aspect of public understanding of local authorities, policymakers concluded that local government hospitals cold not escape from the "general surroundings and atmosphere of the poor law system."[66] The Labour government decided, then, that neither hospital system corresponded with public attitudes or would be appropriate for the new service; the voluntary hospital system had "outlived its usefulness" and the public hospital system had to be "tak[en] out of the field of local government altogether." By 1946, the cabinet agreed that the "time has come to leave [the old system] behind"; starting again with a "clean slate" was preferable to preserving hospital systems that were out of step with public expectations.[67]

Despite serious reservations within the government about overturning established practices, Bevan persuaded his colleagues that establishing hierarchical control over hospital care was a "clean-cut solution" consistent with public sentiment.[68] Although existing local authority arrangements seemed permanently tainted, policymakers emphasized the public's favorable understanding of the central state. Stressing that the "personal experience of...patients would be an important factor in securing public welcome for the scheme," they anticipated that the new system of government administration would be acceptable.[69]

Contrary to Weberian expectations, then, detailed policy decisions focused on, and were determined by, public preferences and understandings. The policy shift from the Coalition to Labour government did not stem from a reassessment of existing administrative capacity. Rather, it was due to a new and more accurate assessment of the public's explicit preference for bold change and the enduring negative meanings attached to continuing local authority provisions; central state involvement seemed necessary and desirable as an alternative.

Administrative arrangements for GP service. Policymakers responded to public opinion toward GP care by reforming the old panel system, by introducing new safeguards that would distance the new service from the

---

65. CAB 128/1, CM (45) 40th, Minutes of cabinet Meeting, 10/11/45, comment by G. A. Isaacs (Minister of Labour and National Service); MH 80/30, NHS (46) 23, "NHS: Meeting with the Representatives of the Voluntary Hospitals," 2/11/46.
66. CAB 129/3, CP (45) 231, Memo, "NHS. The Hospital Services," by Bevan, 10/16/45.
67. MH 80/30, NHS (46) 23, "NHS: Meeting with the Representatives of the Voluntary Hospitals," 2/11/46; CAB 129/3, CP (45) 205, Memo, "NHS: The Future of the Hospital Services," by Bevan, 10/5/45.
68. Pater Interview.
69. CAB 129/3, CP (45) 207, Memo, "NHS," by George Buchanan (Under Secretary of State for Scotland), 10/5/45; Pater Interview.

earlier defects of the capitation system.[70] But Labour's reform of the GP service did not entail the same degree of change as its watershed decision to nationalize hospitals.[71] On the continuum between change and continuity, the GP reforms decidedly tilted toward prewar arrangements.

Labour designed the new service very much aware of strong, sustained public opinion: the country supported such demonstrable changes in the NHI's unpopular panel system as health centers and free doctors' services for all. In response, the government sought to replace highly decentralized prewar arrangements with measures that increased the state's expertise in and control over general medical care.

To "mark" the GP service as something new, Labour established a specialized state administrative arrangement, which assumed responsibility for securing a distribution of doctors that would enable free services to be provided for the entire country. Backed by a popular mandate for change, Bevan confronted doctors' opposition to this expansion of state involvement by noting that "no other professional person could go anywhere he pleased and insist on public remuneration."[72]

Moreover, in place of the highly decentralized and competitive system in which isolated doctors provided treatment, Labour proposed to reorganize the GP service into the highly popular health centers, which would rely on group practice and pooled equipment. The cabinet agreed to "swing [the new service] over to Health Centers" and accepted the Ministry of Health's recommendation to make as large a "show of [their] provision as possible."[73]

Finally, Labour decided that the tradition of unregulated buying and selling of GP practices had to go.[74] This decision reflected the public's expectation of change and its disapproval of a "glorified extension" of the old system. As the BMA's president counseled his members, "in opposing

70. MH 80/32, Memo, "How to Pay Doctors in the GP Service," probably between 7/45 and 2/46.

71. Godber Interview; CAB 129/3, CP (45) 207, Memo, "NHS," by George Buchanan (Under Secretary of State for Scotland), 10/5/45.

72. MH 80/32, NHS (46) 30, Minutes of meeting with representatives of the BMA, 5/13/46. Also see MH 80/30, Memo, "BMA: Notes on Main Points Taken in BMA Council's Report on the Bill," probably 2/46; MH 80/29, NHS (45) 47, Minutes of meetings with medical profession, 12/4/45.

73. MH 80/29, Letter to H. S. Kent (Parliamentary Counsel's Office) from J. Pater, 12/22/45, regarding the drafting of an NHS bill. Also see CAB 129/5, CP (45) 339, "Appendix: Summary of Proposals for a NHS," Bevan, 12/13/45; MH 80/32, Memo, "How to Pay Doctors in the GP Service," probably between 7/45 and 2/46; MH 80/30, "BMA: Notes, on Main Points in BMA Council's Report on Bill," handwritten "February," probably 1946; CAB 128/5, CM (46) 3rd, Minutes of cabinet meeting, 1/8/46.

74. CAB 128/2, CM (45) 58th, Minutes of cabinet meeting, 12/3/45; MH 80/30, "BMA: Notes on Main Points in BMA Council's Report on Bill," handwritten, "February," probably 1946; CAB 129/4, CP (45) 298, Memo, "NHS: Sale and Purchase of Medical Practices," by Bevan, 11/23/45; MH 80/29, NHS (45) 47, Minutes of meetings with medical profession, 12/4/45.

[the] abolition [of purchasing and selling practices] we should have little popular support."[75]

But, even as the government responded to public opinion and extended state involvement in GP care, it pulled back from establishing open and decisive state control; instead, it reacted to the BMA's attempt to draw on the public's lingering wariness over state domination and to dampen support for Labour's entire bill. The BMA portrayed Labour's proposed service as the worst kind of state interference: doctors would be suffocated by rigid state control and humiliated by being put "under" local authorities.[76] To partially defuse these charges, the government guaranteed the continuation of patients' medical "freedom," promising a "greater degree" of patient choice in selecting a doctor.

To underscore that the state's new presence in GP care would not introduce bureaucratization, the cabinet established "professional advice and representation at all levels" to guarantee the medical profession "a voice, in the guiding and providing of the Service." Labour's formal strengthening of the state's authority in the GP branch was compromised, then, by its decision to avoid a firestorm over state control by guaranteeing a "very large measure of self-government."[77]

The cabinet's decision to sacrifice the state's hierarchical control and specialization had the effect of reproducing the medical profession's dominant position in health care. As public authority replaced private control, doctors' participation and privileges were preserved within the service's new administrative structure, institutionalizing existing social relations; other relevant but nonprofessional groups such as health workers were denied comparable representation.[78] The maintenance of the medical profession's privileged position had important repercussions; it contributed to subsequent developments, including the decision to scrap the objective of reorganizing GP care into health centers.

Swept into office on the heels of an upset landslide, Labour formulated major new reforms such as nationalization; unlike the coalition government,

75. MH 77/119, Statement by Souttar to BMA Council, 6/46 (forwarded to Ministry of Health).

76. MH 77/100, Letter to B. Docker (representative of the BHA) from Bevan, 11/9/45; MH 80/32, Memo, "The Minister's Proposals for a NHS: The [BMA] Negotiating Committee's Observations," probably mid-January 1946; MH 80/30, NHS (46) 17, Minutes of meeting with medical profession, 2/4/46; PREM 8/288, Memo to prime minister from N. Brook, 12/19/45; MH 80/32, Memo, "Doctor Hill's Points—Interview with Secretary," 5/10/46; Eckstein 1958.

77. MH 80/30, Memo, "NHS Bill: Lobby Conference.... Notes for Minister," handwritten, 3/21/46; CAB 129/5, CP (45) 339, Memo, "Proposals for a NHS," by Bevan, 12/13/45; MH 80/32, NHS (46) 30, Minutes of meeting with representatives of the BMA, 5/13/46. Also see MH 80/30, NHS (46) 17, Minutes of meeting with medical profession, 2/4/46; MH 80/40, Letter from Bevan to Walter Citrine (Secretary, Trade Union Congress), 7/18/46.

78. CAB 134/697, SS (45) 15th, Minutes of Social Services Committee, 12/17/45.

it also enacted an NHS bill. The country's exceptionally severe circumstances including its dire economic position did not deter policymakers. Rather, Labour's landslide intensified policymakers' preoccupation with public opinion and motivated the government to take the calculated risk of pursuing a bold approach to formulating health policy. Thus, the cabinet accepted Bevan's argument that there could be "no question of postponing ... the operation of the scheme" on the basis that "the resources of the NHS would not be sufficient ... for some years to come."[79] Labour's fundamental commitment to change was nonetheless tempered by the government's devotion to continuity; policymakers sought to avoid a revolutionary rupture from established practices and expectations.

Labour's handling of the NHS sheds light on contending theoretical expectations regarding institutional change. Some government decisions are consistent with Weberian expectations regarding the causal importance of existing organizational capacity. Thus, a state with moderately strong administrative resources did enhance its prewar levels of hierarchical control and specialization in three major areas of health care, especially hospital care. One Ministry of Health administrator credited Labour with significantly strengthening the administrative organization of hospital care: it transformed the prewar system, which was hopelessly "complex and unsuited to the advancing nature of the task," into one that was "managed in a new [and administratively better] way."[80]

Policymakers' decisions on interest group claims and specific institutional changes, however, were not dominated by technical assessments of the state's administrative resources. Rather, interest group influence was tied to policymakers' perception of public opinion. Politicians and bureaucrats explicitly identified salient, popular support for free and universal coverage as their reason for ignoring major interest groups' traditional opposition to these principles. Contrary to Weberian expectations, the moderately strong British state did compromise its autonomy; it granted concessions to medical producers on the less salient issues of private practice and capitation payment. The variation in policymakers' independence from interest group claims was tied, then, not to administrative resources, which remained constant, but to different magnitudes of public sentiment. Moreover, although Weberians would expect the British state's strength to positively prefigure future institutional change, Labour's response to public attitudes was to adopt a fragmented tripartite structure that abandoned coordination across the three services and willingly invited inefficiency.

From the coalition government to the Labour cabinet, there was a sys-

79. CAB 134/697, SS (45) 1st, Minutes of the Social Services Committee, 8/29/45.
80. Godber Interview.

tematic relation between public opinion and policymakers' language and decisions. The public's favoring of a state-run medical service and free, comprehensive coverage repeatedly corresponded with the government's reasons and decisions for defying interest group positions favoring limited coverage. Moreover, deliberation over several issues suggests that it was *after* policymakers' perception of public opinion changed that government policy changed. For instance, Labour fundamentally altered the coalition's policy of preserving the existing hospital systems; this fundamental policy shift followed a change in policymakers' perception of public opinion. Whereas the wartime government inaccurately perceived strong support for preserving voluntary hospitals, the Labour cabinet fully recognized the public's hostility toward the established hospital systems and its support for the state's nationalization of hospitals. The primary focus of and influence on policymakers was their interpretation of public opinion; arguments based on administrative grounds simply failed to dominate policy deliberations.

9 | United States, 1964–1965: Johnson, the 89th Congress, and the Medicare Act

Democratic party candidates won landslide victories in the 1964 presidential and congressional races. Although political observers sensed a dramatic shift in public opinion, Americans' evaluation of public policy actually changed very little: the public continued to support major reform of social welfare arrangements, in particular health care policy. The Democrats' historic landslide did, however, significantly affect the political context of policy making. For politicians and specialists, the transformation of American politics represented an unambiguous shift in public opinion, motivating officeholders to make two bold departures from ongoing discussions and established arrangements: they designed an innovative amalgamation of existing proposals and finally enacted major health legislation that had eluded reformers. But policymakers' pursuit of bold innovation was tempered by a commitment to established arrangements and broad policy goals previously identified by reformers and major politicians such as John Kennedy.

Between November 1964 and July 1965, when the Medicare Bill was signed into law, legislative and executive officials bargained over final authoritative decisions. President Johnson's promotion of Medicare's Social Security approach established it as one of the major subjects of policy debate; members of Congress bargained on policy content. In the comparatively open context of congressional hearings, leading interest groups directly participated in policy discussions. Like their British counterparts, however, American policymakers considered sectional interests a nuisance to be distanced from critical policy decisions.

190

THE STRATEGIC UNIVERSE

The 1964 election linked emerging cultural and political patterns that had previously been developing in separate directions. The fundamental shift in national politics altered policymakers' calculations, intensifying their sensitivity to public opinion and their commitment to bold changes.

Public Opinion

By 1965, the public's preferences and understandings regarding social welfare reform had been evolving for decades but had remained, at least for many political observers, amorphous. The starkly different positions and images of the 1964 presidential candidates, Lyndon Johnson and Barry Goldwater, created a rare opportunity for voters to signal their strong interest in and support for addressing the elderly's health care needs.

From the public's perspective, the 1964 national elections posed a distinct choice between pursuing change or returning to the period before the 1930s and the New Deal. Johnson advocated carrying on the New Deal approach to reform. In particular, he defended Social Security and urged its use to introduce health reform, repeatedly identifying Medicare as a top priority.[1] In contrast, Goldwater had a well-established reputation as an extreme conservative who advocated (among other things) rolling back Social Security to a voluntary system. A private polling organization reported that Americans identified Goldwater with dismantling such New Deal programs as Social Security: despite his attempt to moderate his image, "still many millions of voters ... held to their conviction that Goldwater was a foe of the Social Security system."[2] Similarly, Page's (1978) analysis of public perceptions of Goldwater found that the Republican's efforts to reposition himself toward the center of public opinion had little effect; his image was firmly associated with a return to the pre–New Deal period and with opposition to social welfare reform.

Johnson's landslide victory represented a popular mandate to pursue change, particularly a Medicare approach to health reform. In the period

---

1. Jacobs and Shapiro (1992) have concluded a content analysis of Johnson's policy announcements, as recorded in *The Public Papers of the Presidents* and *The Weekly Compilation of Presidential Documents*. They report a significant jump during the fall campaign in both the strength of Johnson's commitment to Medicare and the amount of time he devoted to the issue.

2. LBJ Library, PR16, Box 346, "Public Opinion Guidelines for the 1965 Business Climate," 2/65, attached to forwarding memo from Jack Valenti to Johnson, 2/8/65. The poll was based on a series of five interviews between August and November 1964; 6,747 respondents ranked twenty-three issues as having a "great deal" to do with their vote for Johnson.

between the election campaign and Medicare's passage in July 1965, the public continued, as it had since the late 1950s, to follow health reform with great interest. A private research organization reported to the White House in February 1965 that among Johnson voters Medicare was a major concern: in addition to foreign policy issues (such as "keeping peace in the world"), it was one of a handful of issues that mattered a "great deal."[3] The White House's private pollster, Oliver Quayle, reported in one of his first postelection surveys that "help for old people" was ranked first in a list of "most important" national issues, with education and other prominent issues not assigned "great importance."[4] Evidence of public interest in Medicare is indirectly corroborated by the *New York Times* coverage; between November 1964 and July 1965, the *Times* devoted more attention to this issue than to other domestic policy areas, such as education.[5] Thus, even amid the feverish policy debates following the 1964 election, health care remained a highly salient issue on the public's agenda.

In addition to remaining salient, Medicare continued to be identified as the public's preferred policy direction. Both published and White House polls echoed the evolution since the 1930s in Americans' understanding and acceptance of government provision of social welfare via the Social Security system. In addition to Quayle's findings, separate published surveys in December 1964 and February 1965 found that nearly two-thirds of the respondents supported use of the Social Security program to finance medical care for the aged. Reflecting the depth of this support, the question wording for the December poll noted that Medicare would include a tax increase: respondents strongly approved of a "medical care program [that] would be financed out of increased social security taxes" (Schiltz 1970, 194).

Forcing respondents to choose among alternative health insurance plans is the most reliable indicator of public preferences toward reform proposals. In a published poll, Harris reported in March 1965 that a significant plurality (46–36%) favored Medicare over a private scheme.[6] Schiltz's exhaustive analysis of public opinion data over time indicates that popular preferences toward Medicare were more "crystallized" and favorable by the 1960s than

---

3. LBJ Library, PR16, Box 346, "Public Opinion Guidelines for the 1965 Business Climate," by Opinion Research Corporation, 2/65, sent to the White House by D. Cook (President, American Electric Power Co.) and forwarded by Jack Valenti to Johnson, 2/8/65.
4. LBJ Library, CF PR16, Box 80, "A Survey of the Political Climate in Minnesota," by Quayle, 6/65.
5. The *Times* devoted 189 articles to the health care issue (19 additional pieces discussed British and Canadian health policy), and 167 articles covered federal policy on education.
6. The wording of the question was the following: "If you had to choose between a federal law which would provide medical care for the aged by a special tax, like Social Security, or a plan of extended private health insurance, which would you choose?" (Erskine 1975, 134).

they had previously been toward Truman's national health insurance schemes (Schiltz 1970, 140).

Medicare's popularity seems to have been grounded in public support for the principle of covering the elderly's health care costs. Below this broad level of support, though, the public's knowledge of the specific provisions of numerous Medicare proposals, which were circulated in Washington, was limited. Discussing the public's incomplete understanding, Schiltz reported that in early 1965, only 40 percent of respondents knew that the administration's Medicare proposal did not cover physicians' fees (1970, 142).

The country's confusion over the White House's hospital-oriented Medicare plan echoed the information provided the public; after all, Americans had been bombarded for half a dozen years by inflated promises to solve the elderly's health care problems. Respondents' reactions in a December 1964 Gallup poll were consistent with the theme of "helping older people" that had persistently surfaced in political debates and media coverage: among those who incorrectly believed that physician fees were covered in the administration's bill, 73 percent approved of Medicare; but among those who understood that the administration's plan did not cover these fees, only 56 percent approved (Schiltz 1970, 144–45). Although socioeconomic characteristics may partly account for this 17 percent difference, this evidence suggests, according to Schiltz, that "failure to include physicians' fees in Medicare's coverage accounted for some degree of opposition among those who might otherwise have supported the proposal" (1970, 145). The public seemed to hold elites to their promise to solve the elderly's health care problems.

The opposite policy approach—public assistance—remained quite unpopular. A series of published polls in the fall of 1964 echoed the humiliation felt by an elderly woman who wrote to the White House that "it hurts to have to take charity."[7] Schiltz's analysis of Americans' reaction to means-tested programs suggests that the " 'dole' [was considered] inimical to self-esteem and to the American way of life" (1970, 158). Polls indicated that the general public continued to harbor suspicions that forcing beneficiaries to take relief somehow broke down their moral character, ultimately encouraging laziness and cheating (Schiltz 1970, 158–59; Katz 1986).

Political Struggles

Labour's victory stunned Britain; but in the United States political observers expected the Democrats, especially the presidential candidate, to win the

---

7. LBJ Library, Gen IS1, Box 2, Letter from Ella Brown to Johnson, 12/19/64.

1964 races. Within the White House, Johnson's closest aides, who had found previous campaigns difficult to predict, concluded quite early in the 1964 race that the outcome was "absolutely certain."[8] With such assurance, Johnson's aides concentrated on shaping the campaign to influence the governing process *after* the election. To win by as large a majority as possible, the Johnson forces portrayed Goldwater as a threatening extremist and gleefully snatched sole possession of the strategically valuable political center. But they concluded that attacks "against Goldwater are almost embarrassingly out of place." Instead, the Democratic ticket focused on a more positive approach to campaigning and on shaping the governing process *after* the election; the point was to create an indisputable symbol of popular support that would propel the White House's policy agenda after November.[9]

By the early summer of 1964, a consensus had formed among senior White House officials that Johnson "has an opportunity . . . to shape the mandate he wants and needs on November 3rd."[10] The general objective was to create a mandate for a "new, creative period [that] . . . clear[ed] up long-hanging domestic business."[11] Not satisfied to win a broad endorsement for "vigorous moves," White House officials sought to capitalize on Johnson's historic "opportunity not only to win a decisive mandate . . . but also to shape that mandate." Thus, nearly half a year before election day, small groups of policy specialists prepared for the campaign by "quietly . . . work[ing] on specific subjects" for Johnson's 1965 legislative program: the administration's projected postelection positions were used to provide specific policy direction for the 1964 campaign.[12] The race, then, offered an opportunity to focus the attention of disparate policymakers on Johnson's agenda and to bolster his postelection influence; connecting with voters outside Washington was expected to unify forces within.

The White House interpretation of public preferences significantly af-

8. LBJ Library, Interview with George Reedy by T. H. Baker (Tape 4), 12/20/68. Also see Interview with Douglas Cater by David McComb, 4/29/69 (Tape 1); Interview with Jack Valenti by J. Frantz, 3/3/71 (Tape 1).

9. LBJ Library, Ex FG1, Box 10, Memo from H. Busty to W. Wirtz, C. Clifford, M. Bundy, D.Cater, D. Goodwin, E. Goldman, 10/14/64. Also see Ex PR16, Box 345, Memo to president from L. O'Brien, 10/4/64; FG100/MC, Box 130, Memo to B. Moyers from H. Busby, approximately 9/64; Interview with Jack Valenti by J. Frantz, 3/3/71 (Tape 1); Gen WE6, Box 16, Letter from C. Roche (Deputy Chairman, Democratic National Committee) to J. Valenti, 7/27/64; Busby Papers, Box 41, Memo to H. Busby from D. Scammon, 9/29/64; LE/IS1, Box 75, Memo to president from B. Moyers, 9/2/64.

10. LBJ Library, CF LE, Box 61, Memo to J. Valenti from B. Moyers, just before 5/30/64.

11. LBJ Library, Ex FG1, Box 10, "Suggested Talking Points: Press Backgrounder Briefing for Sunday 7/5/64," handwritten, "G.E.R[eedy]. Ok to be released. LBJ, 7/4/64." Also see Interview with Jack Valenti by J. Frantz, 3/3/71 (Tape 1); Ex LE, Box 1, Memo to B. Moyers from Ernest Goldstein, 5/29/64.

12. LBJ Library, CF LE, Box 61, Memo to J. Valenti from B. Moyers, just before 5/30/64. Also see Ex FG1, Box 10, Memo to president from D. Cater, 6/3/64; Interview with Jack Valenti by J. Frantz, 3/3/71 (Tape 1).

fected the campaign's selection of a few specific issues for presidential promotion. To pursue an effective strategy, aides recognized that the featured issues must be consistent with the "broad opinions...of the American people."[13] Presidential aide Douglas Cater repeatedly informed Johnson and other White House officials that Medicare was one of the few issues that attracted the largest general interest and support. He suggested that the Quayle state surveys, particularly the voter selections of the "most important" issues, indicated that assisting the elderly was among three issues on which public approval was particularly high.[14] The president and his closest advisers agreed that Medicare was one of the major issues "found to be working for [the president]" and therefore repeatedly ranked health reform during the campaign at the top of Johnson's legislative "must" list.[15] Quantitative analysis confirms this process of responsiveness: Quayle's report of strong public support in July was followed during September and October by a dramatic jump in the strength and extensiveness of Johnson's statements in favor of Medicare (Jacobs and Shapiro 1992). Public opinion, then, was an important reason that Johnson made Medicare, as Mills recalled, "a number one, top priority issue of the 1964 election"; a senior HEW administrator explained that Medicare was not only an issue in the presidential race but also a focus of many congressional contests.[16]

As expected, the Democrats won. The proportion of their victories was, however, surprising. The Party picked up four seats in the Senate and fourteen in the House, where the Democratic majority was the largest in almost three decades and enough to break the previous bipartisan conservative coalition. To Washington elites, voters' resounding rejection of Goldwater in favor of Democratic congressional and presidential candidates seemed to represent a fundamental shift in public opinion toward support of domestic reform. Politicians' and specialists' sense of an attitudinal shift appeared to be confirmed by the House's decision to promote reform by modifying its rules and altering the composition of the powerful Ways and Means Committee (conservative members were removed).

Keeping to the script crafted before the election, Johnson began "whipping his staff into...[a] frenzy" "almost from the very hour that the polls closed." The White House assumed that satisfying Johnson's popular mandate for change required "dynamic" and "decisive" leadership promoting

13. LBJ Library, Ex LE, Box 1, Memo to B. Moyers from Ernest Goldstein, 5/29/64.
14. LBJ Library, Moyers Papers, Box 3, Memo to B. Moyers from D. Cater, 7/21/64; Califano Papers, Box 7, Memo on the Quayle state surveys from D. Cater, 10/7/64 (copies of polls attached); Busby Papers, Box 41, Memo to president from Cater, 10/8/64.
15. LBJ Library, Ex PR16, Box 345, Memo to president from L. O'Brien, 10/4/64. Also see Humphrey Papers, Box 1; Harris 1966, 177; David 1985, 120–21.
16. Mills Interview; LBJ Library, Interview with Robert Ball by David McComb, 11/5/68 (Tape 2).

the "forward thrust of Government." The landslide created, according to HEW administrators, a "singular moment in history" in which "to do whatever was necessary to pass...legislation." Thus, while the deadlock of the early 1960s convinced reformers to avoid frittering away scarce political capital on major battles, the risk now, according to the White House, was that the administration could fall into the "ignominious pitfalls" of pursuing "inaction to avoid rocking the boat."[17]

The White House became immersed in determining the general subject of government policy and completing the "long-neglected agenda of unfinished business" Kennedy had outlined.[18] The political importance attached to setting the government's general direction was reflected in the White House emphasis on the amount of legislation pushed through Congress. Soon after the election, senior White House officials pointed approvingly to polls showing that the president rated high in getting things through Congress, and they emphasized the importance of "totally record[ing] in the public mind" the number of new laws that were being enacted.[19]

The White House's handling of Medicare exemplified the administration's strategy of capitalizing on Johnson's mandate to set the general direction of policy. The White House's private polls before and after election day reinforced the preelection decision to select Medicare for presidential promotion.[20] The White House attempted to convert Johnson's mandate and his specific identification of Medicare during the campaign into political capital for passing legislation. In particular, it used numerous public comments, the State of the Union address, and a special health message to Congress to identify health reform as its top priority.

Compared to its interest in setting the general subject and direction of government policy, the White House was nearly indifferent to the policy content of its Medicare proposals. Even after the 1964 election shocked the political establishment, Johnson pledged to "stick with what we've got and not change horses in the middle of the stream."[21] Accordingly, the admin-

17. LBJ Library, Interview with Jack Valenti by J. Frantz, 3/3/71 (Tape 1); Administrative Histories, HEW, vol. 1, pt. 1, Office of the Assistant Secretary for Legislation, Recollections of Michael Parker (HEW official under Wilbur Cohen), 1968, p. 14; Ex FG1, Box 10, "Memoranda," unauthored, handwritten "12/21/64," possibly initialed by Johnson; Ex FG1, Box 10, Memo from H. A. Knowles to secretary of commerce, 11/6/64, forwarded to B. Moyers, 11/10/64; Busby Papers, Box 18.

18. LBJ Library, Ex FG1, Box 10, "Memoranda," unauthored, handwritten, "12/21/64," possibly initialed by Johnson.

19. LBJ Library, Ex FG1, Box 12, Memo to Johnson and B. Moyers from J. Valenti, 7/14/65. Also see Interview with Anthony Celebrezze by Paige Mulhollan, 1/26/71; Cater Papers, Box 13, Memo to Johnson from Cater, 4/30/65.

20. LBJ Library, CF PR16, Box 80, "A Survey of the Political Climate in Minnesota," by Quayle, 6/65.

21. Cohen Interview. Also see testimony by A. Celebrezze (Secretary, HEW), U.S. Congress, House, Ways and Means Committee, 1965, pp. 4–5.

istration submitted to Congress Medicare legislation that closely followed Kennedy's scheme and was largely the same as the plan the Senate passed in the fall of 1964. The White House's relative disinterest in legislative content reinforced the conservative "incremental philosophy" of Medicare advocates: even after a landslide, they remained determined to minimize the risk of rejection by designing a limited bill. In stark contrast to British policymakers who wanted to "get on board as much as possible," Cohen and others believed that it was necessary to "keep a lot of things out" in order to lay the foundation for future health policy.[22]

Congress followed the president's leadership in charting the broad direction of policy, but it controlled the content of legislation. As the White House projected before the election, Johnson's landslide was interpreted by politicians and political observers as an indisputable expression of popular support for this agenda; this mandate gave the administration tremendous strength in the new Congress.[23] Within Congress, even Republicans accepted Johnson's pursuit of reform: party members in the House installed a more pragmatic minority leader (Gerald Ford) and acknowledged the necessity, as the Republican counsel on Ways and Means suggested, to "face political realities" (Marmor 1973, 63; Harris, 1966).

To members of Congress, voters' choice of Johnson over Goldwater created a "specific mandate" for Medicare whose popularity was no longer denied. According to Mills, the 1964 election enabled Congress to "judge" public opinion. He conceded that before the election members of Congress may not have been in step with the people's thinking on Medicare; but after Johnson campaigned on the issue and won by an unprecedented margin, they "realized that people were for it for the first time."[24]

Mills's reassessment of public opinion was echoed throughout Congress; members viewed the 1964 election as "giving a specific mandate for a series of liberal legislative proposals" and, particularly, as "being favorable to the Medicare program."[25] Members of Congress widely acknowledged that Medicare's passage was now a foregone conclusion; the Democratic leadership's decision to make Medicare legislation the first bill introduced in the House and Senate underscored this message (Marmor 1973, 104–5).

22. Cohen Interview. Also see testimony by Cohen, U.S. Congress, House, Ways and Means Committee, 1965, pp. 78–79; LBJ Library, Ex LE/IS1, Box 75, Memo to Moyers from P. Hughes (BOB, Assistant Director for Legislative Reference), 5/18/65.
23. LBJ Library, Administrative Histories, HEW, vol. 1, pt. 1, Office of the Assistant Secretary for Legislation, Recollections of Michael Parker (HEW official under Wilbur Cohen), 1968, p. 14.
24. Mills Interview; LBJ Library, Ex FG1, Box 10, "Memoranda," unauthored, handwritten, "12/21/64," possibly initialed by Johnson; Interview with Jack Valenti by J. Frantz, 3/3/71 (Tape 1).
25. LBJ Library, Interview with Robert Ball by David McComb, 11/5/68.

Indeed, many Republicans became far more sensitive to public opinion on Medicare, and several groups previously opposed to health reform now accepted Johnson's mandate and the fact that Medicare was going to pass.[26] Accordingly, the Republican congressional leadership abandoned its previous intransigent opposition to reform and proposed its own health insurance bill.

The only serious threat to Johnson's leadership in winning congressional approval of Medicare was the divisive issue of race relations. Administration and congressional officials feared open discussion of the application of the Civil Rights Act of 1964 to Medicare; only this issue had the potential to "jeopardize the bill" by compelling southern supporters of Medicare to reexamine their position.[27]

Although Congress followed Johnson in moving to enact Medicare legislation, it did not merely ratify his proposals. Congress dominated the final formulation of Medicare's content, responding to the election's unambiguous expression of public opinion by pursuing bold innovations. One liberal senator was struck by Congress's newfound enthusiasm for reforming Medicare: a few years earlier proponents of bold alternatives "would have been committed to St. Elizabeth's [mental hospital]," but after the election even "innovation by Republicans and conservative Democrats . . . [became] a sensible strategy."[28]

In particular, the Ways and Means Committee was the focal point of the health policy network's bargaining over Medicare's legislative design; of particular importance were the committee's hearings and executive sessions between January and April, when a bill was reported out. With three opponents of reform on the committee replaced and Mills elevating Medicare to the committee's "first business," Ways and Means sessions were "business-like and deliberate"; they concentrated on formulating specific items for a final bill.[29] Although the committee accepted Johnson's advocacy of the broad Medicare approach, it redesigned his proposal's content be-

26. Harris 1966, 178–79; LBJ Library, CF PR16, Box 80, Memo to Johnson from J. Valenti, 1/11/65, handwritten, "L. Keep in Office"; testimony by William Beaumont (President Emeritus, American Nursing Home Association), U.S. Congress, House, Ways and Means Committee, 1965, pp. 312, 330.

27. The important but largely unexamined relation between Medicare and civil rights legislation is contained in the following documents: LBJ Library, Ex, LE/IS1, Box 75, Letter to H. Byrd from A. Celebrezze, 4/27/65, Memo to Lee White from B. Moyers, 4/27/65, and, Memo to Johnson from Lee White, 4/26/65. Also helpful is Cohen Interview.

28. LBJ Library, Ex IS, Box 1, Letter from L. O'Brien to C. P. Anderson, 8/27/65; Marmor 1973, 76.

29. Marmor 1973, 62. Also see Mills Interview; LBJ Library, Wilson Files, Memo to L. O'Brien from M. Mantos, 1/5/65; Ex LE/IS1, Box 75, Memo to secretary of HEW from Cohen, 1/28/65.

cause it was "too conservative ... [and] too limited" to respond to the election's unambiguous signal of popular expectations.[30]

The bold alternatives generated from Ways and Means' deliberations were largely accepted by the House and Senate and signed into law in July 1965. The only significant attempt to make "radical change" in Mills's scheme was by Russell Long, who chaired the Senate committee responsible for health legislation. But the administration and congressional officials successfully "begged, cajoled and argued" in the Senate to "dissuade ... any kind of frontal attack" on Ways and Means' work; in the end, the upper chamber's changes were "minor and technical."[31] In the first round of votes, Ways and Means' basic package was approved in the House (315–115) and the Senate (68–12), and Mills persuaded (with Cohen's assistance) Senate members of the conference committee to accept the House version.[32] The bill that emerged from the conference committee substantially reflected the decisions reached by Ways and Means and was passed in July 1965 by lopsided margins in the House (307–116) and the Senate (70–24).[33] Thus, Congress followed the broad policy direction charged by Johnson but insisted on reformulating the content of his proposal.

Ways and Means' deliberations organized the policy network in a way that was more open and accessible than that in Britain. Although their bargaining contexts differed, both American and British officials insisted on independence from major interest groups. After the 1964 election, large numbers of doctors threatened to boycott Medicare if it was enacted, and the AMA mobilized its substantial financial and organizational resources, which have traditionally been credited with the defeat of earlier reforms.[34] The AMA's significant material and symbolic resources, however, neither defeated nor dictated Medicare's formulation. Policymakers continued to weigh the

30. Mills Interview. Also see Interview with Thomas Curtis by F. Ingersoll, Former Members of Congress, Inc., 12/9/78; comment by J. Byrne, quoted in David 1985, 130–31; LBJ Library, Interview with Robert Ball by David McComb, 11/5/68; Interview with Mills by J. O'Connor, 4/14/67.

31. LBJ Library, Memo to L. O'Brien from Cohen, 5/6/65. Also see Ex LE/IS1, Box 75, Letter to Johnson from C. P. Anderson, 7/19/65, Memo to Johnson from Cohen, 6/24/65, concerning final action by Finance Committee on Medicare.

32. The critical vote in the House was on whether to recommit the bill for further committee consideration; the 45-vote margin to consider the Ways and Means report on the floor was much closer than the final count. LBJ Library, Ex LE/IS1, Box 75, Memo to Johnson from Cohen 6/24/65, concerning final action by Finance Committee on Medicare; Ex LE/IS1, Box 75, Memo to L. O'Brien from Cohen, 7/19/65; Ex LE, Box 4, Memo to Claude Desautels from Cohen, 7/12/65.

33. For a more detailed discussion of the deliberations in the Senate and the conference committee, see David 1985, chapters 7, 8, and 9.

34. Harris 1966, 175–76, 193–94, 206–8, 216–17; David 1985, 124–25; testimony by Dr. F. Coleman (representative of the AMA), U.S. Congress, House, Ways and Means Committee, 1965, pp. 758–59.

AMA's claims, but Democrats as well as the Republican leadership treated the AMA as a "nuisance" and refused to produce the organization's desired legislative outcome. The AMA suffered, Mills explained, because of its "blind refusal to accept reality": the organization was excluded from unofficial committee deliberations, and its testimony was repeatedly derided for "spout[ing] the usual nonsense" and for ignoring policymakers' narrow concern with the medical profession's technical advice on specific issues.[35]

The Democratically controlled government produced bold Medicare legislation in response to its sense of a shift in public opinion. But this reformist bent coexisted with an attentiveness to continuity and to the avoidance of a radical departure from previous arrangements and policy discussions. Expressing a broad concern within the administration, one official stressed the importance of the word "moderation" as "stand[ing] for all that is ... calm and steady": Johnson and his advisers were the "true moderates" because they were committed to avoiding "excessive, drastic, ... and radical" measures in favor of building a "broad consensus ... [behind] cooperative efforts."[36] Motivated by a similar concern with continuity, Mills decided to "take hold of events and lead them" in order to protect established programs, especially the Social Security system.[37] That the government generated historic new arrangements should not, Marmor reminds us, "obscure the patterns of the preceding decade" (1973, 110).

Policy Discussions

The Medicare approach of using Social Security to finance the elderly's health care was designed by reformers in the early 1950s and had become a salient, popular issue by Kennedy's 1960s presidential campaign. Nevertheless, it was not until the 1964 election gave Johnson a landslide and Congress a new influx of liberal members that this approach was finally adopted. "The only question remaining was the precise form the health insurance legislation would take" (Marmor 1973, 60). Marmor presents a compelling explanation of policymakers' constraints and motivations in coming to accept Medicare as a "statutory certainty," but he does not fully

35. Harris 1966, 179–80, 184–85. Also see Marmor 1973, 62–63; Mills Interview; Cohen Interview; statement by A. Ullman, U.S. Congress, House, Ways and Means Committee, 1965, pp. 758–59.

36. LBJ Library, Ex FG1, Box 10, Memo from H. A. Knowles to secretary of commerce, 11/6/64, forwarded to B. Moyers, 11/10/64.

37. LBJ Library, Interview with Robert Ball by David McComb, 11/5/68. Also see Interview with Thomas Curtis by F. Ingersoll, Former Members of Congress, Inc., 12/9/78; comment by J. Byrne, quoted in David 1985, pp. 130–31.

explain their choice of its precise form or why their relationships with interest groups were alternately defiant and conciliatory.

The final deliberations of Congress and experts primarily occurred in the relatively cloistered confines of the Ways and Means Committee. These deliberations were often shielded from the glare of national attention; nevertheless, public opinion was the central influence on policymakers as they weighed interest group claims for continuing established practices and chose specific changes in administrative arrangements.

State Autonomy and Basic Principles

Politicians and bureaucrats continued to disagree with interest groups over two major Medicare principles, Social Security financing and universal access for the elderly. In the three decades since the New Deal, Americans' understanding of the state gradually changed because of social interaction with new government institutions, especially the Social Security system. The new social understanding of the state was echoed in polling data, which indicated strong, sustained support for Social Security. Thus, the principles of social insurance financing and open access to health care for the elderly were firmly anchored in the state's most popular form of social welfare provision. The alternative approach to providing social welfare, the poor-law approach, was widely resented. In the face of this pattern of public opinion, medical producers in 1965 no longer unambiguously opposed Social Security financing and comprehensive coverage of the elderly; when they did, they exercised little influence.

After the 1964 election, the intense disputes that previously surrounded the issue of Medicare's coverage subsided. The earlier controversy about blanketing-in the aged who had not contributed to Social Security eased; policymakers agreed to provide all elderly citizens with access to Medicare benefits.[38] The only serious dispute concerning coverage involved the age limit that would trigger eligibility. The Senate created a controversy by contradicting Social Security's practice of setting eligibility at sixty-five; it provided an option whereby beneficiaries could become eligible at sixty in exchange for a reduced benefit package.[39]

Senior officials in Congress and the administration successfully objected by emphasizing the future impact of this decision on public opinion. The secretary of HEW warned that soon after Medicare's implementation pop-

38. LBJ Library, Ex LE/IS1, Box 75, Memo to HEW secretary from Cohen, 1/28/65, cc: L. O'Brien, H. Wilson, D. Cater; LE/IS1, Box 75, "Summary of Major Provisions of 'Hospital Insurance and Social Security Act of 1965'," 11/24/64, attached to memo to Johnson from A. Celebrezze, 11/25/64.
39. LBJ Library, Ex LE, Box 4, Memo to Claude Desautels from Cohen, 7/12/65.

ular pressure to expand benefits would accumulate: an individual who opted to become eligible at sixty would later become unhappy at not receiving the full benefits and start urging that benefits be increased.[40] Moreover, Mills strongly opposed the option because it would create the impression among Americans that Medicare was not financially solvent: reducing the retirement age to sixty would make it "appear as if [Medicare]... resulted in starting the social security fund on the road to bankruptcy."[41] The Senate position was inconsistent with the public's understanding of Social Security, and the conference committee abandoned it when finalizing Medicare legislation.

The second issue, adopting Social Security's financing arrangements, attracted significant public attention and was similarly accepted by policymakers. The AMA continued to mistakenly claim that Americans favored limiting government funds to those in need and relying on established poor-law arrangements (albeit the Kerr-Mills program). Insensitive to Americans' changing understanding of state provisions, the AMA charged that there was "no justification for compelling taxpayers and their employers to... buy health care for millions of other people." The AMA predicted that the result of Medicare's unwanted interference would be to waste public funds on those who were able to take care themselves.[42]

The administration and influential members of Congress dismissed the AMA's claims and offered a different (more accurate) interpretation of public opinion. They argued that, although the AMA wanted all government programs to be means tested, the average American wanted a program without means tests. The public detested the "welfare" approach because it forced beneficiaries to submit to the humiliation of a means test; recipients would have to undergo "analyzing, checking, [and] snooping... to find out whether someone is [financially] eligible." Administration and congressional officials readily agreed that the limited appeal of an "Elizabethan poor law" made it impossible to "sell... welfare as your number one political objective"; to win public support for addressing the elderly's health care problem, it was critical not to "confin[e] governmental effort to the relief of poverty among older people." Convinced, then, that the AMA's position in favor of the poor laws was out of touch with Americans' preferences and understandings, Democrats and many Republicans dismissed it as "not even valid at this point."[43]

40. LBJ Library, Ex LE/IS1, Box 75, Memo to Johnson from A. Celebrezze, 7/12/65.
41. LBJ Library, Ex LE/IS1, Box 75, Memo to L. O'Brien from Cohen, 7/19/65.
42. Testimony by Dr. D. Ward (President, AMA), U.S. Congress, House, Ways and Means Committee, 1965, pp. 742–44,748–49.
43. Statement by A. Ullman (member, Ways and Means Committee), U.S. Congress, House, Ways and Means Committee, 1965, pp. 339–41; LBJ Library, Ex LE/IS1, Box 75, Memo to Johnson from Cohen, regarding "Congressmen Herlong and Curtis' 'Eldercare Act of 1965',"

In place of the negatively perceived Kerr-Mills program, Johnson and influential members of Congress continued to insist on an insurance-type program because the "American people...accepted the idea overwhelmingly and enthusiastically."[44] Policy makers were unwilling to rely on the demeaning welfare-type programs; their most decisive consideration was the maintenance of the insurance aspect. Mills and other politicians disregarded interest group opposition and adopted (as designed in the early 1950s) the Medicare approach—making health insurance an extension of the popular and familiar Social Security program. Congress and the administration were confident that the Social Security approach, which "supports the individual's self-reliance and independence," would enjoy enormous popularity.[45]

To visibly fortify Medicare's connection with the popular insurance aspect of the program, Mills insisted that Cohen and other specialists establish a separate trust fund to pay health benefits; isolating the Medicare fund from the Social Security account would ensure that "people can watch" "their own contributions...financing [their care]."[46] Moreover, policymakers significantly increased Social Security taxes to ensure that the program could be " 'sold' and...widely supported" as a self-sustaining program: Mills insisted on being able to tell the House of Representatives that there would be sufficient funds available to pay benefits even in the program's early years.[47] The administration's economic experts unsuccessfully argued against sizable tax increases, which they thought would create a large fiscal drag, stunting consumer purchasing power and economic growth.[48] Mills,

---

2/25/65; Cohen Interview; testimony by A. Celebrezze (Secretary, HEW), U.S. Congress, House, Ways and Means Committee, 1965, pp. 2–3.

44. Testimony by Cohen, U.S. Congress, House, Ways and Means Committee, 1965, pp. 93, 102–3.

45. LBJ Library, Ex LE/IS1, Box 75, Memo to Johnson from Cohen, regarding "Congressmen Herlong and Curtis' 'Eldercare Act of 1965'," 2/25/65. Also see Testimony by K. Gordon (Director, BOB), U.S. Congress, House, Ways and Means Committee, 1965, pp. 802–3; testimony by A. Celebrezze (Secretary, HEW), U.S. Congress, House, Ways and Means Committee, 1965, pp. 2–3; statement by A. Ullman (Member, Ways and Means Committee), U.S. Congress, House, Ways and Means Committee, 1965, pp. 339–41.

46. Mills Interview and Testimony by K. Gordon (Director, BOB), U.S. Congress, House, Ways and Means Committee, 1965, pp. 802–3. Also see LBJ Library, LE/IS1, Box 75, "Summary of Major Provisions of 'Hospital Insurance and Social Security Act of 1965'," 11/24/64, attached to memo to Johnson from A. Celebrezze, 11/25/64; Ex WE6, Box 15, Memo to G. Ackley, 3/13/65; Ex LE/IS1, Box 75, "Summary of Major Provisions of Social Security Amendments of 1965," 3/19/65, attached to memo from Cohen to Johnson, 3/22/65.

47. LBJ Library, Ex WE6, Box 15, Memo to G. Ackley from HEW secretary, 3/13/65, cc: D. Cater, L. O'Brien, K. Gordon. Also see testimony by R. Ball, U.S. Congress, House, Ways and Means Committee, 1965, pp. 82–85; statement by Mills, U.S. Congress, House, Ways and Means Committee, 1965, p. 85; testimony by A. Celebrezze (Secretary, HEW), U.S. Congress, House, Ways and Means Committee, 1965, pp. 4–5, 8–9.

48. LBJ Library, Ex WE6, Box 15, Memo to president from G. Ackley (Chairman, Council of Economic Advisers), 3/12/65; Ex WE6, Box 15, Memo to president from G. Ackley, 3/11/65;

Johnson, and others agreed that adequately financing Medicare in the short term under even the most unfavorable circumstances was necessary to "maintain the confidence of the nation."[49]

The principles of Social Security financing and coverage of the elderly had been outlined more than a decade earlier, but their adoption by authoritative policy makers was not inevitable. Other previously designed arrangements were overturned or threatened with reformulation; for instance, the Senate decided to depart from Social Security's retirement age of sixty-five. Lawmakers approved reformers' original principles in spite of fierce interest group opposition and Senate revisions because they accurately perceived strong, sustained public support for them.

Strong interest group influence. Politicians and specialists sensed that the public was apathetic or potentially supportive of interest group positions on two established principles, the private health insurance practice of including deductibles and the preservation of doctor's autonomy by limiting Medicare's coverage to hospital treatment. In the new political environment, policymakers were willing to compromise with interest groups on these principles but refused to abdicate completely.

Liberal reformers and erstwhile opponents of Medicare awkwardly joined together to oppose the preelection decision to continue the private health insurance practice of charging deductibles. In particular, the AHA and Blue Cross contested the previous interpretation of deductibles and their impact on the public; patient charges would fail to accomplish their intended purpose of deterring beneficiaries from requesting unnecessary care. The charges required to restrain unnecessary hospital use would simply be unaffordable to many genuinely needy beneficiaries. The result, according to hospitals, would be a serious "public relations problem." Hospital administrators presciently anticipated that using patient charges to discourage overutilization of services would incur public scorn; it would fall to hospitals to bear the uncomfortable "onus" of billing elderly patients.[50]

Without public support of free care (comparable to the British reception of Beveridge's recommendation), the administration and Ways and Means Committee reaffirmed their previous decision to include a flat deductible as

---

testimony by K. Gordon (Director, BOB), U.S. Congress, House, Ways and Means Committee, 1965, pp. 793–95.

49. LBJ Library, Ex WE6, Box 15, Memo to G. Ackley from HEW secretary, 3/13/65, cc: D. Cater, L. O'Brien, K. Gordon. Also see Moyers Papers, Box 3, Memo to L. O'Brien from W. Cohen, 3/17/65; Ex FG165, Box 238, Memo to Johnson from J. Valenti, 4/22/65; Ex LE/IS1, Box 75, Memo to HEW secretary from Cohen, 2/3/65, cc: L. O'Brien, H. Wilson, D. Cater, R. Ball; Ex LE/IS1, Box 75, Memo to president from B. Moyers, 4/26/65.

50. Testimony by K. Williamson (representative of AHA), U.S. Congress, House, Ways and Means Committee, 1965, pp. 289. Also see Testimony by W. McNerney (President, Blue Cross Association), U.S. Congress, House, Ways and Means Committee, 1965, pp.168–69, 177.

a concession to medical interest groups and their sympathizers in Congress.[51] Although concluding that it was politic to continue the private health insurance practice of imposing a flat charge, policymakers were alarmed by Senator Long's decision to modify the House bill by pegging the deductible to the beneficiaries' income level. Congress overturned Long's position because members anticipated that the public would perceive an adjustable deductible as a means test: testing beneficiaries' income represented a "complete departure from social insurance concepts" and would result in Medicare becoming "attractive only for very low-income people."[52]

Regarding the second major principle, preserving doctors' autonomy by limiting services covered by the government's new compulsory program, interest groups continued to draw effectively on American's enduring unease toward the state. In particular, the AMA appealed to two related patterns of public understanding: the public's comparative unease with state provision of social welfare and its relative unfamiliarity with doctors' services. In Britain, the long-standing social interactions with hospitals as well as Friendly Societies and NHI panels created overwhelming public expectations of a comprehensive health service, which policymakers could not ignore. American politicians and experts formulated policy in a profoundly different cultural context. Given Americans' ambivalence toward the state and comparatively limited understanding of health care, policymakers naturally did not detect strong public demand; sectional interests were quite effective in bargaining.

The AMA portrayed Medicare as a "dangerous venture." Only an Orwellian future for doctors and patients could result from this "vast new program directed from Washington and financed by tax funds." The traditional independence of doctors would be "restricted by the decisions of untrained Government employees," who would impose rules and regulations. Moreover, the "control and direction of the Secretary of HEW" would force the "voluntary relationship between the patient and his doctor" to "disappear." Summoning Americans' dread of government, the AMA charged that the inescapable outcome of socialized medicine was that "older persons [would become] Federal wards."[53]

51. Testimony by A. Celebrezze (Secretary, HEW), U.S. Congress, House, Ways and Means Committee, 1965, pp. 4–5.

52. LBJ Library, Ex LE/IS1, Box 75, "Two Amendments to Social Security Bill H.R. 6675 Introduced by Senator Russell B. Long and Tentatively Adopted by the Senate Finance Committee on June 17, 1965," attached to memo from Cohen to Johnson, 6/17/65. Also see Ex LE/IS1, Box 75, Memo to L. O'Brien from Cohen, 5/6/65; Ex LE/IS1, Box 75, Memo to HEW secretary from Cohen, 2/3/65, regarding Ways and Means executive sessions, cc: L. O'Brien, H. Wilson, D. Cater, R. Ball...

53. Testimony by Dr. F. Coleman (representative of the AMA), U.S. Congress, House, Ways and Means Committee, 1965, pp. 762–63; testimony by Dr. D. Ward (President, AMA), U.S. Congress, House, Ways and Means Committee, 1965, pp. 742–46, 762–63; testimony by

Administration and congressional officials were acutely sensitive to AMA efforts to invoke Americans' ambivalence toward the state. They worried that "enter[ing] into the 'doctor-patient' arena" would "get [the government]... into the touchy doctor area" and ignite a "massive fight."[54]

To blunt the potential appeal of such interest group warnings, administration and congressional officials acceded to the AMA's argument; they decided to avoid any perception of control of physician services by limiting the coverage of the government's compulsory program. Continuing to use the policy framework that had emerged before the election, they argued for limiting the program to basic hospital coverage, justifying this limitation by stressing that the elderly could not afford to pay the expenses associated with a hospital stay. Far from being dictated by real world problems, government policy was socially constructed: it incorporated the public's understandings and preferences concerning the state and health care.[55]

Medical experts impressed on congressional leaders and Johnson that Medicare should cover doctors who performed specialist services within hospitals—radiologists, anesthetists, pathologists, and physiatrists. To these experts, it seemed irrational to create a program to cover a patient's stay in a technologically advanced hospital while refusing to cover the services of doctors who actually provided the specialized treatments.

But Mills and other members of Congress were far less concerned with what made sense to medical experts than with defusing AMA appeals to the public regarding the independence of doctors from state control. With the AMA charging that inclusion of specialists made it "inevitable... that the entire medical profession will eventually be brought into the province of this bill,"[56] Mills was "totally adamant" that "*all* services rendered by physicians... be excluded from the Social Security–financed [program]." The conference committee and both legislative chambers backed Mills's insistence that no doctor's fees be paid by a compulsory government program; Cohen conceded that the exclusion of hospital specialists was the

---

J. H. Smith (Vice President, Equitable Life Assurance Society), U.S. Congress, House, Ways and Means Committee, 1965, pp. 394–95.

54. LBJ Library, Ex LE/IS1, Box 75, Memo to Moyers from P. Hughes (BOB, Assistant Director for Legislative Reference), 5/18/65.

55. Testimony by A. Celebrezze (Secretary, HEW), U.S. Congress, House, Ways and Means Committee, 1965, p. 14; also see 2–3, 8–9. Also see Testimony by R. Ball (Commissioner of Social Security, HEW), U.S. Congress, House, Ways and Means Committee, 1965, pp. 46–47; testimony by Cohen, U.S. Congress, House, Ways and Means Committee, 1965, pp. 78–79, 241; statement by Mills, U.S. Congress, House, Ways and Means Committee, 1965, pp. 70–71; testimony by Cohen, U.S. Congress, House, Ways and Means Committee, 1965, pp. 68–70, 102–3.

56. Testimony by Dr. D. Ward (President, AMA), U.S. Congress, House, Ways and Means Committee, 1965, pp. 744–45, 762–63.

administration's only important defeat.[57] In contrast, though, to policy-makers' preelection capitulation to AMA criticism, Mills and other officials generated new arrangements that circumvented fears of governmental meddling with doctors' traditional sovereignty. As we see below, they embraced a voluntary insurance program that covered doctors' services—without relying on a compulsory government program.

State Capacity and Administrative Arrangements

During the years of debate, the policy network's deliberations progressed from dissension over whether a problem existed to acknowledgment, even by Medicare's opponents, of the elderly's needs and the existence of a feasible solution. By 1965, politicians' and specialists' main concern was *how* to structure the central state's new administrative organization; particular attention was devoted to two issues—the expansion of the central state into new areas and the significance of such expansion for Medicare's future. Politicians, specialists, and interest groups resumed the ongoing debate over whether and to what degree the state ought to establish hierarchical control over and specialization in the new financing program for the elderly. Their deliberations were framed by the public's ambivalence toward the state: Americans increasingly accepted Social Security while continuing to be suspicious of state provisions of services. On the heels of the Democrats' landslide, Congress stood poised to endorse Medicare advocates' strategy for circumventing this suspicion—"latching" onto the popular Social Security system a new government program for financing the elderly's health care. The critical issue was how to administer this new state role in paying medical providers.

At the outset of Kennedy's term, senior officials in HEW and the Bureau

57. Discussion among administration officials of Mills's position on hospital specialists is contained in the following files in LBJ Library, Ex LE/IS1, Box 75: Memo to HEW secretary from Cohen, 2/3/65, regarding Ways and Means executive sessions, cc: L. O'Brien, H. Wilson, D. Cater, R. Ball . . . ; Memo to O'Brien from Cohen, 3/16/65; Memo to O'Brien from Cohen, 3/17/65; Memo to Johnson from O'Brien, 3/17/65; "Summary of Major Provisions of Social Security Amendments of 1965," 3/19/65, attached to memo from Cohen to Johnson, 3/22/65; Memo to O'Brien from Cohen, 7/19/65; Memo to O'Brien from Cohen, 7/20/65; Letter to Johnson from C. P. Anderson, 7/21/65; Memo to Moyers from P. Hughes (BOB, Assistant Director for Legislative Reference), 5/18/65; Memo to Esther Peterson from R. Mueller (Executive Office of the President, President's Committee on Consumer Interests), 5/5/65. See also Ex LE, Box 4, Memo to Claude Desautels from Cohen, 7/12/65. The views of a prominent medical expert are contained in the following: JFK Library, R. F. Kennedy Papers, Senate Legislation, Box 69, Letter to Mills from Dr. S. Standard (Professor, Clinical Surgery, NYU College of Medicine), 5/7/65, Letter to Adam Molinsky (Robert Kennedy aide) from S. Standard, 4/7/65.

of the Budget had argued for fundamentally strengthening the state's expertise and control in order to create "direct Federal administration" of Medicare's reimbursement of medical providers. By 1965, senior policymakers remained convinced that the state's organizational capacity would have to be strengthened to control Medicare's disbursement of massive sums of money: "We do not want," Mills explained, "to just turn it loose."[58] Indeed, Congress and the president authorized the secretary of HEW (albeit in vague terms) to take overall responsibility for controlling the cost as well as the health and safety standards of Medicare-financed services.

But the president and Congress did not enhance HEW's expertise and hierarchical control to a level commensurate with its new responsibility. The administrative arguments for strengthening the state's organizational capacity were suffocated by decisionmakers' preoccupation with public uneasiness over state interference and by AMA attempts to summon Americans' fear of government meddling.

Administration and congressional officials attempted to defuse or deflect the "considerable furor" over the appearance that the government would "question or interfere in medical practice." Directly contradicting persistent recommendations to enhance the state's administrative control over the cost and quality of Medicare-financed treatment, policymakers actually dispersed the state's authority and ceded specialized functions to private bodies. In particular, they made two changes intended to "protect completely against Federal interference" and to "preserve the doctor-patient relationship": they weakened administrative oversight and ceded control over reimbursement.[59]

Cohen and other administrative officials assisted members of Congress in deliberately compromising Medicare's specialized capacity to oversee the quality of care provided beneficiaries. "The only infringement upon [a patient's] free choice," they assured Mills, would be "limited to matters of health and safety," and those safeguards would be exceptionally permissive—less strict than even those applied by private organizations.[60] Moreover, to discourage HEW from exercising independent judgment and interfering with medical providers, they designed Medicare to ensure leading interests a "voice" in its administration; the HEW secretary was required to consult with the appropriate national and state associations.[61]

58. Statement by Mills, U.S. Congress, House, Ways and Means Committee, 1965, p. 67.
59. Exchange between Mills and Cohen, U.S. Congress, House, Ways and Means Committee, 1965, p. 136, and statement by A. Ullman, U.S. Congress, House, Ways and Means Committee, 1965, pp. 758–59. Also see testimony by K. Williamson (representative of AHA), U.S. Congress, House, Ways and Means Committee, 1965, pp. 222–23, 287.
60. Exchange between Mills and Cohen, U.S. Congress, House, Ways and Means Committee, 1965, p. 138. Also see testimony by R. Ball, U.S. Congress, House, Ways and Means Committee, 1965, pp. 64–65.
61. Testimony by A. Celebrezze (Secretary, HEW), U.S. Congress, House, Ways and Means

Administration and congressional officials' second strategy for defusing potential public unease over the state focused on reimbursement arrangements and on challenging the classic norm of public administration, that state control escalates as the government commits more money. To protect against the charge that the government itself would regulate health care, policymakers decided to pay health providers on a "reasonable cost basis." Instead of imposing control over the expenditure of massive new sums of government money, they adopted permissive reimbursement arrangements that allowed providers to charge what they deemed reasonable. Regardless of the final cost, administration officials allayed congressional fears of socialized medicine by minimizing the state's new role and insisting that Medicare was "not beginning something new": the expenditure of government money would be guided by existing customs.[62]

In another effort to "protect the public from the government," Mills and others decided that the actual reimbursement of medical providers would be performed by a third party outside government. They hoped that allowing private agencies to handle claims, inspect providers, and review billed costs would create a middle ground between the government and the providers of care and avoid confrontation between hospital and government. Given Americans' reservations about the state, administrative and congressional officials were attracted to the fact that using an outside agency like Blue Cross would "get the most out [of] . . . utilization review . . . and the least criticism" for imposing "overall administration by the Federal Government."[63]

Because hospitals would have little or no familiarity with government agencies, providers were expected to be more comfortable dealing with organizations like Blue Cross, with which they had maintained constant contact for years. In addition to satisfying hospitals, relying on a "buffer"

Committee, 1965, p. 7. Also see LBJ Library, Ex LE/IS1, Box 75, "Summary of Major Provisions of Social Security Amendments of 1965," attached to memo to Johnson from Cohen, 3/27/65.

62. Exchange between Mills and R. Ball, U.S. Congress, House, Ways and Means Committee, 1965, pp. 138–45. Also see LBJ Library, Ex LE/IS1, Box 75, "Summary of Major Provisions of Social Security Amendments of 1965," 3/19/65, attached to memo from Cohen to Johnson, 3/22/65; Ex LE/IS1, Box 75, Memo to Moyers from P. Hughes (Assistant Director for Legislative Reference, BOB), 5/18/65; Ex LE/IS1, Box 75, Memo to Esther Peterson from R. Mueller (Executive Office of the President, President's Committee on Consumer Interests), 5/5/65; Ex LE/IS1, Box 75, Memo to O'Brien from Cohen, 3/11/65.

63. Exchanges between Mills and T. Bell (Welfare Director, State of Colorado), U.S. Congress, House, Ways and Means Committee, 1965, pp. 197–222. Also see testimony by W. McNerney (President, Blue Cross Association) and Mills's exchange, U.S. Congress, House, Ways and Means Committee, 1965, pp. 160–61, 174–77, 184–85. Statement by Mills, U.S. Congress, House, Ways and Means Committee, 1965, p. 287; testimony by A. Celebrezze (Secretary, HEW), U.S. Congress, House, Ways and Means Committee, 1965, p. 7; LBJ Library, Ex LE/IS1, Box 75, Memo to O'Brien from Cohen, 3/11/65.

between hospitals and the state was expected to defuse possible public unease about "charge ... that Government was trying ... to intrude in medicine and hospitalization."[64] Thus, as Johnson prepared to sign Medicare into law in July, he emphasized that Medicare carefully "limit[ed] the Secretary's authority on basic control points" in order to prevent "government meddling."[65] In the absence of widespread understanding of state involvement in social welfare, policymakers concluded that introducing strong specialization and hierarchical control was simply not an option.

Politicians and specialists received ample warning about committing massive government funding without a commensurate increase in the state's authority and specialization; dispersing a major portion of HEW's administrative responsibilities would begin, it was said, an irreversible process of rapid cost escalation. In effect, congressional and administration officials decided to sign a check to cover specified services for the elderly but declined to "interfere with the practice of medicine" in order to control the amount on the check and the quality of care it purchased. All reasonable charges would be covered and oversight would be left to private bodies sympathetic to providers.[66] The decision, then, by Mills, Johnson, and other policymakers in favor of a weak hierarchy and specialization continued the American state's tradition of weak administrative capacity.

Administrative arrangements and potential for future development. Medicare's potential for future development was the second major issue in debates over new administrative arrangements; this debate was shaped by American reformers' unusual approach to change. In Britain, the coalition of Labour and Conservative parties was inundated by political division; but on health policy opposing factions agreed on a clear and highly popular objective—comprehensive health services for the entire population. In the wake of its landslide victory, Labour used persistent support for this objective to introduce bold new means like the nationalization of hospitals. In stark contrast, the successive defeats of American health insurance schemes convinced reformers that they could build support for their un-

---

64. Testimony by W. McNerney (President, Blue Cross Association), U.S. Congress, House, Ways and Means Committee, 1965, pp. 174–77, 184–85. Also see testimony by K. Williamson, (representative of AHA), U.S. Congress, House, Ways and Means Committee, 1965, pp. 222–23, 287.

65. Exchanges between Mills and T. Bell (Welfare Director, State of Colorado), U.S. Congress, House, Ways and Means Committee, 1965, pp. 197–222; LBJ Library, Ex LE/IS1, Box 75, Memo to Moyers from P. Hughes (Assistant Director for Legislative Reference, BOB), 5/18/65; LE/IS1, Box 75, Memo to Esther Peterson from R. Mueller (Executive Office of the President, President's Committee on Consumer Interests), 5/5/65; JFK Library, R. F. Kennedy Papers, Senate Legislation, Box 69, Letter to Adam Molinsky (Robert Kennedy aide) from Samuel Standard (Professor, Clinical Surgery, NYU College of Medicine), 4/7/65.

66. LBJ Library, Ex LE/IS1, Box 75, Memo to Moyers from P.Hughes (BOB, Assistant Director for Legislative Reference), 5/18/65.

spoken objective—universal, comprehensive health insurance—only by building on the public's enthusiasm for Social Security. In effect, American policymakers reversed the British approach: the means (Medicare's Social Security approach) was expected to generate support for the unannounced objective. Even after the 1964 election shook Washington's political establishment, longtime reformers like Cohen steadfastly adhered to their incremental philosophy. But the blinders of incrementalism obscured new political opportunities: instead of pressing for innovative means to move boldly toward their objective, reformers treated Medicare as their objective and simply recycled preelection proposals in framing the administration's bill; leadership in aligning Medicare legislation with policymakers' new perception of public opinion fell to reluctant reformers in Congress, particularly Mills.

Under Mills's leadership, members of Congress and policy specialists like Cohen reformulated the administration's Medicare proposal to respond to both existing and anticipated patterns of public opinion. Congressional officials accurately sensed that, after years of promises to solve the elderly's health care problems, the administration's proposal was a "fooler" that failed to respond to the public's existing expectations: the "public does misunderstand [the administration's] program" because "many believe [that] *all* of their medical bills will be paid." Mills and others expected that when the "American people...woke up to the fact that only about 25% of those costs were being paid for," Democrats would face a real storm and would suffer the political effect of this disillusionment. Underscoring the White House's unresponsiveness to existing public opinion, Democrats were "embarrass[ed]...to defend [the administration's] limited [program]"; Republicans and the AMA maneuvered to capitalize on the White House's miscalculation by offering schemes that broadened benefits, though in a constrained form.[67] Mills provided decisive direction: he expanded the administration's benefit package to reflect policymakers' sense of a major shift in public opinion.

In policy discussions, Mills also sought to address the anticipated development of public expectations after Medicare's implementation. Reformers concentrated on appeasing Mills's concern that Medicare was, as its opponents charged, "just the beginning" or "opening wedge"—that reform would unleash inexorable popular pressure for expanding the program's

---

67. LBJ Library, Ex LE/IS1, Box 75, Letter to Johhson from A. Ribicoff, 3/13/65. Also see Ex LE/IS1, Box 75, Memo to L. O'Brien from Cohen, 7/6/65, concerning Senate floor action on the Medicare bill; Ex LE/IS1, Box 75, Memo to Johnson from Cohen, 3/2/65; testimony by Cohen, U.S. Congress, House, Ways and Means Committee, 1965, p. 104; testimony by H. Collier, U.S. Congress, House, Ways and Means Committee, 1965, p. 127; statement by T. Curtis, U.S. Congress, House, Ways and Means Committee, 1965, pp. 58–59; Interview with Mills by C. T. Morrissey, Former Members of Congress, Inc., 4/5/79.

coverage of services and population groups.[68] Thus, Cohen and other reformers joined with Mills to construct a "wall around the spread of these benefits" that would forestall the future growth in the public's expectation.[69] Reformers' renewed efforts to neutralize the "opening wedge" charge meant, in effect, that what was initially considered a means for incrementally achieving a universal, comprehensive program became itself the objective. Erstwhile reformers, then, deliberately—even enthusiastically—assisted Mills to "build into this program some mechanism...to prevent...the spread of the package of benefits to include other services [and groups]."[70]

Mills's dual concern with public opinion, responding to existing public expectations and controlling their future growth, led to two major administrative reforms. Accurately reflecting public preferences and understandings, Mills insisted that Medicare build on Social Security's taxing system: not only was it popular; it would also dampen the public's expectations. If one placed the "whole thing in the general fund of the Treasury...there would never be any end to [the pressures for expansion]." But establishing a "direct financing link between earmarked taxes and particular benefits" would restrain public expectations: the "willingness of people to pay that ...specific tax," administration and congressional officials agreed, "serves to limit the benefit."[71]

In perhaps the boldest action during Medicare's formulation, Mills led an expansion of Medicare's benefit package. This second major administrative change stemmed from Mills's decision to direct the Ways and Means Committee to combine into one bill the three major schemes that had been proposed, the administration's basic hospital insurance proposal, the House Republicans' voluntary insurance plan, and the AMA's call to extend the medical assistance program. Lawmakers adopted this three-prong approach to the design of Medicare's basic framework: the first two components, the compulsory hospital program and the voluntary insurance program for Americans over sixty-five, were enacted as Title 18 of the Social Security Act, and medical relief for the sick poor became Title 19.

Mills's expansion of the benefit package to "tak[e] care of practically all of the [elderly's] needs" reflected his new perception of existing public

68. Statement by T. Curtis, U.S. Congress, House, Ways and Means Committee, 1965, pp. 58, 78.
69. Statement by Mills, U.S. Congress, House, Ways and Means Committee, 1965, pp. 70–71. Also see Marmor 1973.
70. Statement by Mills, U.S. Congress, House, ways and Means Committee, 1965, pp. 70–71.
71. Exchange between Mills and K. Gordon (Director, BOB), U.S. Congress, House, Ways and Means Committee, 1965, pp. 803–5; testimony by Cohen, U.S. Congress, House, Ways and Means Committee, 1965, pp. 124–25.

expectations. As a corrective to their earlier miscalculation, Cohen and the administration wholeheartedly welcomed Mills's "ingenious" proposal for "tak[ing] [Democrats] off the hook from . . . the limitations of the original [administration] bill." The AMA and its congressional supporters were "shocked and opposed" to Mills's response to public opinion but found it "unassailable politically from any serious Republican attack."[72]

Mills's approach was designed not only to respond to existing public opinion but also to contain and deter popular pressure for future expansion of Medicare. In particular, he attempted to use two of the components— the voluntary and poor-law schemes—to erect a "fence" around the new Social Security–financed program for covering hospital costs: these two components would prevent the hospital program from becoming a "wedge" for vast new additions to the Social Security system. Drawing on the Republicans' voluntary insurance approach, Mills proposed that Medicare beneficiaries be offered the option of paying a uniform premium from their Social Security benefits in order to receive supplemental coverage. For Mills, the attractiveness of the voluntary approach was that it would head off "physician coverage in the future under social security by providing it now"; the new program avoided the "touchy doctor area" by not using a compulsory state program.

Finally, the third component of Mills's package borrowed from the AMA: it drew on the enduring negative meanings associated with poor-law arrangements to deter further demands for expanding Medicare. Accurately sensing the public's disapproval of welfare, Cohen assisted Mills in "getting [poor relief] to ride in" as a part of the more favorably perceived Social Security programs.[73] Once established, Mills expected public assistance to represent yet another means of building a fence around Medicare. The negative perceptions of poor relief were expected to undercut future demands to expand Social Security insurance to cover all income groups (Marmor 1973, 79).

Labour's formulation of NHS in Britain approximated the classic pattern by which clear objectives define the administrative means; the formulation of Medicare's administrative structure represented a nearly opposite approach: the means ultimately defined the ends. Erstwhile reformers designed lasting obstacles to achieving their firmly held objective, incremental expansion of Medicare's coverage of services and population. Thus, Cohen

72. LBJ Library, Memo to Johnson from Cohen, 3/2/65; Ex LE/IS1, Box 75, Memo to J. Valenti from Cohen, 3/4/65, Memo to Cater from Cohen, 3/10/65. Also see Memo to Johnson from W. M. Watson, 5/11/65, Memo to L. O'Brien from Cohen, 7/19/65; Mills Interview; interview with Mills by C. T. Morrissey, Former Members of Congress, Inc., 4/5/79.

73. Mills Interview, Cohen Interview.

and other administrative officials could convincingly assure Mills that "in four or six years the medical benefits will [not] be greatly expanded."[74]

The outcome of Medicare's formulation, weak administrative reforms and instances of significant interest group influence, would not surprise Weberians. In a state generally characterized by fragmentation and a comparatively low degree of bureaucratic specialization, American policymakers conceded important principles to interest groups; they also failed to establish direct federal administration over Medicare's cost and quality or to eliminate the decentralized poor laws.

Nonetheless, a Weberian attempt to posit a causal connection between existing administrative resources and institutional change does not hold up if final decisions are disaggregated and the analysis concentrates on the debates and decisions regarding Medicare's details. Public opinion, not organizational capacity, was the primary focus of and influence on policymakers' decisions concerning interest group influence and specific institutional change.

In both the United States and Britain, political struggles altered policymakers' perceptions of public opinion, bringing governmental decision making into line with stable but previously ignored patterns of public preferences and understandings. Thus, the normally fractious Congress widely agreed after the Democrats' landslide that the election expressed a substantial shift in public opinion toward Medicare and members responded by following the president's call for legislation. In the aftermath of the political upheaval in Britain, the Labour government formulated a comprehensive bill and insisted, as Bevan did, that not even financial considerations could prevent major health reform. Moreover, American policymakers' commitment to building on Social Security's taxing system and expanding Medicare's benefits was driven by their perception of public opinion—they wanted to respond to existing preferences and to forestall future expectation of expansion. Despite Weberian expectations, American politicians' adoption of weak arrangements was not dominated by administrative considerations: specialists issued dire warnings but there was relatively little serious discussion of the organizational consequences of preserving decentralized poor-law arrangements and sacrificing the state's specialization and hierarchical control. Rather they reacted to the public's ambivalence to the state by forging a new state role on a weak administrative foundation.

Evidence of culture's impact on policy rests not only on the correspon-

---

74. Testimony by Cohen, U.S. Congress, House, Ways and Means Committee, 1965, pp. 124–25. Also see exchange between Mills and K. Gordon (Director, BOB), U.S. Congress, House, Ways and Means Committee, 1965, pp. 803–5.

dence between public opinion and policy, but also on an important temporal pattern—policymakers changed their decisions *after* they perceived changes in public opinion. It was only after Mills perceived a fundamental shift public opinion that he shifted his position; once ambivalent toward Medicare, he became its bold innovator.

Finally, both NHS and Medicare provide evidence that directly contradicts Weberian expectations. Weberian analysis implies that the moderately weak American state should adopt a conciliatory approach that welcomes significant interest group influence, while the comparatively strong British state should exert independence. But in Britain policymakers designed major concessions to address interest group claims while their American counterparts exercised, on important principles, significant independence. In spite of the AMA's much feared powers, American policymakers adopted a detached view of leading interest groups: the doctors' representatives were derisively dismissed by Mills and others as merely a nuisance, and the Democratically controlled government adopted such popular principles as Social Security financing. Culturalists offer a more plausible explanation for this pattern of interest group influence: the shifts in sectional influence are related to policymakers' perception of strong or weak public sentiment.

In the wake of landslide elections, American and British officials responded to their new perception of public opinion by introducing two bold changes: they formulated major innovative reforms (such as Bevan's hospital nationalization plan and Mills's three-prong approach), and they enacted legislation—an accomplishment that had eluded their predecessors. The pursuit of bold change, though, was firmly rooted in continuity and in a commitment to avoiding radical departures from established arrangements and ongoing discussions. Even Mills's innovative package remained anchored in policy mechanisms, such as insurance, which were firmly established in the public mind. Opponents of reform were left to protest in vain, as one conservative member of the Ways and Means Committee complained, that Medicare advocates were "trading in on" and "utiliz[ing] the terms that have been developed in the private insurance field."[75]

75. Statement by T. Curtis (member, Ways and Means Committee), U.S. Congress, House, Ways and Means Committee, 1965, pp. 34–35.

Conclusion

The formulation of the NHS and Medicare acts shared a common process: public preferences and socially shared understandings substantially affected interest group influence and specific administrative arrangements. The public's role was not limited to identifying broad policy goals, with elite experts free to fashion the means to achieve those goals; rather, the public shaped specific decisions. Despite this common process and shared legal and cultural customs, the distinct nature of the relationship between public opinion and policy making in the United States and Britain produced dramatic differences between the two countries' health policies. Coupling institutional change to public opinion substantially explains how two broadly similar countries evolved dramatically different health care institutions.

I have argued that public preferences and socially shared understandings should be assigned their proper places in institutional analysis; my aim, however, is not to invert the prevailing approach to policy making, replacing institutional analysis at one extreme with cultural analysis at another. Rather, I have argued that policymakers' response to public understandings and preferences is conditioned by political and policy-making processes.

In this concluding chapter, I analyze the uncharted territory between treating public opinion as irrelevant to detailed policy making, on the one hand, and assuming that it is simply ratified in government decisions, on the other. I organized Chapter 1 as an analytic funnel to channel discussion from general arguments to specific empirical cases: with it, we progressed from theories of institutions and culture to focus on the formulation of the NHS and Medicare acts. In this concluding chapter I flip the analytic funnel over, beginning by outlining the evidence on the Medicare and NHS cases and then raising the level of abstraction to encompass evidence from other liberal democracies as well as theories about institutions and culture.

What NHS and Medicare Tell Us

This book's extensive primary evidence on the formulation of Medicare and NHS acts provides the basis for an analysis of public opinion and policy making. In particular, it allows us to examine two types of relationships between public opinion and policy making: the correspondence and the covariation over time of opinion and policy.

For the United States and Britain, I have analyzed public preferences and understandings, as evident in polling data and qualitative studies, and voluminous records (both archival and published) on the deliberations of each country's health policy network. I found that strong, stable patterns of public interest in and support for particular policies corresponded with the outcome of organized bargaining among the legislature, senior executive officials, the bureaucracy, and medical providers. This relationship appears both over time and across issues in the two countries.

By 1942 in Britain and 1960 in the United States, policymakers' agenda paralleled that of the public's on the issue of major health care reform. In Britain, both public understandings, which had gradually evolved through centuries of social interaction with institutions, and more immediate public preferences supported hospital- *and* community-based care, as well as direct state involvement in providing and financing this treatment. By the late 1930s, the level of public expectations was overwhelming the capacity of the prevailing health care system. Even before the completion of the Beveridge Report, the issue of major health care reform was highly salient to the general population; after November 1942, public support for major new policy initiatives intensified, culminating in the widespread backing of sweeping changes in the 1945 election. Policymakers' deliberations in the 1930s and 1940s were consistent with this evolution of public attitudes: politicians and bureaucrats defined the problem in health care as originating in changing public opinion—"hospital-mindedness" and expectations of GP care—and began to devote serious, sustained attention to it.

In the United States, the public's interaction with government and health care institutions generated understandings and preferences that favored hospital care; but the public was comparatively unfamiliar with direct state involvement and with community-based care along the lines of the British panel practices. Historically, Americans had feared and resented orthodox medicine, but by the late 1930s growing segments of the public became attracted to it, especially to sophisticated hospital treatment. As indicated in polls by Louis Harris and others, as well as in media coverage, the issue of major health care reform became salient, as in Britain, approximately half a dozen years before the passage of actual legislation. By the 1960 presidential election, politicians and policy experts perceived a disjuncture between existing health care arrangements and changing public understandings of health care. Major health reform moved from the margins of policy discussions to the mainstream; it was assigned a high priority in the presidential campaign and in Congress.

The American and British governments' treatment of interest groups also corresponded with public opinion. In particular, there was an inverse relationship between alternating levels of opinion and interest group influence: policymakers compromised with relevant interest groups on principles that lacked strong public support, but they defied these groups in cases of unmistakable public enthusiasm. In Britain beginning in the early 1940s, the public supported the free and universal provision of hospital and doctor services; these principles were among the most attractive features of the Beveridge Report. Mirroring public opinion, both the coalition and Labour governments repeatedly defied medical producers' positions and endorsed these principles. As indicated in countless memoranda, minutes, and reports from the Ministry of Health and the cabinet, politicians and bureaucrats successfully made the case for universal and free care by pointing to the great weight of public opinion. Conversely, on the less salient principles of private practice and capitation payment, both the coalition government and the reformist Labour cabinet compromised with relevant producer groups, citing public apathy or potential public support for interest groups' positions.

Like the British, Americans embraced the major principles of health reform six years before legislation was passed. Echoing the public's negative perception of welfare and its acceptance of social insurance, private surveys for Kennedy and Johnson as well as published polls indicated strong, sustained support for the adoption of Social Security's financing mechanism and its coverage of the elderly. Although Americans were comparatively unfamiliar with the state's provision of social welfare, they enthusiastically accepted use of Social Security, which was the most familiar and popular form of state provision. Medicare was, as Harris repeatedly reported to Kennedy, a popular issue in every state he surveyed. Corresponding to strong public support for Social Security's financing and complete coverage of the aged, congressional and administration officials' decisions repeatedly ignored interest group opposition and adopted these social insurance principles. Conversely, on issues that were not particularly salient to the public, interest group influence was strong. In the absence, then, of extensive

Friendly Society or NHI provisions, American policymakers did not perceive—as their British counterparts did—public expectations of doctors' services and free care; in this context, they acceded to sectional pressure and agreed to include deductibles and to exclude medical specialists from the compulsory program.

There is no consistent evidence that the variation in state actors' independence from interest group pressure is related to oscillations in some other critical factor, such as particular health policy areas, the magnitude of interest group pressure, elite culture, or administrative resources. Interest group influence varied across health policies; there appears to be no intrinsic quality about an area of health policy—say, the cost of treatment—that explains the variation in pressure group influence. Interest groups influenced the adoption of deductibles in the United States, for example, whereas British policymakers disregarded sectional claims for patient charges and adopted free care. Moreover, the cross-sectional variations in interest group influence are unrelated to fluctuations in the pressure applied by these groups. Relevant producer groups opposed all major changes (with remarkably little discrimination) and their organizational and financial resources remained constant over time. In addition, the cross-sectional variations in interest group influence did not coincide with changes in elite culture; government decisions regarding interest group positions were staked out during periods of consensus building *and* were maintained after landslide elections. Finally, the variations in pressure group effectiveness were not associated with fluctuations in administrative resources.

The only critical factor that consistently varied with fluctuations in interest group influence is public opinion: high and low levels of public sentiment were inversely related to state actors' independence from interest groups. This association holds in spite of both differences between the two countries (i.e., the issues raised and the wartime context in Britain) and changes within each country, such as shifts from political deadlock to political receptiveness following electoral landslides. Systematic evidence that policymakers' decisions corresponded with public opinion suggests that elites had relatively little discretion or leeway on issues that attracted strong, sustained, and focused public support.

Public opinion was also broadly consistent with policymakers' deliberations over administrative arrangements. In Britain, quantitative and qualitative studies of public preferences echoed the more general evolution of socially shared understandings: the public widely resented the existing hospital and GP care and favored a greater state role in its provision. The existing municipal hospitals bore the stigma of the poor laws, and the voluntary hospitals were tainted by their incessant requests for contributions; GP care was widely disliked for providing "second-class treatment" and then only for a small section of the population. As an alternative the public, after 1939, strongly supported state ownership and control of hospitals. It also favored reorganizing GP care, not to create a glorified extension of the existing system but to establish a state-run medical service and a system of health centers. The language and decisions of policymakers paralleled these patterns in public opinion. In particular, successive British cabinets endorsed group practice and other reforms to mark the GP service as new, as when they imposed state control over the geographic distribution of doctors. Moreover, and perhaps most significant, Labour decided to nationalize hospitals.

In contrast to the British, who wanted to make medical services a state matter, Americans held far more ambivalent attitudes toward the state. In particular, the American public's acceptance of state involvement via Social Security coexisted with its traditional uneasiness over the prospect of excessive interference. As a private pollster reported to Kennedy, "most people want something done but have doubts about the method." Americans' ambivalence toward the state coincided with policymakers' incipient approach to institutional change: politicians and experts expanded the Social Security system but protected the nation against state control by dispersing the new program's authority and hamstringing the development of administrative specialization. Thus, presidents Kennedy and Johnson, as well as influential members of Congress, decided to demonstrate Medicare's protections against government meddling by adopting, among other measures, the use of private agencies such as Blue Cross to administer the expenditure of government funds. Moreover, they decided to prevent state interference in the future both by including social safeguards like linking earmarked taxes to benefits and by expanding Medicare's benefits via voluntary and poor-law approaches.

Dramatic differences, then, in American and British policymakers' handling of administrative arrangements coincided with important variations in public understandings and preferences in the two countries. In the United States, the decision to minimize direct state involvement and to rely on nonstate arrangements echoed the public's comparative unfamiliarity with state provisions. In Britain, introduction of a significantly larger and stronger state role reflected the British public's more favorable understanding of state provisions; instead of ceding important administrative functions to nonstate bodies, British policymakers assumed that the state would play a major role in financing and providing health care.

In contrast to public opinion toward major principles, American and British attitudes toward administrative arrangements were more ambiguous and less clear. The British issues of hospital nationalization and health centers were clear exceptions; public support for these administrative arrangements was strong and focused. In general, though, the British design of the GP branch and Washington's response to Americans' ambivalence show that the correspondence of opinion and policy was evident but relatively broad gauged. When the public was not attentive to detailed administrative arrangements like the nationalization of hospitals, elite decisionmakers had greater discretion or leeway than they did when handling basic principles.

In short, the NHS and Medicare acts were the products of deliberations over the policy agenda as well as interest group claims and administrative capacity. A clear pattern emerged: the language and decisions of politicians and experts repeatedly and explicitly coincided with strong, stable patterns of public opinion.

Public opinion and policy making corresponded, then, but correspondence alone does not establish a causal connection between the two. It might be asserted that the strong association of public opinion and health policy making is spurious; references to public opinion by policymakers and interest groups could merely be a tactical ploy that does not represent a genuinely significant influence on policy deliberations. Moreover, the causal connection may not involve the public's impact on policy as much as the reverse: elites may manipulate public preferences to coincide with desired policies and then respond to this manufactured opinion. Indeed, politicians can devote significant resources to shaping public opinion, as illustrated by Johnson's mandate-shaping efforts during the 1964 election and by Kennedy's promotional activities in the 1960 campaign and in the 1962 crusade for Medicare.

Two related arguments, however, suggest that relatively autonomous public preferences and understandings drove the formulation of the NHS and Medicare acts. First, public opinion is not easily or regularly manipulated. Elites may pummel their society with self-serving messages—and achieve occasional, important successes—but there is no systematic evidence that government officials (whether presidents or demagogues like Senator Joseph McCarthy) can persistently orchestrate large swings in public opinion (Page and Shapiro 1992). Public understandings have an enduring quality because they are embedded in institutions and in social relations—the actions and interactions of ordinary people; elites do not possess the capacity to override the extensive (explicit and tacit) knowledge of ordinary people.

Indeed, evidence on the institutional and political developments associated with the NHS and Medicare acts suggests that policymakers fully appreciated the opacity and resiliency of public understandings. Presidential appeals as well as the formation of the American and British public opinion apparatus were driven by policymakers' preoccupation with responding to, rather than manipulating, public opinion. Kennedy's and Johnson's efforts to lead Americans, for instance, were informed by existing public opinion; they chose Medicare because it *already* enjoyed high public interest and support.

A second reason for suggesting that relatively autonomous public sentiment drives government decisions involves the temporal ordering of policymakers' decisions and their perception of public opinion. Pivotal instances of policy change occurred after policymakers sensed that public opinion had changed. In Britain during the 1930s and early 1940s, policymakers rejected major health reform as impractical. The onset, though, of the coalition's political upheavals prompted policymakers' perception of public opinion to shift. After this perceived change in public sentiment, politicians and bureaucrats changed their policy toward major health reform: it was now practical politics to devote sustained attention to specifying comprehensive alternatives.

The changes in American and British policy after the 1964 and 1945 elections are especially important. Unambiguous political events, like the lopsided victories of the Labour and Democratic parties, enable large numbers of individuals in fragmented governmental institutions to reevaluate public sentiment. After the 1945 British election's indisputable signal, Labour fundamentally changed the coalition policy concerning hospital care: it rejected the wartime government's decision to preserve the existing and widely disliked hospital system and responded to public opinion by using the state to openly and decisively take over hospitals. Similarly, it was only after Wilbur Mills perceived a fundamental shift in American public opinion following the 1964 election that his ambivalence toward Medicare was transformed into a bold and successful advocacy of a three-prong approach. In short, pivotal policy shifts occurred after politicians and specialists reached a new and more accurate assessment of public opinion. This sequence provides support for the argument that the opinion-policy relationship is neither spurious nor manipulated outright. Despite, then, significant variations within and between the United States and Britain, public opinion both corresponded *and* covaried over time with policymakers' decisions on the NHS and Medicare acts.

POLICY MEETS THEORY

Prevailing approaches to policy making, such as those associated with the pluralists and Max Weber as well as with most research on health care, tend to emphasize the role of elites and institutional processes. I have argued that institutional approaches, and in particular a variant of Weberian research, neglects or altogether ignores the impact of public understandings and preferences. I have offered instead strong but qualified support for culturalist interpretations of institutional change. Assigning public opinion its proper analytic place, though, should not obscure the contributions of Weberian and other prevailing analyses of policy making; they have helped to shift the study of politics from the system's functions toward processes that help account for specific institutional changes, namely, policy networks and political struggle.

Institutions without Subjects

The prevailing institutional approach to policy making convincingly argues that institutions do not automatically change to fulfill presumably required functions of an overarching system. This approach usefully emphasizes that institutional changes are refracted through political conflict and policy networks. According to Weberian accounts, politicians' and bureaucrats' motivatation to enter the fray are based on their calculations concerning how to advance their power and position. Moreover, Weberians draw on research on policy networks to suggest that proposals for institutional change emerge from organized patterns of bargaining, which transcend the boundaries between the legislature, the executive branch, and nongovernmental experts and groups. It is suggested that policy networks structure interactions between the experts and informed politicians who specify and choose alternatives. In particular, elected officeholders' attraction to publicity encourages them to use their authoritative position to set the broad direction of policy; professional policy experts, whether bureaucrats or nongovernmental specialists, generate or specify the content of policy proposals.

Weberian research suggests that two characteristics of policy networks are especially important. First, their organization of ongoing interactions ensures a significant degree of continuity and cohesion. Politicians and experts share and pass on "policy learning" based on past experiences (Heclo 1974); this shared perspective forms the basis for common approaches to policy making (e.g., American officials' incremental philosophy). Second, the access and attention granted to nongovernmental groups is not equal. In the context of private control over economic activity, politicians and bureaucrats incorporate producers of critical goods and services into the state's decision making. Representatives of relevant producer groups, then, gain privileged positions, enjoying disproportionate access to authoritative policymakers.

Weberians use research on policy networks and political contestation to claim that the state's objective administrative capacity is the primary focus and determinant of institutional change. In particular, they develop two theoretical expectations: state actors' autonomy from interest groups is a function of the state's organizational capacity, and existing administrative resources prefigure new institutional changes.

The outcome of American and British health policy formulation could reasonably be interpreted as consistent in important respects with Weberian analysis. For example, the moderately weak American state is associated both with instances of strong interest group influence and with the construction of administrative arrangements characterized by low levels of hierarchy and specialization. Conversely, the British state's comparatively more extensive administrative resources coincide both with instances of weak sectional influence and with decisions to enhance the state's capacity within each of the health service's three branches (especially its hospital branch).

The outcome of American and British health care deliberations may be somewhat expected, but the story behind them is surprising. Evidence from the NHS and Medicare acts indicates that Weberian analysis of state autonomy and specific institutional changes is misspecified and contradicted by counterevidence. Initially, Weberians claimed that the state's overall weakness or strength explains the degree to which politicians and bureaucrats can take initiatives that are independent from or opposed by major producer groups. More recent research by Weberians suggests that fluctuations in state capacity within a single state mean that the autonomy of government actors can also vary across individual policy areas, from agricultural to labor policy (Skocpol and Finegold 1982; Ikenberry 1988). The NHS and Medicare acts raise a difficult analytic puzzle for Weberians: policy deliberations in one policy area (and therefore under uniform administrative conditions) were characterized by variations in interest group influence. In the cases of Medicare and NHS, the variation in sectional influence was not consistently related to policymakers' differential assessment of administrative resources.

In this book I have challenged Weberian analysis of state actors' relation to major interest groups, indicating that state autonomy varies not only across policy areas but also within an area. Moreover, the systematic correspondence between public opinion and policymakers' handling of interest group pressure suggests that Weberian analysis of state autonomy is misspecified. The alternating weakness and strength of medical providers is explained not by administrative capacity, which remained constant, but by policymakers' perceptions of strong or weak public opinion.

A second major Weberian expectation is that state actors' decisions to adopt new administrative arrangements are dominated by their consideration of objective organizational capacity. Indeed, during the formulation of the NHS's and Medicare's administrative arrangements, clusters of bureaucrats and politicians did, on occasion, discuss the state's organizational capacity: American officials advocated direct federal administration to control the cost and quality of Medicare, and Britain's Ministry of Health championed unified administration. Authoritative policymakers reacted to arguments for enhancing administrative capacity in a straightforward fashion: they either summarily overturned them or treated them, in an equally humbling way, as irrelevant. Conceding that new institutional arrangements would be weak, they concentrated not on what works best but on what *mattered* and would be acceptable in terms of public preferences and understandings. The correspondence and covariation of public opinion and administrative changes suggest that Weberians misspecify the causal process behind institutional development.

Weberians' claim for a causal connection between administrative capacity and policy making is further undermined by significant counterevidence. American and British treatment of interest group claims contradicts Weberian theoretical expectations: instances of high state autonomy coincided with the American state's moderately weak administrative resources, and Britain's comparatively more extensive capacity was associated with government concessions to medical producers.

Moreover, senior American officials did have high confidence in their administrative capacity, as evident by the aggressive campaign to persuade President Kennedy to adopt direct federal administration. Contrary to Weberian expectations, these officials did not turn away from establishing hierarchical control because it was too much for the government machinery. Rather, the White House and members of Congress did not seriously consider these capacity-enhancing arguments because they were primarily concerned with Americans' enduring ambivalence toward the state and their support for building on Social Security. The Medicare case, then, is characterized by the coexistence of strong confidence in state capacity and institutional changes that established weak administrative arrangements.

Finally, after identifying a reform approach that was consistent with public preferences and understandings, American policymakers (despite their comparatively weak institutions) significantly expanded government involvement in health care. Although the degree of future cost escalation was unintended, the Medicare legislation nonetheless was intended as a historic enlargement of both the state's area of responsibility (i.e. expanding access to health care) and its budgetary commitment, which for the first time made "the federal government . . . a major financier of medical services" (Marmor et al. 1990, 179). In this respect, policymakers' responsiveness to public demand for reform actually prompted them to overcome the historic weakness of the American state.

Culturalism Confirmed

The NHS and Medicare acts confirm two central aspects of cultural analysis, its conclusions about culture and its implications for policy analysis. Investigation of public opinion in the immediate decades after World War II concluded that the preferences of ordinary people were unstable and incoherent (Campbell et al. 1960). The recent, multidisciplinary investigation of culture has significantly revised this postwar analysis. This investigation proceeds on the assumption that the interaction of social beings produces meanings that are both embedded in institutions and widely shared and transmitted down generations. Enduring public understandings pattern or organize individuals' more specific (and at times transitory) preferences.

My analysis here suggests that enduring social understandings and more immediate public preferences toward health care and the state are stable and coherent. For instance, I have found, as previous studies suggested, that Americans harbor a persistent ambivalence toward state involvement in social welfare: enduring unease of state interference awkwardly coexists with an acceptance of state involvement in specific social welfare programs (Page and Shapiro 1992; Feldman and Zaller 1992).

Evidence of British and American public competence may appear to be contradicted by instances in which the public was unclear or confused about some details regarding health policy. On detailed (often nonsalient) policy issues, Americans and Britons repeatedly displayed low levels of knowledge; moreover, Americans failed to correctly identify features of the numerous, competing health care proposals that emerged after Johnson's landslide 1964 victory. These limits on public knowledge regarding nonsalient items are reasonable and certainly do not indicate incompetence on the part of ordinary people. After all, most people are consumed by their occupational and private lives and can devote only limited time and resources to politics. Moreover, Americans' confusion regarding the details of different Medicare proposals echoes the information and choices presented them by politicians: as members of Congress readily conceded, politicians' inflated rhetoric fooled Americans.

The key issue is that during the formulation of the NHS and Medicare acts, the public, though not mastering all policy details, did develop consistent, reasonable patterns of understandings and preferences. It is this kind of knowledge that allows ordinary people, not unlike legislators and chief executives, to guide authoritative choices among alternatives.

The formulation of the NHS and Medicare acts substantiates a second aspect of culturalist analysis, that public preferences and socially shared understandings significantly influence institutional changes and elite negotiations with interest groups. According to culturalists, no activity exists outside socially shared meanings and public preferences. Indeed, the evidence on correspondence and covariation demonstrates that these understandings and preferences are a primary determinant of specific changes in administrative capacity. The public's impact can involve promoting a particular policy, such as the focused support for nationalizing hospitals; or it can entail setting the more general context for policy formulation. The distinct patterns of public opinion in the United States and Britain "loaded the dice," making certain institutional changes conceivable while barring others. Policy options that were conceivable in Britain (e.g., a massive state role and the establishment of community-based care for the entire population) were simply unfathomable during Medicare's formulation.

Culturalist expectations are also confirmed by the variation in the American and British state's autonomy. For culturalists, public preferences and understandings are the medium for (and therefore an influence on) state actors' assessment of interest group demands. The systematic correspondence between public opinion and state actors' relationships to interest groups suggests that government bargaining with sectional interests cannot simply be reflective of self-evident administrative capacity. Rather, the state's autonomy from interest group pressures is substantially affected by enduring cultural patterns and strong public preferences.

The culturalist conclusion, that interest group influence is connected to socially shared understandings and public preferences, runs counter to prevailing conceptions of pressure group politics. It makes perfect sense that governments would defy interest groups and incur their vociferous attacks for good material reasons—reasons, for instance, linked to controlling government expenditures. It is much harder to comprehend that they would be willing to enter protracted battles in the name of something as seemingly abstract as socially shared meanings and public preferences. Yet the perception of strong public expectations led policymakers to defy fierce interest group pressure on major principles (free and universal care in Britain and complete coverage of the elderly in the United States), principles that promised to *increase* costs.

Culturalism, Politics, and Policy Making

Although authoritative decisions are significantly affected by public opinion, policy should not be treated as an epiphenomenon of culture. Indeed, a central weakness of culturalist analysis is precisely the tendency to exaggerate the causal significance of public attitudes, to reduce decisions on specific policies and on interest group influence to subjectivity. The making of the NHS and Medicare acts indicates that the public's impact on policy making is more contingent and variable than typically suggested by culturalist accounts; of particular importance are policy networks and state actors' strategic calculations.

Culture is not encoded into policy, with government officials serving as latter-day scribes. Rather, American and British health reform suggests that policymakers' response to the public was refracted through the organized deliberations of policy networks. These deliberations indicate that, although power was shared, it was not shared equally. Producer groups' bargaining position gave them a privileged vantage point denied others: American and British medical producers could not dictate their desired policies, but their disproportionate access enabled them to seize the initiative—an especially decisive advantage in cases of nonsalient issues. Even in the aftermath of the Labour and Democratic parties' electoral landslides, ardent reformers continued to weigh long-standing interest group positions and to offer concessions on such nonsalient but nonetheless important issues as remuneration and professional representation in the new program. As a result, the new NHS and Medicare programs partially reproduced the dominant position of medical providers and the subordinate position of such non-professional groups as health workers. Even the Labour government rejected the pleas of Britain's largest unions for representation of health workers in the new service.

Culture's impact on policy formulation is shaped or distorted not only by sectional interests but also by the character of a policy network's deliberations. The process of designing new institutions involves aligning policy proposals with public understandings and preferences; in this cumbersome process, politicians and experts detach public understandings and preferences from their prevailing points of reference and reposition them. Policymakers' earliest and easiest decisions involved adopting highly salient and popular principles or administrative arrangements. For instance, in the early 1950s, Wilbur Cohen and other reformers intentionally designed the Medicare approach to reposition the public's support for Social Security toward support for expanding state involvement in health care.

Policymakers are, however, required to exercise more discretion when specifying less salient administrative arrangements: their most difficult and time-consuming tasks involve formulating specific arrangements that will induce the public to perceive and accept a new program in terms of its prevailing repertoire of understandings and preferences. American and British policymakers specified these alternative arrangements in ways that were guided by "policy learning." The successful track record of British politicians and bureaucrats in enacting and administering NHI and other social welfare programs encouraged them, as one administrator explained, to "get as much as possible" when designing NHS. American officials operated, in the wake of successive defeats, on the basis of the conservative philosophy of incrementalism; this minimalist approach emphasized both rejecting new powerful administrative structures to control government expenditures and using voluntary insurance and welfare assistance to forestall or deter future demands on the Social Security system. Bludgeoned by past failures, erstwhile reformers willingly exercised their discretion in repositioning American attitudes in order to erect lasting obstacles to achieving their objective of a universal, comprehensive insurance program.

Moreover, the contested nature of policymakers' attempts to align policy and public attitudes further ensures that institutional changes are not simply epiphenomena of culture. Elections are an important component of the strategic calculations of politicians and, by extension, bureaucrats. The decisiveness of policy issues in electoral contests is mitigated by voters' reliance on political party labels and candidates' personal characteristics or images; in addition, the advantages of incumbency and, specifically, constituency service insulate many members of Congress and Parliament from serious electoral challenge (Cain et al. 1987).

Nonetheless, politicians are sensitive to highly salient, well-supported issues because they may attract independent voters who swing elections and because candidates as a rule are risk averse (bending to mood shifts is less dangerous than courting revolt) (Downs 1957; Page 1978; Mayhew 1974).[1] Politicians' sensitivity to public attitudes has also been encouraged by the development of a public opinion apparatus; this apparatus educated policymakers to be, as one British administrator explained, "publicity minded and not merely keep their noses hard down to the administrative grindstone." The palpable pressure on policymakers to respond to the public's policy preferences is illustrated by the Conservative party's decision not to release its health reform; it feared damaging criticism for abandoning the coalition's promises. The desire to echo public sentiment also convinced Kennedy and Johnson to campaign for Medicare and persuaded a divided Labour cabinet to adopt a bold NHS plan.

State actors' strategic calculations are critical because they explain, in large part, the timing of and motivation for their interest in reform; these calculations determine how and whether politicians and bureaucrats view responsiveness to public opinion as serving their interests. Dramatic shifts in the American and British policy-making environment were prompted by the changing character of political struggle: political changes after 1942 in Britain and 1960 in the United States convinced policymakers to attempt to respond to public opinion but stalemated their efforts; the electoral land-

---

1. Elected officials may also be motivated to follow strong, sustained public opinion because of a sense of duty or because they share their constituents' disposition (e.g., they have the same reaction to new circumstances or information) (Erikson et al. 1991).

slides of 1945 and 1964 fueled a bold approach to health care reform. When policy experts defied politicians' calculations and threatened to become independent entrepreneurs, officeholders struck their proposals down and insisted on setting the goals.

In terms of culturalist analysis, strategic calculations are especially significant when they predispose policymakers to misperceive or to refuse to respond to public opinion. The NHS and Medicare acts are checkered with illustrations: political deadlock blocked legislation after Kennedy's 1960 electoral victory and the British coalition government's formation; it also encouraged the coalition's misperception of public attitudes toward the panel system and voluntary hospitals.

Because of the role of state actors' strategic calculations, culture's impact on policy formulation is neither automatic nor consensual. Further, analysis of the timing and motivation of policymakers does not tell us very much about the *nature* of political contestation.

The nature of political conflict is often equated with self-interested scrambles for material goods. The NHS and Medicare acts suggest that political contestation involves not only material goods but also public understandings and preferences, and policymakers attempting to detach and reattach meanings (Hall 1988). Advocates of policy change attempted to detach such powerful symbols as Social Security, which was tied to one set of historical associations, and rearticulate it in a different direction; provider groups and their allies countered by summoning opposing meanings and preferences. For instance, although the AMA stood to gain financially from Medicare's passage, it steadfastly opposed the program, framing its arguments in terms of the poor-law stigma or antistatism. Members of policy networks struggled to gain ascendancy in the framing of health policy; they simultaneously attempted to win public interest and support for a particular proposal and to construct alliances with other politicians. Leadership can be critical in battles for tactical advantage. Resourceful policy specialists (like American reformers who designed the Social Security approach in the 1950s) can initiate debate in a way that establishes the terms of negotiations; effective politicians (like Wilbur Mills and Aneurin Bevan) construct alliances that negotiate the shoals of public opinion and contending sectional and political pressures.

In short, coupling cultural analysis with the investigation of politics and policy-making processes makes it clear that institutional change is sufficiently contingent and variable that no outcome is guaranteed; culture predisposes but cannot, in a straightforward manner, determine any single outcome. The gradual, contested process of floating and redefining policies to coincide with public opinion and with what is possible politically may explain the similar policy processes by which the NHS and Medicare acts were formulated. In both countries, health reform followed parallel progressions: once discovered as an agenda item, health reform was subsequently pursued through consensual and then bold approaches.

THE CONDITIONAL RELEVANCE OF PUBLIC OPINION

The NHS and Medicare acts challenge social scientists' tendency to study public opinion and policy making as two separate, largely unconnected phenomena. This bifurcation has been facilitated by each research tradition's narrow assumptions: survey research has assumed that public opinion is ratified into policy, and institutional analysis is conducted as if public opinion were virtually irrelevant. There is uncharted territory, though, between the extremes of irrelevance and ratification. Whether and how public opinion influences policy making can be affected by a number of conditions.

A high magnitude of public support for a particular policy direction is generally necessary for public opinion to affect policymaking. Research in the United States and Western Europe on a range of issues, from national security to education and social security, suggests that public opinion is systematically related to government decisions when it is of a high magnitude for a sustained duration.[2] In addition, time-series analysis of a similar range of domestic and foreign policy issues suggests that changes in public opinion are also related to changes in government actions. For instance, monthly troop withdrawals from Vietnam were related to growth in public opposition to the Vietnam War and to support for troop withdrawals (Farkas et al. 1990; Page and Shapiro 1992, chap. 6; Bartels 1991).[3] On issues that are absent from national debate or are not part of social actors' repertoire of understandings, the public is unlikely to exert significant influence; government policy is most likely to respond to sectional interests.

Nevertheless, even ideal conditions (i.e., strong or changing public preferences) are not sufficient for the public to exercise influence. Congruence

2. Research on public opinion's relevance to policy making has been conducted at three levels: the broad relation between the ideological character of public opinion and policy making (Stimson 1991; Schlesinger 1986; Smith 1982); the collective opinion-policy relation in numerous areas of government activity (Page and Shapiro 1983 and 1992; Farkas et al. 1990; Monroe 1979; Weissberg 1976); and in-depth investigation of public opinion's impact on the formulation of specific policies (Jacobs 1992b; Risse-Kappen 1991; Jasper 1990; Eichenberg 1989; Russett 1990; Graham 1989; Kusnitz 1984; Bartels 1991; Burstein 1985; Cook and Barrett 1992).

3. In terms of the NHS and Medicare acts, the most critical characteristics of public opinion seem to have been the public's sustained high level of support and policymakers' *perception* of a change. The possibility of substantial change in public opinion toward major health reform was mitigated because of the already high levels of aggregate support. The political relevance of changes in public opinion seems to be especially pertinent in new areas of government activity, where public support has not already reached high levels.

between the values and preferences of elites and those of the mass public is neither natural nor inevitable in liberal democracies; a disjuncture can develop because politicians and bureaucrats misperceive, defy, or are unable to respond to the public. In particular, three factors determine the impact of strong or changing public opinion on detailed policy making: bargaining context, political dynamics, and policy networks.

Public opinion's relevance can be significantly affected by two variations in the bargaining context, variations across issue areas and cross-national differences. "High and quiet politics," in which senior policymakers conduct quick, hidden discussions concerning emergencies or national security issues, can prevent the impact of public opinion. For instance, on such issues as the Cuban missile crisis or the early decisions on nuclear energy, the president or a small group of senior congressional and bureaucratic officials used their monopoly over information to reach decisions secretly; other elites were prevented from speaking out, and the public was kept ignorant and, in some cases, deceived. Conversely, public opinion is especially relevant on issues that attract "high and loud politics," for example, on policies that attract sustained debate in the media and among major politicians and in which the public has long-standing experience.

The bargaining context can also vary across countries. In Britain and to a much greater extent in the United States, fragmented policy-making institutions encourage fluid, ongoing coalition building; this relatively open policy-making environment creates ample opportunities for public support of policy issues to find advocates. In contrast, in France's corporatist bargaining system, characterized by a centralized political system and a professional bureaucracy, there are comparatively fewer opportunities for public opinion to influence policy making. Risse-Kappen (1991) suggests, for example, that similar patterns of public opinion toward Gorbachev had quite different impacts on American and French foreign policy; this divergence is attributed to each country's different bargaining context.

In terms of policy innovation, then, corporatist arrangements tend to obstruct public influence, whereas pluralist bargaining patterns encourage it; the long-term impact of these different bargaining contexts is not, however, clear. For instance, the corporatist integration of major producer groups (including labor) into central political institutions may encourage more enduring representation of strong public support for welfare state policies (Risse-Kappen 1991; Crockett and Wlezien 1987). Conversely, the fluid and open nature of pluralist bargaining contexts may mitigate the long-term effect of public opinion; in the end, the possibility of implementing enduring public understandings and preferences is less likely given the lack of sustained organizational pressure by broad-based mass movements. Indeed, Morone persuasively argues that upsurges in Americans' support for political reform and government innovations prompt institutional changes, which in the long run become unresponsive to public opinion; they "advantage some citizens, disadvantage others, and seem almost invisible to all" (1990, 323).

A second condition affecting the relevance of public opinion to policy making is political context. Political stalemate can entrap policies that enjoy even strong support. As evident in the American and British shift from consensus to bold approaches to health reform, change in the electoral landscape and in the political leadership creates nearly irresistible incentives for politicians and bureaucrats to respond to strong public support for particular policies.

A third set of influences on the political relevance of public opinion are policy networks, the experts and informed politicians who specify and choose alternatives. Two norms may lead politicians and specialists to exercise maximum discretion when aligning proposals with strong or changing public opinion. Members of policy networks may discount public opinion on complex issues like actuarial projections for Social Security or arms control (Cook and Barrett 1992; Russett 1990). Moreover, although members of the legislative branch are notoriously preoccupied with their district's parochial concerns, they do regularly discount narrow public preferences in order to emphasize the country's overall interests: officials insist on being responsible *for* (rather than *to*) the public (Vogler and Waldman 1985; Maass 1983).

RETHINKING DEMOCRATIC POLICY MAKING

The argument that public understandings and preferences have extensively influenced detailed policy making, under certain conditions, challenges a long-standing tendency in the analyses of liberal democracy. From Madison to Schumpeter, a persistent thrust of liberal democratic theory has been to downplay the citizenry's participation in government decision making; the emphasis has been on maintaining and enhancing protections for individual liberty and the quality of government policy.

Weberian research is consistent with this tradition's emphasis on elites and their judgments. In their analysis of the New Deal, for example, Skocpol and Finegold (1982) report that the Agricultural Adjustment Administration equipped an insulated group of elites with a body of experts and the authoritative lines of control to formulate and implement effective policies. They conclude that this agency's relatively strong capacity was necessary to produce desirable (albeit administratively "workable") policies. In contrast, the National Recovery Administration's weak administrative resources, which made elite domination vulnerable to interference, were doomed to produce undesirable policies that were ineffective and self-defeating. Morone more recently renews the claim that the making of effective policies is tied to strong hierarchical control and specialization. Reversing John Dewey's dictum regarding the remedy for the afflictions of democracy, Morone argues that the cure for America's ineffective policies is a "stronger, more competent government" (1990, 334).

Under the cover of ensuring that "[normative] reflection ... do[es] not cut short analysis and understanding," the Weberians implicitly bolster a top-heavy and technocratic notion of policy making: empirical findings—that strong state structures operated by expert elites ensure greater government effectiveness—become accepted as desirable objectives (Evans et al. 1985, 364).

A comparison of the health policies produced by the American and British states seemingly confirms the long-standing fear of the mass public (rather than competent, suitably equipped elites) playing a major role in making policy. In the comparatively stronger British state, policymakers enacted health care legislation that significantly enhanced the government's administrative capacity, especially in terms of its hospital service. In the fragmented American state, though, politicians and policy experts compromised Medicare's organizational integrity in order to circumvent the public's enduring suspicion of the state; introducing a massive and visible change in the state's organizational capacity was inconceivable. Lacking the administrative competence possessed by their British counterparts, American policymakers built a major new state program without the presence of a major state; indeed, they willingly ceded control over Medicare's cost and administration to nonstate bodies.

Administratively weak American policymakers, it would seem, echoed the public's ambivalence toward the state: they expanded benefits but avoided even the appearance of strong state control. As anticipated by the Kennedy administration's advocates of direct federal administration, the result of weak hierarchical control over a government system of retrospective, third-party reimbursement has been rapid and nearly uncontrollable cost escalation since Medicare was implemented. Here seems to be a classic case in which smart policies were identified but policymakers were unable to free themselves from the harness of popular prejudices regarding socialized medicine and government meddling.

The evidence from American and British health policy, however, is far more ambiguous than this top-heavy interpretation would imply. Indeed, the theoretical implications of the NHS and Medicare acts suggest a nearly opposite conclusion: taking the public's understandings and preferences into account did make a substantial difference in the well-being of the public; errors in policy design were at least as much the fault of elites as that of the public. The most favorable developments introduced by the NHS and Medicare acts were associated with weak state autonomy and strong, sustained public opinion. The basic principles of American and British reform meaningfully enlarged social rights: regardless of their income, citizens were granted—without stigma—dramatically expanded access to health care. Success in legislating these social rights over the fierce opposition of medical groups illustrates precisely the positive influence of public attitudes on insulated policy networks. The public's infringement on state autonomy was necessary and desirable.

American and British design of future administrative arrangements for health care was, in important respects, positively aided by public influence as well. In both countries, the impact of public opinion led politicians to abandon compromise arrangements that were excessively faithful to the concerns of producer groups: Henry Willink's hodge-podge of arrangements and Cohen's package with Senator Jacob Javits. Policymakers concluded that these compromise arrangements were out of touch with public opinion and decided to abandon them; in doing so, they dodged an administrative nightmare that would have required a "staff of archangels to work." In addition, Labour's response to public expectations for nationalizing hospitals dramatically enhanced the NHS's administrative capacity in this branch.

Clearly, public opinion favorably influenced the expansion of social rights and the generation of some strong administrative arrangements. But what is to be made of Medicare's remarkably weak administrative foundation? After all, the public's unease regarding the state framed politicians' choice of private organizations like Blue Cross and other administratively emasculating arrangements.

In contrast to their focused reactions to basic principles, Americans' understandings and preferences toward administrative arrangements were hazy; it was on these matters that elite discretion was greatest. The decision to establish a massive funding program without sufficient governmental controls can be attributed, to a significant extent, to elites. The misuse of elite discretion is illustrated by the unrelenting commitment of politicians and experts, even after the 1964 landslide, to incrementalism, and by the willingness of reformers to cede political leadership to a conservative southern Democratic (Mills). Prevailing research and theoretical inquiry neglects or ignores both these errors on the part of elites as well as the public's positive impact on government decision making.

The NHS and Medicare acts challenge the basic theoretical assumption of elitist interpretations of policy making, that the knowledge of elites is inevitably far superior to that of the mass public. To expect even properly trained elites to master scientifically obtainable knowledge places inhuman demands on state actors' instrumental (and moral) knowledge. Even if elites are especially competent to assess administrative feasibility, major institutional changes require them to weigh risks, assess uncertainties, and trade off the relative desirability of competing moral values; these decisions defy expert answers (Dahl 1989). Conversely, so-called ordinary people—not unlike legislators and chief executives—have sufficient knowledge, if not to master all policy details, then to coherently identify and consistently support general principles that can positively guide policy making. Far from representing an unwanted intrusion, the influence of a competent public can, as the NHS and Medicare cases attest, defeat unworkable or unfair proposals and identify policies that advance citizenship and administrative competence.

Bibliography

Abel-Smith, Brian. 1964. *Hospitals, 1800–1948*. London: Heinemann.

Addison, Paul. 1977. *The Road to 1945*. London: Quartet.

Alford, Robert. 1975. *Health Care Politics*. Chicago: University of Chicago Press.

Allison, Graham. 1971. *Essence of Decision*. Boston: Little, Brown.

Almond, Gabriel, and G. Bingham Powell. 1966. *Comparative Politics: A Developmental Approach*. Boston: Little, Brown.

Almond, Gabriel, and Sidney Verba. 1963. *The Civic Culture: Political Attitudes and Democracy in Five Nations*. Princeton: Princeton University Press.

Atkinson, Michael, and William Coleman. 1989. "Strong States and Weak States: Sectoral Policy Networks in Advanced Capitalist Economies." *British Journal of Political Science* 19:47–67.

Axinn, June, and Herman Levin. 1975. *Social Welfare: A History of the American Response to Need*. New York: Dodd, Mead.

Barber, Benjamin. 1988. *The Politics of Conquest*. Princeton: Princeton University Press.

Bartels, Larry. 1991. "Constituency Opinion and Congressional Policy Making: The Reagan Defense Buildup." *American Political Science Review* 85 (June): 457–74.

Beard, Charles. 1913. *An Economic Interpretation of the Constitution of the United States*. Boston: MacMillan.

Beer, Samuel. 1965. *British Politics in the Collectivist Age*. New York: Alfred A. Knopf.

Berger, Peter, and Thomas Luckman. 1967. *The Social Construction of Reality*. New York: Doubleday.

Berkowitz, Edward, and Kim McQuaid. 1980. *Creating the Welfare State*. New York: Praeger.

Beveridge, William. 1953. *Power and Influence*. London: Hodder and Stoughton.

Billington, Monroe. 1972. "Roosevelt, the New Deal, and the Clergy." *Mid-America* 54:20–33.

Blank, Robert. 1988. *Rationing Medicine*. New York: Columbia University.

Bornet, Vaughn D. 1983. *The Presidency of Lyndon B. Johnson*. Lawrence: University of Kansas Press.

Briggs, Asa. 1961. "The Welfare State in Historical Perspective." *Achives Europeanes de Sociologie* 2:221–58.

British Institute of Public Opinion [BIPO]. 1943. *The Beveridge Report and the Public.* London.

Brooks, Joel. 1987. "The Opinion-Policy Nexus in France: Do Institutions and Ideology Make a Difference?" *The Journal of Politics* 49:465–80.

——. 1985. "Democratic Frustration in the Anglo-American Polities: A Quantification of Inconsistency between Mass Public Opinion and Public Policy." *The Western Political Science Quarterly* 38:250–61.

Brown, Steve. 1980. *Political Subjectivity.* New Haven: Yale University Press.

Burridge, Trevor, 1985. *Clement Attlee: A Political Biography.* London: Jonathan Cape.

Burstein, Paul. 1985. *Discrimination, Jobs, Politics.* Chicago: University of Chicago Press.

Cain, Bruce, John Ferejohn, and Morris Fiorina. 1987. *Personal Vote.* Cambridge: Harvard University Press.

Calder, Angus. 1968. *A People's War.* London: Jonathan Cape.

Calder, Angus, and Dorothy Sheridan. 1984. *Speak for Yourself: A Mass-Observation Anthology, 1937–49.* London: J. Cape.

Callahan, Daniel. 1990. *What Kind of Life: The Limits of Medical Progress.* New York: Simon and Schuster.

Campbell, Angus, Phil Converse, Warren Miller, and Donald Stokes. 1960. *The American Voter.* New York: Wiley.

Cantril, Hadley. 1967. *The Human Dimension: Experiences in Policy Research.* New Brunswick, N.J.: Rutgers University Press.

Clark, Sir Fife. 1970. *The Central Office of Information.* London: Allen and Unwin.

Clark, P. F. 1971. *Lancashire and the New Liberalism.* Cambridge: Cambridge University Press.

Cobb, Roger, and Charles Elder. 1972. *Participation in American Politics.* Boston: Allyn and Bacon.

Cockerell, Michael, Peter Hennessy, and David Walker. 1984. *Sources Close to the Prime Minister: Inside the Hidden World of News Manipulation.* London: Macmillan.

Cohen, Wilbur. 1968. "Communication in a Democratic Society." In *The Voice of Government,* ed. Ray Hiebert and Carlton Spitzer. New York: Wiley.

Cohen, Wilbur, Charles Poskanzer, and Harry Sharp. 1960. "Attitudes toward Governmental Participation in Medical Care." Hearings before Subcommittee on Problems of the Aged and Aging, Committee on Labor and Public Welfare, U.S. Senate, 86th Congress, 2d Session, April.

Collins, Doreen. 1965. "The Introduction of Old Age Pensions in Great Britain." *Historical Journal* 8:246–59.

Collins, Randall. 1980. "Weber's Last Theory of Capitalism: A Systematization." *American Sociological Review* 45 (December): 925–42.

Conover, Pamela, and Stanley Feldman. 1984. "How People Organize the Political World." *American Journal of Political Science* 28:93–126.

Cook, Fay Lomax, and Edith Barrett. 1992. *Support for the American Welfare State: Views of Congress and the Public.* New York: Columbia University Press.

Crockett, Laura, and Christopher Wlezien. 1987. "Corporatism, Pluralism, and Representation: Public Opinion and Social Welfare Policy in the European Economic Community." Paper presented at the annual meeting of the Midwest Political Science Association, Chicago.

Crossman, Richard. 1981. *Backbench Diaries.* Ed. J. Morgan. London: Jonathan Cape.

Crowther, M. Anne. 1986. "Medicine and the End of the Poor Law." *Society for the Social History of Medicine,* bulletin 38 (June): 74–76.

Cunningham, Hugh. 1981. "The Language of Patriotism, 1750–1914." *History Workshop* 12 (Autumn): 8–33.

Dahl, Robert. 1989. *Democracy and Its Critics*. New Haven: Yale University Press.

——. 1985. *A Preface to Economic Democracy*. Berkeley: University of California Press.

——. 1956. *A Preface to Democratic Theory*. Chicago: University of Chicago Press.

Dalton, Russell. 1985. "Political Parties and Political Representation: Party Supporters and Party Elites in Nine Nations." *Comparative Political Studies* 18:267–99.

Dangerfield, George. 1970. *The Strange Death of Liberal England*. London: Macgibbon and Kee.

David, Sheri. 1985. *With Dignity: The Search for Medicare and Medicaid*. Westport, Conn.: Greenwood Press.

Derthick, Martha. 1979. *Policymaking for Social Security*. Washington, D.C.: Brookings Institution.

Devine, Donald. 1970. *The Attentive Public: Polyarchical Democracy*. Chicago: Rand McNally.

Digby, Anne. 1982. *The Poor Law in 19th Century England and Wales*. London: Chameleon Press.

Douglas, Mary. 1982. *In Active Voice*. London: Routledge and Kegan Paul.

——. 1970. *Natural Symbols*. Hammmondworth: Penguin.

Downs, Anthony. 1957. *An Economic Theory of Democracy*. New York: Harper.

Doyal, Lesley. 1983. *The Political Economy of Health*. Boston: South End Press.

Easton, David. 1957. "An Approach to the Analysis of the Political System." *World Politics* 11 (April): 383–400.

Eatwell, Roger. 1979. *The 1945–51 Labour Governments*. London: B. T. Batsford.

Eckstein, Harry. 1988. "A Culturalist Theory of Political Change." *American Political Science Review* 82:789–804.

——. 1960. *Pressure Group Politics: The Case of the British Medical Association*. London: Allen and Unwin.

——. 1958. *The English Health Service*. Cambridge: Harvard University Press.

Edwards, George, III. 1981. "Congressional Responsiveness to Public Opinion: The Case of Presidential Popularity." In *Public Opinion and Public Policy*, ed. Norman Luttbeg. Itasca, Ill.: R. E. Peacock.

Eichenberg, Richard. 1989. *Public Opinion and National Security in Western Europe*. Ithaca: Cornell University Press.

Emy, H. V. 1973. *Liberals, Radicals, and Social Politics: 1892–1914*. Cambridge: Cambridge University Press.

Erikson, Robert. 1978. "Constituency Opinion and Congressional Behavior: A Reexamination of the Miller-Stokes Representation Data." *American Journal of Political Science.* 22:511–35.

——. 1976. "The Relationship between Public Opinion and State Policy: A New Look at Some Forgotten Data." *American Journal of Political Science* 22:25–36.

Erikson, Robert, and Norman Luttbeg. 1973. *American Public Opinion: Its Origins, Content, and Impact*. New York: Wiley.

Erikson, Robert, Norman Luttbeg, and Kent Tedin. 1991. *American Public Opinion: Its Origins, Content, and Impact*. 4th ed. New York: Macmillan.

——. 1980. *American Public Opinion: Its Origins, Content, and Impact*. 2d ed. New York: Wiley.

Erskine, Hazel. 1975. "The Polls: Health Insurance." *Public Opinion Quarterly* 39: 128–41.

Esping-Andersen, Gosta. 1985. *Politics against Markets*. Princeton: Princeton University Press.

Esping-Anderson, Gosta, Roger Friedland, and E.O. Wright. 1976. "Modes of Class Struggle and the Capitalist State." *Kapitalistate* 3:186–219.

Evans, Peter, Dietrich Rueschemeyer, and Theda Skocpol. 1985. *Bringing the State Back In*. Cambridge: Cambridge University Press.

Farkas, Steve, Robert Shapiro, and Benjamin Page. 1990. "The Dynamics of Public Opinion and Policy." Paper presented at the annual meeting of the American Association for Public Opinion Research, Lancaster, Pa.

Feldman, Stanley. 1988. "Structure and Consistency in Public Opinion," *American Journal of Political Science* 32 (May): 416–40.

Feldman, Stanley, and John Zaller. 1992. "The Political Culture of Ambivalence: Ideological Responses to the Welfare State," *American Journal of Political Science* 36 (February): 268–307.

Flinn, M. W. 1976. "Medical Services under the New Poor Law." In *The New Poor Law in the 19th Century*, ed. Derek Fraser. New York: St. Martin's Press, 1976.

Foner, Eric. 1970. *Free Soil, Free Labor, Free Men: The Ideology of the Republican Party before the Civil War*. New York: Oxford University Press.

Foot, Michael. 1973. *Aneurin Bevan*, vol. 2. London: Davis-Poynter.

Former Members of Congress, Inc. *Former Members of Congress Oral History Collection*. Sanford, N.C.: Microfilming Corporation of America.

Fox, Daniel. 1986. *Health Policies, Health Politics: The British and American Experience, 1911–1965*. Princeton: Princeton University Press.

Fraser, Derek. 1976. *The New Poor Law in the Nineteenth*. New York: St. Martin's Press.

Galambos, Louis. 1970. "The Emerging Organization Synthesis in Modern American History." *Business History Review* 44:279–90.

Gallup, George, ed. 1976. *The Gallup International Public Opinion Polls, Great Britain 1937–75*. New York: Random House.

Geertz, Clifford. 1973. *The Interpretation of Culture: Selected Essays*. New York: Basic Books.

Giddens, Anthony. 1981. "Agency, Institution, and Time-Space Analysis." In *Advances in Social Theory and Methodology*, ed. K. Knorr-Cetina and A. Cicourel. Boston: Routledge and Kegan Paul.

——. 1979. *Central Problems in Social Theory*. Berkeley: University of California Press.

Gilbert, Bentley. 1966. *The Evolution of National Insurance in Great Britain: The Origins of the Welfare State*. London: Michael Joseph.

——. 1964. "The Decay of Nineteenth-Century Provident Institutions and the Coming of Old Age Pensions in Great Britain." *Economic Historic Review* 17:551–63.

Ginsberg, Benjamin. 1986. *The Captive Public*. New York: Basic Books.

Graham, Thomas. 1989. *American Public Opinion on NATO, Extended Deterrence, and Use of Nuclear Weapons*. SIA Occasional Paper no.4. Lanham, Md.: University Press of America.

Greenstein, Fred I. 1982. *The Hidden Hand Presidency: Eisenhower as Leader*. New York: Basic Books.

Grossman, Michael Baruch, and Martha Joynt Kumar. 1981. *Portraying the President: The White House and the News Media*. Baltimore: Johns Hopkins University Press.

Gutman, Herbert. 1975. *Work, Culture, and Society in Industrialising America*. Oxford: Oxford University Press.

Haley, Bruce. 1978. *The Healthy Body and Victorian Culture*. Cambridge: Harvard University Press.

Hall, Stuart. 1988. "The Toad in the Garden: Thatcherism among The Theorists." In *Marxism and the Interpretation of Culture*, ed. C. Nelson and L. Grossberg. Urbana: University of Illinois Press.

Harris, José. 1986. "Political Ideas and the Debate on State Welfare, 1940–45." In *War and Social Change*, ed. Harold Smith. Manchester: Manchester University Press.

———. 1983. "Did British Workers Want the Welfare State? G. D. H. Cole's Survey of 1942." In *The Working Class in Modern British History*, ed. J. M. Winter. Cambridge: Cambridge University Press.

———. 1977. *William Beveridge*. Oxford: Clarendon Press.

Harris, Louis. 1973. *The Anguish of Change*. New York: Norton.

Harris, Richard. 1966. *A Sacred Trust*. New York: New American Library.

Harrisson, Tom. 1944. "Who'll Win." *Political Quarterly* 15:21–32.

Hartz, Louis. 1955. *The Liberal Tradition in America*. New York: Harcourt Brace Jovanovich.

Hawley, Ellis. 1978. "The Discovery and Study of a 'Corporate Liberalism'." *Business History Review* 52:309–20.

Heclo, Hugh. 1974. *Modern Social Politics in Britain and Sweden*. New Haven: Yale University Press.

Heidenheimer, Arnold, Hugh Heclo, and Carolyn Adams. 1983. *Comparative Public Policy*. 2d ed. New York: St. Martin's Press.

Held, David. 1987. *Models of Democracy*. Stanford: Stanford University Press.

Hess, Stephen. 1984. *The Government/Press Connection: Press Officers and Their Offices*. Washington, D.C.: The Brookings Institution.

Hewitt, Christopher. 1974. "Policy Making in Postwar Britain: A National-Level Test of Elitist and Pluralist Hypotheses." *British Journal of Political Science* 4:187–216.

Hilderbrand, Robert C. 1981. *People and Power: Executive Management of Public Opinion in Foreign Affairs, 1897–1921*. Chapel Hill: University of North Carolina Press.

Hill, Charles. 1964. *Both Sides of the Hill*. London: Heinmann.

Hinkley, Barbara. 1983. *Stability and Change in Congress*. New York: Harper and Row.

Hirshfield, Daniel. 1970. *The Lost Reform: The Campaign for Compulsory Health Insurance in the United States*. Boston: Harvard University Press.

Hochschild, Jennifer. 1981. *What's Fair? American Beliefs about Distributive Justice*. Cambridge: Harvard University Press.

Hodgkinson, Ruth. 1967. *The Origins of the National Health Service: The Medical Services of the New Poor Law, 1834–71*. Berkeley: University of California Press.

Hofstadter, Richard. 1955. *The Age of Reform*. New York: Random House.

———. 1948. *The American Political Tradition*. New York: Knopf.

Hollingsworth, J. Rogers. 1986. *A Political Economy of Medicine: Great Britain and the United States*. Baltimore: Johns Hopkins University Press.

Hollingsworth, J. Rogers, Jerald Hage, and Robert Hanneman. 1990. *State Intervention in Medical Care: Consequences for Britain, France, Sweden, and the U.S., 1890–1970*. Ithaca: Cornell University Press.

Honigsbaum, Frank. 1979. *The Division of British Medicine: A History of the Separation of General Practice from Hospital Care, 1911–1968*. New York: St. Martin's Press.

Howkins, Alun. 1977. "Edwardian Liberalism and Industrial Unrest: A Class View of the Decline of Liberalism." *History Workshop* 4 (Autumn): 143–61.

Hunt, E.H. 1981. *British Labor History, 1815–1914,* Atlantic Highlands, N.J.: Humanities Press.

Hunt, Lynn, ed. 1989. *The New Cultural History.* Berkeley: University of California Press.

——. 1984. *Politics, Culture, and Class in the French Revolution.* Berkeley: University of California Press.

Hyde, David, et al. 1954. "AMA: Power, Purpose, and Politics in Organized Medicine." *Yale Law Journal* 63:938–1022.

Ikenberry, John. 1988. "Market Solutions for State Problems," and "Conclusion: An Institutional Approach to American Foreign Economic Policy." *International Organization* 42:219–43.

Inglehart, Ronald. 1990. *Culture Shift in Advanced Industrial Society.* Princeton: Princeton University Press.

——. 1977. *The Silent Revolution: Changing Values and Political Styles among Western Publics.* Princeton: Princeton University Press.

Iyengar, S., and D. Kinder. 1987. *News That Matters.* Chicago: University of Chicago Press.

Jacobs, Lawrence. 1992a. "The Recoil Effect: Public Opinion and Policy Making in the U.S. and Britain." *Comparative Politics* 24 (January): 199–217.

——. 1992b. "Institutions and Culture: Public Opinion and Health Policy in the U.S. and Britain," *World Politics* 44 (January): 179–209.

——. 1990. "A Social Interpretation of Institutional Change: Public Opinion and Policy Making in the Enactment of the British National Health Service Act of 1946 and the American Medicare Act of 1965." Ph.D. diss., Columbia University.

Jacobs, Lawrence, and Robert Shapiro. 1992. "Leadership and Responsiveness: Some New Evidence on the Johnson Presidency." Paper presented at the annual meeting of the American Political Science Association, Washington, D.C.

——. 1991. "Democracy, Leadership, and the Private Polls of Kennedy and Johnson." Paper presented at the annual meeting of the American Political Science Association, Washington, D.C.

——. 1989. "Public Opinion and the New Social History: Some Lessons for the Study of Public Opinion and Democratic Policy Making." *Social Science History* 13:1–24.

Jameson, Fredric. 1981. *The Political Unconscious.* Ithaca: Cornell University Press.

Jasper, James. 1990. *Nuclear Politics: Energy and the State in the United States, Sweden, and France.* Princeton: Princeton University Press.

Jeffrey, Tom. 1980. "Mass Observation and Health," Paper presented at the annual conference of the Society for the Social History of Medicine, University of Liverpool.

——. 1978. "Mass Observation—A Short History." Occasional paper No. 55, Center for Contemporary Cultural Studies. University of Birmingham, England.

Jensen, Richard. 1980. "Polls and Politics: Democracy by the Numbers." *Public Opinion* (February/March): 53–59.

Jewell, Malcolm. 1983. "Legislator-Constituency Relations and the Representative Process." *Legislative Studies Quarterly* 8 (August): 303–37.

Johnson, Richard. 1978. "Edward Thompson, Eugene Genovese, and Socialist-Humanist History." *History Workshop Journal* 6 (Autumn): 79–100.

Jones, Gareth Stedman. 1983. *Languages of Class: Studies in English Working Class History.* Cambridge: Cambridge University Press.

Kammen, Michael. 1986. *A Machine That Would Go of Itself: The Constitution in American Culture.* New York: Alfred A. Knopf.

Katz, Michael. 1986. *In the Shadow of the Poorhouse: A Social History of Welfare in America*. New York: Basic Books.

Katzenstein, Peter, ed. 1978. *Between Power and Plenty: The Foreign Economic Policies of Advanced Industrial States*. Madison: University of Wisconsin Press.

Katznelson, Ira. 1986. "Working-Class Formation: Constructing Cases and Comparisons" In *Working Class Formation*, ed. I. Katznelson and A. Zolberg. (Princeton: Princeton University Press).

———. 1985. "Working-Class Formation and the State: Nineteenth-Century Britain in American Perspective." In *Bringing the State Back In*, ed. P. Evans, D. Rueschemeyer, and T. Skocpol. Cambridge: Cambridge University Press.

———. 1981. *City Trenches: Urban Politics and the Patterning of Class in the United States*. New York: Pantheon Books.

Kemler, Edgar. 1947. *The Deflation of American Ideals: An Ethical Guide for New Dealers*. Seattle: University of Washington Press.

Kernell, Samuel. 1986. *Going Public: New Strategies of Presidential Leadership*. Washington, D.C.: Congressional Quarterly Press.

Kervasdoue, Jean de, John Kimberly, and Victor Rodwin. 1984. *The End of an Illusion: The Future of Health Policy in Western Industrialized Nations*. Berkeley: University of California Press.

Key, V. O. 1961. *Public Opinion and American Democracy* New York: Alfred A. Knopf.

Kingdon, John. 1984. *Agendas, Alternatives, and Public Policies*. Boston: Little, Brown.

Klein, Rudolf. 1983. *The Politics of the National Health Service*. London: Longman.

Korpi, Walter. 1983. *The Democratic Class Struggle*. London: Routledge and Kegan Paul.

Koss, Stephen. 1984. *The Rise and Fall of the Political Press in Britain: The Twentieth Century*, vol. 2. Chapel Hill: University of North Carolina Press.

———. 1981. *The Rise and Fall of the Political Press in Britain: The Nineteenth Century*, vol. 1. Chapel Hill: University of North Carolina Press.

Krasner, Stephen. 1978. *Defending the National Interest: Raw Materials Investments and U.S. Foreign Policy*. Princeton: Princeton University Press.

Krosnick, Jon, and Donald Kinder. "Research Notes: Altering the Foundations of Support for the President through Priming." *American Political Science Review* 84 (June): 497–512.

Kusnitz, Leonard. 1984. *Public Opinion and Foreign Policy: America's China Policy, 1949–1979*. Westport, Conn.: Greenwood.

Leavitt, Judith, and Ronald Numbers, eds. 1985. *Sickness and Health in America*. Madison: University of Wisconsin Press.

Leiby, James. 1978. *A History of Social Welfare and Social Work in the United States*. New York: Columbia University Press.

Leuchtenburg, William. 1963. *Franklin D. Roosevelt and The New Deal, 1932–1940*. New York: Harper and Row.

Light, Paul. 1991. *The President's Agenda: Domestic Policy Choice from Kennedy to Reagan*. Baltimore: Johns Hopkins University Press.

Lockridge, Kenneth. 1970. *A New England Town: The First Hundred Years*. New York: Norton.

Lowi, Theodore. 1979. *The End of Liberalism*. 2d ed. New York: Norton.

Lubove, Roy. 1968. *The Struggle for Social Security, 1900–1935*. Cambridge: Harvard University Press.

Luttbeg, Norman, ed. 1981. *Public Opinion and Public Policy: Models of Political Linkage*. 3d ed. Itasca, Ill: F. E. Peacock.

Maass, Arthur. 1983. *Congress and the Common Good*. New York: Basic Books.

MacIntyre, Alasdair. 1971. "Is a Science of Comparative Politics Possible." In *Against the Self-Images of the Age*. New York: Schocken Books.

Mackintosh, J. M. 1953. *Trends of Opinion about Public Health: 1901–51*. London: Oxford University Press.

Macpherson, C. B. 1977. *The Life and Times of Liberal Democracy*. New York: Oxford University Press.

Margach, James. 1979. *The Anatomy of Power: An Enquiry into the Personality of Leadership*. London: W. H. Allen.

———. 1978. *The Abuse of Power: The War between Downing Street and the Media from Lloyd George to Callaghan*. London: W. H. Allen.

Marmor, Theodore. 1983. *Political Analysis and American Medical Care*. New York: Cambridge University Press.

———. 1973. *The Politics of Medicare*. Chicago: Aldine.

Marmor, Theodore, Jerry Mashaw, and Philip Harvey. 1990. *America's Misunderstood Welfare State: Presistent Myths, Enduring Realities*. New York: Basic Books.

Marmor, Theodore, and David Thomas. 1972. "Doctors, Politics, and Pay Disputes: 'Pressure Group Politics' Revisited." *British Journal of Political Science* 2:421–42.

Marwick, Arthur. 1970. *Britain in the Century of Total War: War, Peace, and Social Change, 1900–67*. Middlesex: Penguin Books.

———. 1964. "Middle Opinion in the Thirties: Planning, Progress and Political 'Agreement'." *English Historical Review* 79:285–98.

Matusow, Allen. 1984. *The Unravelling of America: A History of Liberalism in the 1960s*. New York: Harper and Row.

Mayhew, David. 1974. *Congress: The Electoral Connection*. New Haven: Yale University Press.

McConnell, Grant. 1966. *Private Power and American Democracy*. New York: Knopf.

McLaine, Ian. 1979. *Ministry of Morale: Home Front Morale and the Ministry of Information in World War Two*. London: Allen and Unwin.

Meacham, Staudish. 1977. *A Life Apart: The English Working Class, 1890–1914*. Cambridge: Harvard University Press.

Miliband, Ralph. 1972. "Reply to Nicos Poulantzas." In *Ideology in Social Science*, ed. Robin Blackburn. New York: Vintage Books.

———. 1969. *The State in Capitalist Society*. New York: Basic Books.

Miller, Warren, and Donald Stokes. 1963. "Constituency Influence in Congress." *American Political Science Review* 57:45–56.

Monroe, Alan. 1979. "Consistency between Public Preferences and National Policy Decisions." *American Political Quarterly*, 7:3–19.

Monroe, Alan, and Paul Gardner, Jr. 1987. "Public Policy Linkages." In *Research in Micropolitics*, vol. 2. ed. Samuel Long. Boulder, Colo.: Westview Press.

Morgan, Kenneth O. 1984. *Labour in Power: 1945–1951*. Oxford: Oxford University Press.

———. 1971. *The Age of Lloyd George*. New York: Barnes and Noble.

Morone, James. 1990. *The Democratic Wish: Popular Participation and the Limits of American Government*. New York: Basic Books.

Myles, John. 1989. *Old Age in the Welfare State: The Political Economy of Public Pensions*. Lawrence: University Press of Kansas.

———. 1988. "Postwar Capitalism and the Extension of Social Security into a Retirement Wage." In *The Politics of Social Policy in the United States*, ed. M. Weir, A. Orloff, and T. Skocpol. (Princeton: Princeton University Press).

Nadel, Mark. 1972. "Public Policy and Public Opinion." In *American Democracy: Theory and Reality,* ed. Robert Weisberg and Mark Nadel. New York: Wiley.

Nelson, Barbara. 1984. *Making an Issue of Child Abuse.* Chicago: University of Chicago Press.

Neustadt, Richard. 1960. *Presidential Power.* New York: Wiley.

Nozick, Robert. 1974. *Anarchy, State, and Utopia.* New York: Basic Books.

Numbers, Ronald. 1985. "The Fall and Rise of the American Medical Profession." In *Sickness and Health in America,* ed. Judith Leavitt and Ronald Numbers. Madison: University of Wisconsin Press.

———. 1979. "The Third Party: Health Insurance in America." In *The Therapeutic Revolution,* ed. Morris Vogel and Charles Rosenberg. Philadelphia: University of Pennsylvania Press.

O'Connor, James. 1973. *The Fiscal Crisis of the State.* New York: St. Martin's Press.

Offe, Claus. 1984. *Contradictions of the Welfare State.* ed. J. Keane. Cambridge: MIT Press.

———. 1973. "The Capitalist State and the Problem of Policy Formation." In *Stress and Contradiction in Modern Capitalism,* ed. L. Lindberg, R. Alford, C. Crouch, and C. Offe. Lexington, Mass.: Heath.

Offer, Avner. 1981. *Property and Politics, 1870–1914: Landownership, Law, Ideology, and Urban Development in England.* Cambridge: Cambridge University Press.

Ogilvy-Webb, Marjorie. 1965. *The Government Explains: A Study of the Information Services.* A Report of the Royal Institute of Public Administration. London: Allen and Unwin.

Orloff, Ann. 1988. "The Political Origins of America's Belated Welfare State." In *The Politics of Social Policy in the United States,* ed. M. Weir, A. Orloff, and T. Skocpol. Princeton: Princeton University Press.

Orloff, Ann, and Theda Skocpol. 1984. "Why Not Equal Protection? Explaining the Politics of Public Social Spending in Britain, 1900–1911, and the United States, 1880s–1920." *American Sociological Review* 49:726–50.

Ortner, Sherry. 1984. "Theory in Anthropology since the Sixties." *Comparative Studies in Society and History* 26:126–66.

Ostrogorski, M. Y. 1902. *Democracy and the Organization of Political Parties.* 2 vols. London: Macmillan.

Page, Benjamin. 1978. *Choices and Echoes in Presidential Elections.* Chicago: University of Chicago Press.

Page, Benjamin, and Robert Shapiro. 1992. *The Rational Public.* Chicago: University of Chicago Press.

———. 1983. "Effects of Public Opinion on Policy." *American Political Science Review* 77:175–90.

———. 1982. "Changes in Americans' Policy Preferences." *Public Opinion Quarterly* 46:24–42.

Page, Benjamin, Robert Shapiro, and Glenn Dempsey. 1987. "What Moves Public Opinion." *American Political Science Review* 81 (March): 23–43.

Pateman, Carole. 1970. *Participation and Democratic Theory.* Cambridge: Cambridge University Press.

Pater, John. 1981. *The Making of the National Health Service.* London: Pitman Press.

Payne, Stanley. 1946. "Some Opinion Research Principles Developed through Studies of Social Medicine." *Political Opinion Quarterly* 10:93–98.

Pelling, Henry. 1968. "The Working Class and the Origins of the Welfare State." In

Popular Politics and Society in Late Victorian Britain, ed. Henry Pelling. London: Macmillan.

Pious, Richard. 1979. *The American Presidency.* New York: Basic Books.

Poen, Monte M. 1979. *Harry S. Truman versus the Medical Lobby: The Genius of Medicare.* Columbia: University of Missouri Press.

Political and Economic Planning. 1933. "Government Public Relations." *Planning Broadsheet,* no. 14, November 21, 1933.

Pomper, G. M. 1980. *Elections in America.* 2d ed. New York: Longman.

Poulantzas, Nicos. 1978. *State, Power, Socialism.* London: NLB.

Pryor, Frederic. 1988. "Corporatism as an Economic System: A Review Essay." *Journal of Comparative Economics* 12:317–44.

Przeworski, Adam. 1986. *Capitalism and Social Democracy.* Cambridge: Cambridge University Press.

Quadagno, Jill. 1988. *The Transformation of Old Age Security: Class and Politics in the American Welfare State.* Chicago: Chicago University Press.

——. 1982. *Aging in Early Industrial Society: Work, Family, and Social Policy in Nineteenth-Century England.* New York: Academic Press.

Reverby, Susan and David Rosner. 1979. *Health Care in America: Essays in Social History.* Philadelphia: Temple University Press.

Rimlinger, Gaston. 1971. *Welfare Policy and Industrialization in Europe, America, and Russia.* New York: Wiley.

Risse-Kappen, Thomas. 1991. "Public Opinion, Domestic Structure, and Foreign Policy in Liberal Democracies." *World Politics* 43 (July): 479–512.

Rodwin, Victor. 1984. *The Health Planning Predicament.* Berkeley: University of California Press.

Rosen, George. 1971. "The First Neighborhood Health Center." *American Journal of Public Health* 61:1620–35.

Rosenberg, Charles. 1987. *The Care of Strangers: The Rise of America's Hospital System.* New York: Basic Books.

——. 1979a. "Inward Vision." *Bulletin of History of Medicine* 53:346.

——. 1979b. "The Therapeutic Revolution: Medicine, Meaning, and Social Change in 19th Century America." In *The Therapeutic Revolution,* ed. Morris Vogel and Charles Rosenberg. Philadelphia: University of Pennsylvania.

——. 1979c. "Florence Nightingale on Contagion: The Hospital as a Moral Universe." In *Healing and History: Essays For George Rosen,* ed. Charles Rosenberg. New York: Science History Publications.

——, ed. 1979d. *Healing and History: Essays for George Rosen.* New York: Science History Publications.

——. 1979e. "George Rosen and the Social History of Medicine." In *Healing and History: Essays For George Rosen,* ed. Charles Rosenberg. New York: Science History Publications.

——. 1977. "And Heal the Sick." *Journal of Social History* 10:448

——. 1974. "Social Class and Medical Class in 19th Century America: The Rise and Fall of the Dispensary." *Journal of the History of Medicine and Allied Sciences* 29:32–54.

Rosenkrantz, Barbara Gutman. 1985. "The Search for Professional Order in Nineteenth Century American Medicine." In *Sickness and Health in America,* ed. Judith Leavitt and Ronald Numbers. Madison: University of Wisconsin Press.

——. 1979. "Damaged Goods: Dilemmas of Responsibility for Risk." *Milibank Memorial Fund Quarterly.* 57:1–37.

———. 1972. *Public Health and the State: Changing Views in Massachusetts*. Cambridge: Harvard University Press.

Rosner, David. 1982. *A Once Charitable Enterprise: Hospitals and Health Care in Brooklyn and New York, 1885–1915*. New York: Cambridge University Press.

Ross, Dorothy. 1979. "The Liberal Tradition Revisited and the Republican Tradition Addressed." In *New Directions in American Intellectual History*, ed. John Higham and Paul Conkin. Baltimore: Johns Hopkins University Press.

Russett, Bruce. 1990. *Controlling the Sword: The Democratic Governance of National Security*. Cambridge: Harvard University Press.

Salinger, Pierre. 1966. *With Kennedy*. Garden City, N.Y.: Doubleday.

Sartori, Giovanni. 1987. *The Theory of Democracy Revisited*. Chatham, N.J.: Chatham House.

Schattschneider, E. E. 1960. *The Semi-Sovereign People*. Hinsdale, Ill.: Dryden Press.

———. 1948. *The Struggle for Party Government*. College Park:, Md.: French-Bray Printing.

Schiltz, Michael. 1970. *Public Attitudes toward Social Security, 1935–65*. Washington, D.C.: GPO.

Schlesinger, Arthur, Jr. 1986. *The Cycles of American History*. Boston: Houghton Mifflin.

———. 1960. *The Age of Roosevelt: The Politics of Upheaval*. Boston: Houghton Mifflin.

Schudson, Michael. 1989. "How Culture Works: Perspectives from Media Studies on the Efficacy of Symbols." *Theory and Society* 18:153–80.

Schumpeter, Joseph. 1976. *Capitalism, Socialisms, and Democracy*. London: Allen and Unwin.

Searle, Geoffrey. 1979. *Eugenics and Politics in Britain, 1900–14*. Leyden: Noordoff International Press.

———. 1971. *The Quest for National Efficiency*. Oxford: Blackwell.

Seymour-Ure, Colin. 1968. *The Press, Politics, and the Public: An Essay on the Role of the National Press in the British Political System*. London: Methuen.

Shapiro, Robert. 1982. *The Dynamics of Public Opinion and Public Policy*. Ph.D. diss., University of Chicago.

Shapiro, Robert, and John Young. 1988. "Public Opinion toward Social Welfare Issues: The United State in Comparative Perspective." In *Research in Micropolitics*, vol.3, ed. Samuel Long. Greenwich, Conn: JAI Press.

Shonick, W. 1984. "Early Developments and Recent Trends in the Evolution of Local Public Hospitals." *Annual Review of Public Health* 5:53–81.

Sicherman, Barbara. 1979. "The New Mission of Doctors." In *Nourishing the Humanistic in Medicine*, ed. W. Roger and D. Barnard. Pittsburgh: University of Pittsburgh Press.

Skocpol, Theda. 1985. "Bringing the State Back In: Strategies of Analysis in Current Research." In *Bringing the State Back In*, ed. P. Evans, D. Rueschemeyer, and T. Skocpol. Cambridge: Cambridge University Press.

———. 1979. *States and Social Revolutions*. New York: Cambridge University Press.

———, ed. 1984. *Vision and Method in Historical Sociology*. New York: Cambridge University Press.

———. 1992. *Protecting Soldiers and Mothers*. Cambridge: Harvard University Press.

Skocpol, Theda, and Kenneth Finegold. 1982. "State Capacity and Economic Intervention in the Early New Deal." *Political Science Quarterly* 97:255–77.

Skocpol, Theda, and John Ikenberry. 1983. "The Political Formation of the American Welfare State in Historical and Comparative Context." *Comparative Social Research* 6:87–148.

Skowronek, Stephen. 1984. "Political Time." In *The Political Presidency,* ed. Michael Nelson. Washington: Congressional Quarterly Press.

——. 1982. *Building a New American State: The Expansion of National Administrative Capacities.* New York: Cambridge University Press.

Smith, F. B. 1979. *The People's Health, 1830–1900.* New York: Holmes and Meier.

Smith, Geoffrey. 1986. "The Prime Minister and the Press: Britain." In *Presidents, Prime Ministers, and the Press,* ed. Kenneth Thompson. Lanham, MD: University Press of America.

Smith, Tom. 1982. "General Liberalism and Social Change in Post World War II America: A Summary of Trends." *Social Indicators Research* 10:1–28.

Sorensen, Theodore. 1965. *Kennedy.* New York: Bantam Books.

Starr, Paul. 1982. *The Social Transformation of American Medicine.* New York: Basic Books.

Steele, Richard W. 1985a. *Propaganda in an Open Society: The Roosevelt Administration and the Media, 1933–41.* Westport, Conn.: Greenwood Press.

——. 1985b. "News of the 'Good War': World War II News Management." *Journalism Quarterly* (Winter): 707–16

——. 1978. "American Popular Opinion and the War against Germany: The Issue of the Negotiated Peace, 1942." *Journal of American History* 65 (December): 704–23.

——. 1974. "The Pulse of the People: Franklin D. Roosevelt and the Gauging of American Public Opinion." *Journal of Contemporary History* 9 (October): 195–216.

Stepan, Alfred. 1978. *The State and Society: Peru in Comparative Perspective.* Princeton: Princeton University Press.

Stevens, Rosemary. 1989. *In Sickness and in Wealth: American Hospitals in the 20th Century.* New York: Basic Books.

——. 1976. *American Medicine and the Public Interest.* New Haven: Yale University Press.

Stimson, James. 1991. *Public Opinion in America: Moods, Cycles, and Swings.* Boulder, Colo.: Westview Press.

Sudman, Seymour. 1982. "The Presidents and the Polls." *Public Opinion Quarterly* 46:301–10.

Sundquist, James. 1968. *Politics and Policy: The Eisenhower, Kennedy, and Johnson Years.* Washington, D.C.: The Brookings Institution.

Swift, Roy. 1968. "Using Special Events." In *The Voice of Government,* ed. Ray Hiebert and Carlton Spitzer. New York: Wiley.

Taylor, Stephen. 1978. "The Birth of a Service: 1. Before the War." *Update,* November 15, 1978.

——. 1979a. "The Birth of a Service: 2. Blast of War." *Update,* January 15, 1979.

——. 1979b. "The Birth of a Service: 3. Role of Public Opinion." *Update,* February 1, 1979.

Thompson, Dorothy. 1984. *The Chartists: Popular Politics in the Industrial Revolution.* New York: Pantheon Books.

Thompson, E. P. 1978a. "The Poverty of Theory or an Orrey of Errors." In *The Poverty of Theory and Other Essays.* New York: Monthly Review Press.

——. 1978b. "The Peculiarities of the English." In *The Poverty of Theory and Other Essays.* New York: Monthly Review Press.

——. 1966. *The Making of the English Working Class.* London: Vintage Books.

Tilly, Charles. 1981. *As Sociology Meets History.* New York: Academic Press.

——, ed. 1975. *The Formation of National States in Western Europe.* Princeton: Princeton University Press.

Titmuss, Richard. 1950. *History of the Second World War: Problems of Social Policy.* London: HMSO.

Tocqueville, Alexis de. 1969. *Democracy in America,* ed. J. P. Mayer. New York: Anchor Books.

Tulis, Jeffrey. 1987. *The Rhetorical Presidency.* Princeton: Princeton University Press.

Tunstall, Jeremy. 1970. *The Westminster Lobby Correspondents: A Sociological Study of National Political Journalism.* London: Routledge and Kegan Paul.

United Kingdom. 1944. *A National Health Service.* London: HMSO, cmd 6502.

U.S. Congress. House. Ways and Means Committee. 1965. *Hearings on HR1.* 89th Cong., 1st sess. Washington, D.C.: GPO.

——. 1964. *Hearings on HR11865.* 88th Cong., 2d sess. Washington, D.C.: GPO.

——. 1963. *Hearings on HR3920.* 88th Cong., 1st sess. Washington, D.C.: GPO.

——. 1961. *Hearings on HR4222.* 87th Cong., 1st sess. Washington, D.C.: GPO.

——. 1959. *Hearings on HR4700,* 86th Cong., 1st sess. Washington, D.C.: GPO.

——. 1958. *Hearings on Unemployment Insurance Amendment,* 85th Cong, 2d sess. Washington, D.C.: GPO.

Vogel, Morris J. 1980. *Invention of Modern Hospital: Boston, 1870–1930.* Chicago: University of Chicago Press.

——. 1976. "Patrons, Pactitioners, and Patients: The Voluntary Hospital in Mid-Victorian Britain." In *Victorian America,* ed. Daniel Howe. Philadelphia: University of Pennsylvania.

Vogler, David, and Sidney Waldman. 1985. *Congress and Democracy.* Washington, D.C.: Congressional Quarterly.

Walcott, Charles, and Karen Hult. 1989. "Management Science and the Great Engineer: Governing the White House during the Hoover Administration." Manuscript, Virginia Polytechnic Insitute.

Weber, Max. 1978. *Economy and Society,* ed. Guenther Roth and Claus Wittich. Berkeley: University of California.

——. 1958. *The Protestant Ethic.* New York: Charles Scribner's Sons.

Webster, Charles. 1988. *The Health Services since the War,* vol. 1. London: HMO.

——. 1987. "Labour and the Origins of the NHS." In *Science, Politics, and the Public Good,* ed. N. Rupke. London: Macmillan.

——. 1982. "Healthy or Hungry Thirties?" *History Workshop* 13 (Spring): 110–28.

Weir, Margaret, and Theda Skocpol. 1985. "State Structures and the Possibilities for 'Keynesian' Responses to the Great Depression in Sweden, Britain, and the United States." In *Bringing the State Back In,* ed. P. Evans, D. Rueschemeyer, and T. Skocpol. Cambridge: Cambridge University Press.

Weissberg, Robert. 1979. "Assessing Legislator-Constituency Policy Agreements." *Legislative Studies Quarterly* 4:605–22.

——. 1976. *Public Opinion and Popular Government.* Englewood Cliffs, N.J.: Prentice-Hall.

Whitley, Paul. 1981. Public Opinion and the Demand for Social Welfare in Britain." *Journal of Social Policy* 10:453–75.

Wiebe, Robert. 1967. *The Search for Order: 1877–1920.* New York: Hill and Wang.

Wildavsky, Aaron. 1987. "Choosing Preferences by Constructing Institutions," *American Political Science Review* 81:3–21.

Wilensky, Harold. 1975. *The Welfare State and Equality: Structural and Industrial Roots of Public Expenditure.* Berkeley: University of California Press.

Williams, Francis. 1970. *Nothing So Strange: An Autobiography.* London: Cassell.

Wilsford, David. 1990. *Doctors and the State: The Politics of Health Care in France and the United States*. Durham, N.C.: Duke University Press.

Winfield, Betty Houchin. 1984. "The New Deal Publicity Operation: Foundation for the Modern Presidency." *Journalism Quarterly* 61 (Spring): 40–48.

Wood, Gordon. 1984. "Politics without Parties." *New York Review of Books*, October 11, 1984.

——. 1969. *The Creation of the American Republic*. Chapel Hill: University of North Carolina Press.

Woodward, John. 1974. *To Do the Sick Harm: A Study of the British Voluntary Hospital System to 1875*. London: Routledge and Kegan Paul.

Woodward, John, and David Richards. 1977. *Health Care and Popular Medicine in Nineteenth Century England: Essays in the Social History of Medicine*. London: Croom Helm.

Young, James Harvey. 1977. "Patient Medicine and the Self-Help Syndrome." In *Medicine Without Doctors*, ed. G. Risse, R. Numbers, and J. Leavitt. New York: Science History Publications.

| Index

Abel-Smith, Brian, 40, 42, 45, 50–51, 61–62
Addison, Paul, 69, 71, 122, 167n, 169, 171
Administration of Medicare. *See* Medicare: state expansion
Administrative design. *See* State capacity; United States
Agenda setting:
  culturalist analysis of, 60
  emergence of problem (Britain), 60–63, 75–78, 82, 217
  emergence of problem (U.S.), 85–88, 99–101, 217–18
  process of, 59–60, 106
  role of public opinion, 106–7
  Weberian analysis of, 60, 63, 82–84, 106
  See also Britain; United States
Agricultural Adjustment Administration, 6, 233
Allison, Graham, 3
Almond, Gabriel, 3, 8, 12
American Hospital Association (AHA), 14, 87–88, 204. *See also* Hospitals; State autonomy
American Medical Association (AMA), 14, 55, 88–89, 100, 102, 104–5, 148–49, 151–54, 157, 159, 161, 163, 199–200, 202, 205–8, 211–13, 215. *See also* Hospitals; State autonomy
American Political Science Review, 9n

Apothecaries. *See* Medical profession organization
Atkinson, Michael, 6
Attlee, Clement, 30–31, 170, 172–73
Axinn, June, 47

Ball, Robert, 90n
Bargaining, by government officials and interest groups, 232. *See also* State autonomy
Barrett, Edith, 231n, 233
Bartels, Larry, 231
Beard, Charles, 167n
Beer, Samuel, 141, 144
Berger, Peter, 7
Berkowitz, Edward, 46
Bevan, Aneurin, 172, 174–75, 177–86, 215, 230
Beveridge, William, 67–70, 72–73, 77
Beveridge committee, 76
Beveridge Report, 9, 17, 29, 66–67, 111–20, 122, 129, 134–35, 143, 160, 169, 176, 204, 217–18
Bevin, Ernest, 173
Blue Cross, 54–55, 87n, 158–60, 204, 209, 220, 235
Briggs, Asa, 51
Britain:
  Central Office of Information, 30
  Chartists, 46
  coalition government, 13, 18, 120–23, 129, 185

Library of Congress Cataloging-in-Publication Data

Jacobs, Lawrence R.
    The health of nations : public opinion and the making of American
and British health policy / Lawrence R. Jacobs.
        p.   cm.
    Includes bibliographical references and index.
    ISBN 0–8014–2761–4 (alk. paper).
    1. Medical policy—United States—History—20th century.
2. Medical policy—Great Britain—History—20th century.   3. Medical
policy—United States—Public opinion.   4. Medical policy—Great
Britain—Public opinion.   5. Medicare—History.   6. National Health
Service (Great Britain)—History.   7. Health planning—United
States—Citizen participation.   8. Health planning—Great Britain—
Citizen participation.   I. Title.
RA395.A3J33   1993
362.1′0973′0904—dc20

                                                            92–54967